Lecture Notes of the Institute
for Computer Sciences, Social Informatics
and Telecommunications Engineering   288

More information about this series at http://www.springer.com/series/8197

Pietro Cipresso · Silvia Serino ·
Daniela Villani (Eds.)

Pervasive Computing Paradigms for Mental Health

9th International Conference, MindCare 2019
Buenos Aires, Argentina, April 23–24, 2019
Proceedings

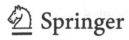 Springer

Editors
Pietro Cipresso ⓘ
IRCCS Istituto Auxologico Italiano
Milan, Italy

Daniela Villani ⓘ
Catholic University of the Sacred Heart
Milan, Italy

Silvia Serino ⓘ
Department of Clinical Neurosciences
University of Lausanne
Lausanne, Switzerland

ISSN 1867-8211 ISSN 1867-822X (electronic)
Lecture Notes of the Institute for Computer Sciences, Social Informatics
and Telecommunications Engineering
ISBN 978-3-030-25871-9 ISBN 978-3-030-25872-6 (eBook)
https://doi.org/10.1007/978-3-030-25872-6

This Springer imprint is published by the registered company Springer Nature Switzerland AG
The registered company address is: Gewerbestrasse 11, 6330 Cham, Switzerland

Preface

We are delighted to introduce the proceedings of the ninth edition of MindCare—EAI International Conference on Pervasive Computing Paradigms for Mental Health, which took place at Belgrano University, Buenos Aires (April 23–24, 2019). In its nine editions, MindCare has gathered scientists and clinicians from more than 30 countries allowing for the creation of a multidisciplinary community that shares a common interest: understanding and advancing the state of the art by building innovative ideas in mental health care.

The emerging interface between technology and psychological research and practice has led to new opportunities for building new paradigms in mental health care, in parallel with compelling questions about how it is possible to promote and structure these changes to improve psychological well-being. The MindCare Conference discussed the use of innovative technologies for sustaining individual and social well-being in both healthy and clinical populations and it brought together a growing community of researchers and practitioners from different domains, including computer engineering, psychiatry, and psychology.

Thanks to the collaboration with the Aiglé Foundation, MindCare 2019 focused on the exploitation of the technological advancements to provide improved diagnosis and a better support to both healthy individuals and patients, as well as to extend the theoretical knowledge, grasping the interest of an extraordinary audience of 200 registered participants.

The technical program of MindCare 2019 consisted of 22 full papers. Aside from the high-quality paper presentations, the technical program also featured three keynote speakers—Prof. Cristina Botella from Jaume I University, Spain; Prof. Giuseppe Riva from Catholic University of the Sacred Heart, Italy; and Prof. Pim Cuijpers from Vrije University, The Netherlands—who proposed three meaningful and inspiring theoretical proposals to highlight how to use technologies for monitoring and maintaining mental health.

Coordination with the steering chair, Prof. Imrich Chlamtac, and with the local chair, Beatriz Gómez, was fundamental for the success of the conference. It was also a great pleasure to work with an excellent Technical Program Committee led by Dr. Daniela Villani, which provided a high-quality peer-review process for all the submitted papers.

We would like to warmly thank Prof. Hector Fernandez-Alvarez, Emeritus Professor at Universidad de Belgrano, and Prof. Andres Roussos, Professor at Universidad de Buenos Aires, for their active participation and discussion during the conference. We also acknowledge the European-funded project "BodyPass" – API-ecosystem for cross-sectorial exchange of 3D personal data (H2020-779780)—for supporting the event.

We strongly believe that MindCare 2019 provided a good forum for all researchers, developers, and practitioners to discuss all technological aspects that are relevant to mental health, as indicated by the contributions presented in this volume.

June 2019

Pietro Cipresso
Silvia Serino
Daniela Villani

Organization

Steering Committee

Imrich Chlamtac   University of Trento, Trento, Italy

Organizing Committee

General Chairs

Pietro Cipresso   Istituto Auxologico Italiano, Milan, Italy
and Università Cattolica del Sacro Cuore, Milan,
Italy

Silvia Serino   CHUV/Centre Hospitalier Universitaire Vaudois,
Lausanne, Switzerland

Daniela Villani   Università Cattolica del Sacro Cuore, Milan, Italy

Local Chair

Beatriz Gómez   Fundación Aiglé, Buenos Aires, Argentina

Workshops Chair

Alice Chirico   Università Cattolica del Sacro Cuore, Milan, Italy

Publicity and Social Media Chair

Javier Fernández Alvarez   Università Cattolica del Sacro Cuore, Milan, Italy

Publications Chair

Desirée Colombo   Jaume I University, Castellón, Spain

Web Chair

Giulia Corno   Universidad de Valencia, Valencia, Spain

Posters and PhD Track Chair

Elisa Pedroli   Istituto Auxologico Italiano, Milan, Italy

Panels Chair

Elisa Pedroli   Istituto Auxologico Italiano, Milan, Italy

Tutorials Chair

Alice Chirico   Università Cattolica del Sacro Cuore, Milan, Italy

Technical Program Committee

Chair

Daniela Villani   Università Cattolica del Sacro Cuore, Italy

Members

Carissoli Claudia   Università Cattolica del Sacro Cuore di Milano, Milan, Italy
Chirico Alice   Università Cattolica del Sacro Cuore di Milano, Milan, Italy
Cipresso Pietro   Istituto Auxologico Italiano, Milan, Italy
Colombo Desirée   Jaume I University, Castellón, Spain
De Pasquale Carolina   Dublin Institute of Technology, Dublin, Ireland
Di Lernia Daniele   Università Cattolica del Sacro Cuore di Milano, Milan, Italy
Fernández-Álvarez Javier   Università Cattolica del Sacro Cuore di Milano, Milan, Italy
Gaggioli Andrea   Università Cattolica del Sacro Cuore di Milano, Milan, Italy
Higuchi Masakazu   University of Tokyo, Tokyo, Japan
Jaén Irene   Jaume I University, Castellón, Spain
Maldonato Nelson Mauro   Federico II University, Naples, Italy
Malighetti Clelia   Università Cattolica del Sacro Cuore di Milano, Milan, Italy
Mantovani Fabrizia   Università degli Studi di Milano Bicocca, Milan, Italy
Martinez-Borba Veronica   University of Zaragoza, Teruel, Spain
Mitsuteru Nakamura   University of Tokyo, Tokyo, Japan
Molinari Guadalupe   Instituto de Salud Carlos III, Madrid, Spain
Morganti Francesca   University of Bergamo, Bergamo, Italy
O'Nell Jack   Dublin Institute of Technology, Dublin, Ireland
Osma Jorge   University of Zaragoza, Zaragoza, Spain
Pedroli Elisa   Istituto Auxologico Italiano, Milan, Italy
Repetto Claudia   Università Cattolica del Sacro Cuore di Milano, Milan, Italy
Serino Silvia   University Hospital Lausanne, Lausanne, Switzerland
Suso-Ribera Carlos   Jaume I University, Castellón, Spain
Triberti Stefan   University of Milan, Milan, Italy
Tuena Cosimo   Istituto Auxologico Italiano, Milan, Italy

Contents

Virtual-Reality Music-Based Elicitation of Awe: When Silence
Is Better Than Thousands Sounds.......................... 1
   Alice Chirico and Andrea Gaggioli

Clara: Design of a New System for Passive Sensing of Depression,
Stress and Anxiety in the Workplace....................... 12
   Juwon Lee, Megan Lam, and Caleb Chiu

System of Nudge Theory-Based ICT Applications for Older Citizens:
The SENIOR Project....................................... 29
   Giada Pietrabissa, Italo Zoppis, Giancarlo Mauri, Roberta Ghiretti,
   Emanuele Maria Giusti, Roberto Cattivelli, Chiara Spatola,
   Gian Mauro Manzoni, and Gianluca Castelnuovo

Virtual Reality for Anxiety and Stress-Related Disorders:
A SWOT Analysis 43
   Javier Fernández-Alvarez, Desirée Colombo, Cristina Botella,
   Azucena García-Palacios, and Giuseppe Riva

Experiencing Dementia from Inside: The Expediency
of Immersive Presence.................................... 55
   Francesca Morganti

Psychological Correlates of Interoceptive Perception in Healthy Population. ... 71
   Daniele Di Lernia, Silvia Serino, and Giuseppe Riva

Development of a Computational Platform to Support the Screening,
Surveillance, Prevention and Detection of Suicidal Behaviours 83
   Juan Martínez-Miranda, Antonio Palacios-Isaac, Fernando López-Flores,
   Ariadna Martínez, Héctor Aguilar, Liliana Jiménez, Roberto Ramos,
   Giovanni Rosales, and Luis Altamirano

Anthropometry and Scan: A Computational Exploration on Measuring
and Imaging... 102
   Michelle Toti, Cosimo Tuena, Michelle Semonella, Elisa Pedroli,
   Giuseppe Riva, and Pietro Cipresso

Immersive Episodic Memory Assessment with 360° Videos: The Protocol
and a Case Study 117
   Claudia Repetto, Silvia Serino, Mauro Maldonato, Teresa Longobardi,
   Raffaele Sperandeo, Daniela Iennaco, and Giuseppe Riva

An Internet-Based Intervention for Depressive Symptoms: Preliminary Data
on the Contribution of Behavioral Activation and Positive Psychotherapy
Strategies.   129
    Sonia Romero, Adriana Mira, Juana Bretón-Lopez, Amanda Díaz-García,
    Laura Díaz-Sanahuja, Azucena García-Palacios, and Cristina Botella

Usability of a Transdiagnostic Internet-Delivered Protocol for Anxiety
and Depression in Community Patients   147
    Amanda Díaz-García, Alberto González-Robles, Javier Fernández-Álvarez,
    Diana Castilla, Adriana Mira, Juana María Bretón,
    Azucena García-Palacios, and Cristina Botella

How Can We Implement Single-Case Experimental Designs in Group
Therapy and Using Digital Technologies: A Study with
Fibromyalgia Patients   157
    Carlos Suso-Ribera, Guadalupe Molinari, and Azucena García-Palacios

An Attempt to Estimate Depressive Status from Voice.   168
    Yasuhiro Omiya, Takeshi Takano, Tomotaka Uraguchi,
    Mitsuteru Nakamura, Masakazu Higuchi, Shuji Shinohara,
    Shunji Mitsuyoshi, Mirai So, and Shinichi Tokuno

Usability, Acceptability, and Feasibility of Two Technology-Based Devices
for Mental Health Screening in Perinatal Care: A Comparison
of Web Versus App   176
    Verónica Martínez-Borba, Carlos Suso-Ribera, and Jorge Osma

Feasibility and Utility of Pain Monitor: A Smartphone Application
for Daily Monitoring Chronic Pain   190
    Irene Jaén, Carlos Suso-Ribera, Diana Castilla, Irene Zaragoza,
    and Azucena García-Palacios

Discrimination of Bipolar Disorders Using Voice   199
    Masakazu Higuchi, Mitsuteru Nakamura, Shuji Shinohara,
    Yasuhiro Omiya, Takeshi Takano, Hiroyuki Toda, Taku Saito,
    Aihide Yoshino, Shunji Mitsuyoshi, and Shinichi Tokuno

Exploring Affect Recall Bias and the Impact of Mild Depressive
Symptoms: An Ecological Momentary Study   208
    Desirée Colombo, Carlos Suso-Ribera, Javier Fernandez-Álvarez,
    Isabel Fernandez Felipe, Pietro Cipresso, Azucena Garcia Palacios,
    Giuseppe Riva, and Cristina Botella

Full Body Immersive Virtual Reality System with Motion Recognition
Camera Targeting the Treatment of Spider Phobia.   216
    Jacob Kritikos, Stavroula Poulopoulou, Chara Zoitaki,
    Marilina Douloudi, and Dimitris Koutsouris

Evaluation of a Self-report System for Assessing Mood Using Facial
Expressions   231
  Hristo Valev, Tim Leufkens, Corina Sas, Joyce Westerink,
  and Ron Dotsch

Testing a Deactivated Virtual Environment in Pathological Gamblers'
Anxiety   242
  Michelle Semonella, Pietro Cipresso, Cosimo Tuena, Alessandra Parisi,
  Michelle Toti, Aurora Elena Bobocea, Pier Giovanni Mazzoli,
  and Giuseppe Riva

Promoting Wellbeing in Pregnancy: A Multi-component Positive
Psychology and Mindfulness-Based Mobile App   250
  Claudia Carissoli, Giulia Corno, Stefano Montanelli,
  and Daniela Villani

Beyond Cognitive Rehabilitation: Immersive but Noninvasive Treatment
for Elderly   263
  Elisa Pedroli, Pietro Cipresso, Silvia Serino, Michelle Toti,
  Karine Goulen, Mauro Grigioni, Marco Stramba-Badiale,
  Andrea Gaggioli, and Giuseppe Riva

Correction to: Full Body Immersive Virtual Reality System with Motion
Recognition Camera Targeting the Treatment of Spider Phobia C1
  Jacob Kritikos, Stavroula Poulopoulou, Chara Zoitaki,
  Marilina Douloudi, and Dimitris Koutsouris

Author Index   275

Virtual-Reality Music-Based Elicitation of Awe: When Silence Is Better Than Thousands Sounds

Alice Chirico[1]($\boxtimes$) and Andrea Gaggioli[1,2]

[1] Department of Psychology, Università Cattolica Del Sacro Cuore, Milan, Italy
alice.chirico@unicatt.it
[2] Applied Technology for Neuro-Psychology Lab, Istituto Auxologico Italiano, Milan, Italy
a.gaggioli@auxologico.it

Abstract. Several researches have revealed the potential of awe, a complex emotion arising from vast stimuli able to prompt for a restructuration of people' mental schema, on wellbeing and health. Despite a lot has been revealed about awe, researchers still face the challenge of eliciting intense instances of awe in a controlled way. A combination of two or more emotion-induction techniques can enhance the intensity of the resulting emotion. VR has resulted as one of the best techniques to elicit awe, but it has never been tested in combination with other effective awe-inducing methods, such as music. Here, we tested the combined effect of VR and music on the resulting awe's intensity. We randomly assigned 76 healthy participants to one of these four conditions: (i) VR with background sounds (ii) VR and Music, (iii) only Music; (iv) VR without sounds. VR environments and music have been validated in previous studies on awe. Before the exposure to each stimulus, we asked participants to rate the extent to which they *felt* (i.e., experienced) seven emotions. After the exposure, we measured also how much participants *perceived* (i.e., they "read" it into the emotional material) each of the seven emotions, as well as their general affect (Positive and Negative Affective Schedule), their sense of presence (i.e., how much participants felt to be "*present*" within a scene) (ITC-SOPI Inventory), the sense of perceived vastness and need for accommodation associated to the stimulus material (Brief Awe-Scale). We also assessed also participants' disposition to live seven discrete positive emotions (Dispositional Positive Emotions Scale) and musical preferences (STOMP). "VR with Music" condition elicited a higher (even not significant) sense of ecological validity compared to Music condition. All conditions elicited significantly higher sense of felt awe, joy, and fear compared to the baseline and a significantly lower anger after each condition. Participants in the Music condition felt a lowest sense of amusement after the exposure. We found no effect of condition on felt awe. Conversely, perceived awe was significantly higher in the "VR and Music" condition compared to the Music condition. "VR without sounds" condition elicited significantly higher sense of fear compared to Music condition, and significantly lower sense of pride and sadness compared to Music condition. We found no significant effect for any covariate variable. These results have relevant implications for fundamental research on awe and to design awe-based training enhancing wellbeing health, or targeting severe emotional disorders, such as Depression.

P. Cipresso et al. (Eds.): MindCare 2019, LNICST 288, pp. 1–11, 2019.
https://doi.org/10.1007/978-3-030-25872-6_1

Keywords: Awe · Emotion-induction · Virtual reality · Music · Wellbeing · Perceived emotions · Felt emotions · Silence

1 Introduction

Emotions are pervasive phenomena shaping most aspects of people life [1–8]. Since William James' seminal work [9], several researchers have dedicated an entire life to define what emotions are and how they are made [10], to understand and predict their impact on our life. At the heart of this question dwells another issue, that is, how to study emotions in a controlled way [11–15]. A wide array of emotion-induction techniques has been developed to address this issue [13–17] and several meta-analytical works [18–20] have been carried out to find out the best technique to use, in order to obtain the most intense emotional impact. However, one aspect emerged. Not all techniques are equally effective in inducing a target mood, affect or emotion [21]. Thus, most research focused on identifying the best technique for a target emotion (e.g., [12]). Far more recent is the research on the best emotion-induction techniques for complex emotions, such as awe [1, 22–27]. Despite awe has been mostly labelled as a "positive" emotion (e.g., [28–30]), recent studies demonstrated that this phenomenon is closer to a mixed, ambiguous state [25–27, 31]. Thus, awe results as an unusual emotion [23]. The uniqueness of awe is reflected also in the way it shapes our life. Awe might be conceived as a sort of "interference" into the quiet flow of life since it can deeply and enduringly change people' perspective towards life, themselves and other people [23, 32, 33]. Awe emerges when we face something much bigger than us (conceptually or visually) that can question us and our accustomed way to process stimuli, or to make predictions [34]. This emotion can expand our perception of time available to live [35], thus decreasing also our level of distress, when we are repeatedly exposed to it [36], and enhancing the satisfaction with our life [37]. Awe makes us more generous [29], prone to help other people [38, 39], less aggressive [40]. Finally, a key point on awe is the effect on the self. Awe leads to a self-diminishment (less attention/importance towards the self), which has been found beneficial for several reasons, above all, recently, for ameliorating depressive symptoms. Tarani [41] showed that awe could decrease the degree of ruminative thoughts on the self and the contingent feeling of hopelessness.

Given all this complexity associated to awe, researchers still struggle to reproduce intense experiences of awe in a controlled setting [22]. Several awe-eliciting techniques have been developed to address these issue but Virtual Reality (VR) resulted among the most effective ones [1, 22, 26, 27]. Virtual Reality can be defined as a 3-D computer generated environment users can also interact with [22]. One key asset provided by VR is resembling even complex phenomena in a controlled setting, thus placing VR nearer reality. Recently, it has been demonstrated that VR and an equivalent scenario in real life do no significantly differ in terms of resulting affective intensity, including awe [42]. However, even in real life, highly intense experiences of awe are extremely rare. Therefore, the question becomes how to enhance the intensity of awe using VR. One solution is provided by the literature on emotion-induction [43]. Combining techniques, which have already resulted effective in eliciting a target emotion, can enhance the intensity of the resulting affect [18, 43]. With this regard, another understudied awe-inspiring technique is music, which has been tested only in few studies to date [44, 45]. The aim of this study was to test the combined effect of VR and Music for the elicitation of highly intense instances of awe in the lab. We disambiguated the effect of Music and VR alone (without background sounds), as well as VR with music or with background sounds, using pre-validated stimuli. We chose only one excerpt of awe-inspiring music taken from Silvia [44], and a awe-inducing VR environment that has been tested by the Authors in a previous study [27].

Moreover, since the effect of awe-inspiring music resulted mediated by Openness to Experience personality trait [44] as well as by musical preferences [45], we considered also musical preferences [46], Big Five personality traits [47], and the disposition to live positive emotions (Positive Emotion Dispositions) [48], including awe, Finally, the emotion-music link is often questioned since it has been frequently suggested that music can only "mimic" emotions and not make people feel authentic emotional states [49]. Therefore, also in this study, we disentangled this aspect by distinguishing between emotions perceived by participants into the musical material and really felt.

2 Methodology

2.1 Sample and Procedure

The study sample comprised 76 adults (42 women) volunteers from Italy. Their mean age was 23.14 (S.D. = 4.01). We chose a between-design in which each participant was randomly assigned either to one of these conditions: (i) VR with background sounds (ii) VR and Music, (iii) only Music; (iv) VR without sounds.

Upon arrival to the lab, participants signed formed consent, the VR and musical equipment was settled. Each emotional induction lasted 5 min. Before each session, participants were required to rate the extent to which they felt (i.e., really experienced) seven emotions (joy, anger, pride, disgust, sadness, amusement and awe) on a 7-point likert scale (1 = not at all; 7 = extremely). Only after the exposure, we measured also their general contingent Affect (Positive and Negative Affective Schedule, PANAS [50]), how much they perceived (i.e., they "read" this emotion into the emotional material) each of the seven emotions (joy, content, pride, love, amusement, compassion and awe), their sense of presence (i.e., how much participants felt to be "present" within the scene depicted in VR or through music) (ITC-SOPI Inventory [51]), as well as the sense of perceived vastness and need for accommodation associated to the stimulus material (Brief Awe-Scale [26]). Finally, since awe elicitation has resulted modulated by trait variables and music effectiveness depends also on people musical preferences, we assessed also participants disposition to live seven discrete positive emotions (Dispositional Positive Emotions Scale [48]) and musical preferences (STOMP [46]). Participants in the VRE conditions received the same instructions provided by [27] (Fig. 1).

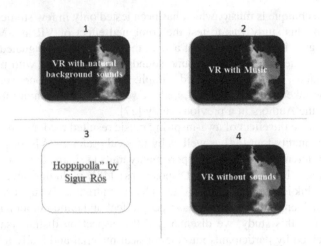

Fig. 1. Research matrix representing the four experimental conditions: 1. VR with natural background sounds; 2. VR with Music; 3. only Music; 4. VR without sounds.

2.2 Measures and Instruments

Self-reported state measures: we measured three main categories of state variables:

(i) Discrete emotions: we assessed the extent to which participants *felt* (i.e., really experienced) vs. *experienced* (i.e., only perceive it into the emotional stimuli) seven distinct emotions (joy, anger, pride, disgust, sadness, amusement and awe) on a 7-point likert scale (1 = not at all; 7 = extremely), as We did in [27].

(ii) General Affect: we adopted the Italian PANAS version [50] that encloses the two main categories of the affective experience. This self-reported instrument is composed of 20 adjectives measuring the positive (PA) (10 adjectives) and the negative (NA) (10 adjectives) dimension of affective experience.

(iii) Sense of presence: we chose the Italian version of the ITC-SOPI Sense of Presence Inventory to rate the extent to which each participant experiences a sense of being "really" present within the emotional stimulus on four dimensions (Engagement, Physical Presence, Ecological Validity, Negative Effects). This self-reported scale is composed of 36-item on a 5-point likert scale (1 = strongly disagree to 5 = strongly disagree).

(vi) Awe sub-dimensions: we assessed awe-related sub-components with a scale that we validated in a previous study, which is called "Brief Awe-scale" [26]. This self-reported instrument is composed of seven items rating the two main dimensions of awe on a 7 point likert scale (1 = not at all; 7 = extremely): perceived vastness (4 items) and need for accommodation (3 items).

Self-reported Dispositional Measures. Besides state measure of affect, emotion and sense of presence, we also assessed:

(i) Disposition to live Positive Emotions: this scale has been developed by Shiota et al. [48] and it is a 38-item instrument on a 7point likert scale (1 = strongly disagree; 7 = strongly agree) to measure the intensity of seven different discrete positive emotions (joy, contentment, pride, love, compassion, amusement), including awe.

(ii) Musical Preferences: this self-reported instrument is a widely used 14-item scale measuring people' preferences for musical genres. It is composed of four scales referring to four general music-preference components: (i) Reflective & Complex; (ii) Intense & Rebellious; (iii) Upbeat & Conventional; (iv) Energetic & Rhythmic.

Stimuli. The selected music was ("Hoppípolla" by Sigur Rós), which has already validated by Silvia [44] and selected in order not to be familiar to our participants.

The VR environment was taken from [27] as the most awe-inspiring scenario.

3 Data Analysis

We carried out nine separated mixed ANOVAs 4 (between condition: VR with natural background sounds; VR with music; Music; VR with no sounds) x 2 (time: pre vs. post exposure) for each of the state discrete *felt* emotions (joy, anger, pride, disgust, sadness, amusement and awe) and affect variables (positive and negative affect). Moreover, we carried out eleven between ANOVAs (between condition: VR with natural background sounds; VR with music; Music; VR with no sounds) for each of the state discrete *perceived* emotions (joy, anger, pride, disgust, sadness, amusement and awe) and dimensions of presence (Engagement, Physical Presence, Ecological Validity, Negative Effects).

4 Results

Results showed no significant differences for positive or negative affect across conditions. We found only a significant effect of time (pre-post exposure) for *felt* anger $[F(1,68) = 9.852; p = .003; \eta^2_{partial} = .127]$, fear $[F(1,68) = 4.223; p = .044; \eta_{partial}^2 = .058]$, joy $[F(1,68) = 100.380; p < .0001; \eta^2_{partial} = .251$ awe $[F(1,68) = 100.380; p < .0001; \eta^2_{partial} = .596]$, which were all significantly increased after the exposure to each condition. We did not find a significant effect of condition on felt awe. Finally, we found a significant interaction effect between time and condition for amusement $[F(3,68) = 3.64; p = .017; \eta^2_{partial} = .138]$: participants in the Music condition felt a lower sense of amusement (even if not significantly) after the exposure compared to other conditions.

Regarding *perceived* awe, Bonferroni post hoc comparisons showed that only "VR with music" condition $[F(3,68) = 3.129; p < .0001; \eta^2_{partial} = .121]$ induced a significantly higher level of awe compared to the "Music" condition. Moreover, data revealed a significant effect of condition on perceived pride $[F (3,68) = 5.593; p < .05; \eta^2_{partial} = .198]$ (Post hoc with Bonferroni showed that "Music" elicited a significantly higher pride than "VR without sounds" condition), perceived sadness $[F (3,68) = 4.904; p < .05; \eta^2_{partial} = .178]$ (post hoc with Bonferroni showed that "Music" elicited the

Table 1. Descriptive statistics for each state variable in the four conditions before and after emotion induction (M = mean; SD = Standard Deviation)

| | Pre-experimental | | | | | | | | Post-experimental | | | | | | | |
| | VR with natural background sounds | | VR with music | | Music | | VR with no sounds | | VR with natural background sounds | | VR with music | | Music | | VR with no sounds | |
	M	SD	M	SD	M	SD	M	SD	M	SD	M	SD	M	SD	M	SD
Felt_Anger	2.45	1.572	1.78	1.060	2.22	1.437	1.93	1.385	1.91	1.221	1.61	1.461	1.17	.383	1.29	.469
Felt fear	2.45	1.036	2.11	1.278	2.67	1.572	2.86	1.834	3.18	1.537	2.83	1.505	2.17	1.724	3.71	1.729
Felt joy	3.55	0.522	3.56	1.617	3.61	1.614	3.57	1.651	5.00	1.000	4.72	1.674	5.17	1.689	4.36	1.692
Felt sadness	2.36	1.859	2.17	1.425	2.56	1.886	2.00	0.961	2.27	1.737	2.06	1.731	2.89	1.811	1.79	1.369
felt Pride	3.73	1.348	3.78	1.927	3.67	1.749	3.36	1.447	3.82	1.471	3.61	1.819	4.50	1.790	3.00	1.797
Felt amusement	4.64	1.206	4.00	1.495	4.28	1.274	3.36	1.336	4.18	2.089	4.50	1.823	3.56	1.723	4.79	1.626
Felt awe	3.73	1.421	2.83	1.855	2.67	1.283	3.14	1.460	5.45	1.508	5.56	1.653	4.61	1.819	5.64	1.865
Perceived Anger									2.09	1.640	1.06	.236	1.39	.979	1.14	.363
Perceived fear									4.00	1.342	3.06	1.514	2.17	1.383	3.57	1.869
Perceived joy									4.64	.924	4.67	1.372	5.17	1.383	3.14	1.791
Perceived sadness									2.36	1.206	1.89	1.079	3.56	1.653	1.86	1.406
Perceived pride									3.45	1.508	3.06	1.765	4.28	1.602	1.86	1.610
Perceived amusement									4.18	1.834	4.61	1.754	3.78	1.396	3.43	1.950
Perceived awe									5.91	1.446	5.89	1.811	4.44	1.790	5.43	1.742
Positive affect									2.61	0.32193	2.74	.51930	2.85	.45794	2.81	.43828
Negative affect									2.46	.26934	2.45	.42179	2.60	.38267	2.60	.38122
Physical presence									58.64	6.577	56.94	12.698	57.61	8.311	60.64	13.821
Engagement									48.55	6.251	49.44	8.618	47.00	7.436	50.86	6.993
Ecological validity									17.00	2.530	19.06	3.638	15.50	4.475	18.93	5.903
Negative effect									13.64	4.675	11.94	4.425	10.00	5.099	12.43	4.433
Vastness									17.18	3.99545	19.89	5.37849	16.67	4.08728	19.28	5.97982
Need for accommodation									8.18	2.96034	7.67	3.88057	8.44	3.61731	9.14	5.41873

significantly lowest sadness) and perceived fear [F (3,68) = 2.762; p < .05; $\eta^2_{partial}$ = .109] (Bonferroni's post hoc revealed no significant differences), and joy [F(3,68) =5.405; p = .002; $\eta^2_{partial}$ = .193] (post hoc revealed that "VR without sounds" elicited a significantly lower perceived joy compared to "VR with sounds" and "Music" condition). Pride and Sadness were significantly lower in the "VR without sounds" condition compared to the Musical one, while fear was significantly higher in the "VR without sounds" condition compared to the Music condition.

We did not find any significant differences across condition for the dimension of perceived vastness and need for accommodation, awe sub-components. However, "VR with music" conditions showed the highest level of perceived vastness compared to other conditions, while "VR without sounds" elicited the higher need for accommodation compared to the remaining conditions.

With regard to the sense of presence, we found only an almost significant difference between Music and "VR with Music" in terms of Ecological Validity [F (3) = 2.613; p = .058; $\eta^2_{partial}$ = .103] ("VR and Music" condition elicited a higher, but not significant, sense of ecological validity compared to "Music" condition).

To deepen the analysis of perceived and felt awe across conditions, we conducted twenty-one mixed ANCOVAs 4 (between condition: VR with natural background sounds; VR with music; Music; VR with no sounds) x 2 (time: pre vs. post exposure) on *felt* awe, and twenty-one one-way between-measures ANCOVAs 4 (between condition: VR with natural background sounds; VR with music; Music; VR with no sounds) on *perceived* awe. We entered each trait variable as a covariate separately in each model. None of these models resulted significant. For descriptive statistic, please, see Table 1.

Finally, we carried out not parametrical Pearson's correlations between the disposition to live awe and each dimension of musical preferences for each condition separately. We fund only a significant positive correlation between disposition to live awe and preference for "Reflective and complex" dimension of musical preferences (r = .479; p = .033).

5 Discussion and Conclusion

Emotion-induction studies can provide two main guidelines for researchers interested in intensifying specific emotions or affect in the lab: (i) To choose emotion-elicitation techniques that have already proved as effective for the target emotion; (ii) To test a combination or two or more of these techniques to increase the intensity of the resulting emotion. In this study, we advanced this field in two ways. First, we tested these guidelines on a complex ambiguous emotion, that is, awe. Secondly, we provided the first empirical evidence of a joint induction through Virtual Reality and Music in the lab. Our results showed that for complex emotions such as awe, the combination of two or more emotion-elicitation techniques shaped the resulting emotional experience differently in the case of a perceived vs. felt emotion. Specifically, we showed that while inducing higher intensity perceived awe in the lab was a function of a combination between VR and music, this did not occur for felt awe. Curiously, felt awe was not differently affected by none of our variables (both condition and trait variables considered as covariates). These results are only partially in line with previous findings from [44, 45]. Specifically, Pilgrim et al. [45] showed that preferences for several musical genres interacted with stable personality and cognitive dispositions (e.g., need for cognition) include the subsequent awe experience, for instance, country music was positively and significantly correlated with cognitive closure, which is associated with discomfort with ambiguity and difficulty to adapt to the environment, thus should be negatively related to awe. However, Pilgrim et al. [45] focused on dispositional awe, while, in this study, we initially concentrated on a combination of state and trait awe. therefore, we also carried out several correlations between disposition to live awe and each dimension of musical preferences. Interestingly, we found only a positive linear link with "Reflective and complex" dimension of musical preferences, which includes blues, jazz, classical, and folk music. Also, Pilgrim et al. found that reflective and complex music was associated with greater experienced awe if controlled for need for cognition. Therefore, in future studies, we should also consider the role of personality and cognitive stable factors to explain differences across conditions. Moreover, as suggested by Pilgrim et al., since people experience awe in relation of their preferred music (e.g., [52, 53]), maybe, our selected music did not meet the preferences of participants. Another possible explanation could be that awe can act differently from a "conventional" emotion, thus requiring a higher degree of perceived salience and relevance of music to be elicited. Future studies should manipulate or disambiguate the role of perceived relevance of music in inducing awe. Curiously, while the preference for country music enhanced the resulting perceived awe after the "VR and music" more than the "Music" condition, it was the condition without sounds that was affected more by this musical preference compared to the Musical one. *Sometimes, silence wins against visual and vestibular stimulation* (VR) for eliciting intense awe.

A possible future step to deepen the differences between perceived and felt emotions, could be to use psychophysiological measures during the ongoing emotional experience [54]. Indeed, felt and perceived awe acted differently in this study, showing diverse pattern of results concerning the induction of this emotion in the lab.

All these findings help gain new knowledge about the elicitation of ambiguous emotions, such as awe, in a controlled setting, which is a suitable procedure for designing valid and effective evidence-based trainings or treatment based on these emotions. A crucial implication concerns the use of VR and musical stimuli for the treatment of severe disorders, such as Major Depression, or simply, for the promotion of wellbeing and health of a wide population.

References

1. Chirico, A., et al.: Awe enhances creative thinking: an experimental study. Creat. Res. J. **30**, 123–131 (2018)
2. Lench, H.C., Flores, S.A., Bench, S.W.: Discrete emotions predict changes in cognition, judgment, experience, behavior, and physiology: a meta-analysis of experimental emotion elicitations. Psychol. Bull. **137**(5), 834 (2011)
3. DeSteno, D., et al.: Discrete emotions and persuasion: the role of emotion-induced expectancies. J. Pers. Soc. Psychol. **86**(1), 43 (2004)

4. Nabi, R.L.: Exploring the framing effects of emotion: do discrete emotions differentially influence information accessibility, information seeking, and policy preference? Commun. Res. **30**(2), 224–247 (2003)
5. Frijda, N.H.: Emotions and action. In: Feelings and emotions: the Amsterdam symposium (2004)
6. Lewis, M., Haviland-Jones, J.M., Barrett, L.F.: Handbook of Emotions. Guilford Press, New York (2010)
7. Dalgleish, T., Power, M.: Handbook of Cognition and Emotion. Wiley, New York (2000)
8. Bradley, M.M., Lang, P.J.: Emotion and motivation. Handb. Psychophysiol. **2**, 602–642 (2000)
9. James, W.: What is an Emotion? Mind **9**(34), 188–205 (1884)
10. Barrett, L.F.: How Emotions are Made: The Secret Life of the Brain. Houghton Mifflin Harcourt, Boston (2017)
11. Nummenmaa, L., Niemi, P.: Inducing affective states with success-failure manipulations: A meta-analysis. Emotion **4**(2), 207 (2004)
12. Ellard, K.K., Farchione, T.J., Barlow, D.H.: Relative effectiveness of emotion induction procedures and the role of personal relevance in a clinical sample: a comparison of film, images, and music. J. Psychopathol. Behav. Assess. **34**(2), 232–243 (2012)
13. Fakhrhosseini, S.M., Jeon, M.: Affect/emotion induction methods. In: Emotions and Affect in Human Factors and Human-Computer Interaction, pp. 235–253. Elsevier (2017)
14. Mills, C., D'Mello, S.: On the validity of the autobiographical emotional memory task for emotion induction. PLoS ONE **9**(4), e95837 (2014)
15. Västfjäll, D.: Emotion induction through music: a review of the musical mood induction procedure. Musicae Sci. **5**(1_suppl), 173–211 (2001)
16. Gerrards-Hesse, A., Spies, K., Hesse, F.W.: Experimental inductions of emotional states and their effectiveness: a review. Br. J. Psychol. **85**(1), 55–78 (1994)
17. Park, B.-J., et al.: Emotion induction and emotion recognition using their physiological signals. In: 2012 7th International Conference on Computing and Convergence Technology (ICCCT). IEEE (2012)
18. Westermann, R., Stahl, G., Hesse, F.: Relative effectiveness and validity of mood induction procedures: analysis. Eur. J. Soc. Psychol. **26**, 557–580 (1996)
19. Lench, H.C., Flores, S.A., Bench, S.W.: Discrete Emotions Predict Changes in Cognition, Judgment, Experience, Behavior, and Physiology: A Meta-Analysis of Experimental Emotion Elicitations. American Psychological Association (2011)
20. Ferrer, R.A., Grenen, E.G., Taber, J.M.: Effectiveness of internet-based affect induction procedures: a systematic review and meta-analysis. Emotion **15**(6), 752 (2015)
21. Jallais, C., Gilet, A.-L.: Inducing changes in arousal and valence: comparison of two mood induction procedures. Behav. Res. Methods **42**(1), 318–325 (2010)
22. Chirico, A., et al.: The potential of virtual reality for the investigation of awe. Front. Psychol. **7**, 1766 (2016)
23. Chirico, A., Gaggioli, A.: Awe: more than a feeling. Humanistic Psychol. **46**, 274–280 (2018)
24. Chirico, A., Cipresso, P., Riva, G., Gaggioli, A.: A process for selecting and validating awe-inducing audio-visual stimuli. In: Oliver, N., Serino, S., Matic, A., Cipresso, P., Filipovic, N., Gavrilovska, L. (eds.) MindCare/FABULOUS/IIOT 2015-2016. LNICST, vol. 207, pp. 19–27. Springer, Cham (2018). https://doi.org/10.1007/978-3-319-74935-8_3
25. Chirico, A., Cipresso, P., Gaggioli, A.: Psychophysiological correlate of compex spherical awe stimuli. Neuropsychol. Trends **33**, 79–80 (2016)
26. Chirico, A., et al.: Effectiveness of immersive videos in inducing awe: an experimental study. Sci. Rep. **7**(1), 1218 (2017)

27. Chirico, A., et al.: designing awe in virtual reality: an experimental study. Front. Psychol. **8**, 2351 (2018)
28. Ballew, M.T., Omoto, A.M.: Absorption: how nature experiences promote awe and other positive emotions. Ecopsychology **10**(1), 26–35 (2018)
29. Prade, C., Saroglou, V.: Awe's effects on generosity and helping. J. Posit. Psychol. **11**, 1–9 (2016)
30. Yaden, D.B., et al.: The development of the awe experience scale (AWE-S): a multifactorial measure for a complex emotion. J. Posit. Psychol. **14**, 1–15 (2018)
31. Gordon, A.M., et al.: The dark side of the sublime: distinguishing a threat-based variant of awe. J. Pers. Soc. Psychol. **102**, 70–717 (2016)
32. Bonner, E., Friedman, H.: A conceptual clarification of the experience of awe: an interpretative phenomenological analysis. Humanist. Psychol. **39**(3), 222–235 (2011)
33. Schneider, K.: The resurgence of awe in psychology: Promise, hope, and perils. Humanistic Psychol. **45**(2), 103 (2017)
34. Chirico, A., Yaden, David B.: Awe: a self-transcendent and sometimes transformative emotion. In: Lench, Heather C. (ed.) The Function of Emotions, pp. 221–233. Springer, Cham (2018). https://doi.org/10.1007/978-3-319-77619-4_11
35. Rudd, M., Vohs, K.D., Aaker, J.: Awe expands people's perception of time, alters decision making, and enhances well-being. Psychol. Sci. **23**(10), 1130–1136 (2012)
36. Stellar, J.E., et al.: Positive affect and markers of inflammation: discrete positive emotions predict lower levels of inflammatory cytokines. Emotion **15**(2), 129 (2015)
37. Krause, N., Hayward, R.D.: Assessing whether practical wisdom and awe of god are associated with life satisfaction. Psychol. Relig. Spirit. **7**(1), 51 (2015)
38. Piff, P.K., et al.: Awe, the small self, and prosocial behavior. J. Pers. Soc. Psychol. **108**(6), 883 (2015)
39. Stegemoeller, B.: Collective Awe and Prosocial Behavior, p. 27. DePaul University Honors Program (2016)
40. Yang, Y., et al.: Elicited awe decreases aggression. J. Pac. Rim Psychol. **10** (2016)
41. Tarani, E.: Affective and Cognitive Effects of Awe in Predicting Hopelessness and Brooding Rumination (2017). Master's Theses. p. 4824. https://doi.org/10.31979/etd.v6td-4d7s, https://scholarworks.sjsu.edu/etd_theses/4824
42. Chirico, A., Gaggioli, A.: When virtual feels real: comparing emotional responses and presence in virtual and natural environments. Cyberpsychol., Behav. Soci. Netw. **22**, 82–96 (2019)
43. Baumgartner, T., et al.: The emotional power of music: how music enhances the feeling of affective pictures. Brain Res. **1075**(1), 151–164 (2006)
44. Silvia, P.J., et al.: Openness to experience and awe in response to nature and music: personality and profound aesthetic experiences. Psychol. Aesthet. Creat. Arts **9**(4), 376–384 (2015)
45. Pilgrim, L., Norris, J.I., Hackathorn, J.: Music is awesome: influences of emotion, personality, and preference on experienced awe. J. Consum. Behav. **16**, 442–451 (2017)
46. Rentfrow, P.J., Gosling, S.D.: The do re mi's of everyday life: the structure and personality correlates of music preferences. J. Pers. Soc. Psychol. **84**(6), 1236 (2003)
47. Ubbiali, A., Carlo, C., Hampton, P., Deborah, D.: Italian big five inventory. Psychometric properties of the italian adaptation of the big five inventory (BFI). Appl. Psychol. Bull. **59**(266), 37 (2013)
48. Shiota, M.N., Keltner, D., John, O.P.: Positive emotion dispositions differentially associated with big five personality and attachment style. J. Posit. Psychol. **1**(2), 61–71 (2006)
49. Gabrielsson, A.: Emotion perceived and emotion felt: Same or different? Musicae Sci. **5**(1 suppl), 123–147 (2002)

50. Terraciano, A., McCrae, R.R., Costa Jr., P.T.: Factorial and construct validity of the Italian positive and negative affect schedule (PANAS). Eur. J. Psychol. Assess. **19**(2), 131 (2003)
51. Lessiter, J., et al.: A cross-media presence questionnaire: the ITC-sense of presence inventory. Presence **10**(3), 282–297 (2001)
52. Liljeström, S., Juslin, P.N.: The roles of music choice, social context, and listener personality in emotional reactions to music: A listening experiment (2011)
53. Schubert, E.: Emotion felt by the listener and expressed by the music: literature review and theoretical perspectives. Front. Psychol. **4**, 837 (2013)
54. Chirico, A., Cipresso, P., Gaggioli, A.: Psychophysiological specificity of four basic emotions through autobiographical recall and videos. In: 7th EAI International Symposium on Pervasive Computing Paradigms for Mental Health 2018, 9–10 January 2018, Boston, USA

Clara: Design of a New System for Passive Sensing of Depression, Stress and Anxiety in the Workplace

Juwon Lee[1(✉)], Megan Lam[2], and Caleb Chiu[2]

[1] The University of Hong Kong, Pokfulam, Hong Kong
u3534591@connect.hku.hk
[2] Neurum Health, Room 1405, 135 Bonham Strand Trade Centre,
135 Bonham Strand, Sheung Wan, Hong Kong
{meg, caleb}@neurumhealth.com

Abstract. Collective evidence from research on the detriment of mental ill-health in the workplace consistently points to the need for better management of workplace mental health. However, difficulty in making a reliable, unobtrusive measurement of an employee's mental health remains an obstacle in the way of effective interventions at an organizational level. In this paper, a system named Clara is proposed with aims to enable passive measurement, and hence effective management, of workplace mental health. A literature review of different approaches to measure depression, stress, and anxiety is presented, followed by a discussion on the design principles that guided the development of Clara. The overarching system architecture is then outlined, and individual components of the system are explored in finer details. The paper illustrates how Clara, with its passive measurement techniques, has the potential to enable objective assessment of workplace depression, stress and anxiety, allowing for delivery of timely interventions.

Keywords: Workplace mental health · Passive sensing · Machine learning · Depression · Stress · Anxiety

1 Introduction

In recent years, mental health problems in the workplace have been among the top concerns for organizations of varying sizes. In a survey conducted by Mental Health America (MHA) on 17000 workers of different industries, over 35% answered they "always" miss 3–5 days a month because of workplace stress [1]. In the same survey, over 80% answered their personal relationships are being negatively affected by workplace stress [1].

Despite the prevalence of the problem, many suffer in silence. A survey-based study conducted on 44000 employees in America showed that only about half of the people experiencing mental health problems have talked to their employers about their problems [2]. This lack of openness that arises from the stigma associated with mental illnesses makes them altogether a more trying challenge to tackle.

© ICST Institute for Computer Sciences, Social Informatics and Telecommunications Engineering 2019
Published by Springer Nature Switzerland AG 2019. All Rights Reserved
P. Cipresso et al. (Eds.): MindCare 2019, LNICST 288, pp. 12–28, 2019.
https://doi.org/10.1007/978-3-030-25872-6_2

Some attempts have been made to put a price tag to this debilitating phenomenon, and one of such examples is the return on investment analysis report created by PwC on "creating a mentally healthy workplace" [3]. The report, which measured the cost of mental health problems in the workplace as the sum of costs of absenteeism, presenteeism and compensation claims, showed that per year, employers in a single developed country loses on average $11 billion - $4.7 billion in absenteeism, $6.1 billion in presenteeism and $146 million in compensation claims [3]. In [4], the authors measured the cost of poor mental health in the workplace by exploring the association of depressive episodes and work productivity, effectively illustrating that about one-third of the annual $51 billion cost of mental illnesses in America is related to productivity losses.

Incentivized by such tangible implications of mental health problems in the workplace, a growing number of employers have started taking initiatives to improve mental wellbeing of its employees. For example, based on the findings from the American Psychological Association (APA) study [5] that highlighted the importance of support from managerial positions on the mental wellbeing of employees, Unilever began to encourage managers through their global health initiatives to take workshops to recognize signs of mental health distress [6]. Similarly, Delta Air Lines has set up early and active intervention programs to support employees with mental health issues. The programs include the employee assistance program (EAP) that provides employees with unlimited phone consultations with master's-level clinicians, three free face-to-face counseling visits per issue per year and behavioral health leaves [7].

A number of studies have been conducted to evaluate the efficacy of such measures taken by employers at an organizational level. A comprehensive literature review of such studies was provided by [8], which presented comparisons of evaluations on three separate categories of workplace mental health initiatives, namely universal interventions, secondary preventions and tertiary preventions. Universal interventions refer to strategies for improving mental health that are delivered to all employees in a work setting without regard to individual risk factors. On the other hand, secondary preventions and tertiary preventions are targeted to subgroups of employees determined to be at risk [8].

A meta-synthesis of qualitative research suggests that both secondary and tertiary prevention have strong evidence for robust effects and reduced symptoms [8]. However, as these intervention strategies require preliminary identification of target subgroups characterized by high levels of risk factors, a key challenge to delivery of interventions lies in the early detection of such risk factors. The subtlety of mental ailments, which are difficult to detect from an external observation, makes accurate measurement of their presence and severity an extremely challenging task.

The costly harms of workplace mental health problems and the heightened interest around initiatives to address them justify the need for a better employee mental-health management tool with enhanced risk detection capabilities. With aims to deliver more timely, targeted interventions at an organizational level, a new system named Clara is proposed.

In this paper, a literature review on multimodal measurement techniques of mental health is presented, with a focus on measurement of depression, anxiety and stress levels. The literature review is followed by an in-depth description of Clara, covering its design principles, overall system architecture and individual components. The paper concludes with a discussion on Clara's limitations, areas of future research as well as implications on the betterment of workplace mental health management.

2 Literature Review on Measurement of Mental Health

The past studies on measurement of affective states including depression, anxiety and stress have often been categorized into three modalities: psychological, physiological and behavioral. Though psychological assessments carried out via questionnaires make up the most widely used method for evaluating such state of mental health [9], their reliability and relevance outside the laboratory setting were often called to question, mainly with regards to the subjectivity introduced from self-report nature. On the other hand, the growing accessibility of digital devices such as mobile phones and smart watches have sparked a noticeable trend in augmenting such self-reported inputs with verifiable data of physiological and behavioral modalities [10].

2.1 Questionnaire-Based Psychological Assessments

Assessment of depression and anxiety have commonly been done in tandem through psychometric instruments including DASS-21 [11], PHQ-9 [12] and GHQ-28 [13]. Likewise, several questionnaire-based assessment methods have been developed for measurement of stress levels. Examples include the Standard Stress Scale (SSS) [14], the Perceived Stress Scale (PSS) [15] and the Stress Response Inventory (SRI) [16]. Together, these questionnaire-based instruments offer clinicians and researchers a standardized means to screen for depression, anxiety and stress. Notably, DASS-21 delivers a set of subscales for each of the three scales it measures, depression, anxiety and stress, allowing for simultaneous yet thorough measurements on the three spectra [11]. For a comprehensive analysis on these measures, their theoretical foci and validation results, we refer to a review by Sakakibara et al. [17].

Despite the widespread usage of such assessment methods, the clinical relevance of their outcomes has often been a source of debate in the psychology community. Concerns frequently raised include reliance on introspective ability of participants, systematic response distortions, and lapses in memory of participants when asked to recall their state from the past [9]. These questionnaire-based assessments have also been criticized for their inability to capture a continuous evolution, and hence subtle changes, of affective states [18].

2.2 Digital Biomarker-Enabled Measurements

With the flux of different sensor-equipped digital devices entering the market, the term "digital biomarker" was introduced to the lexicon of clinical medicine. Its definition is given as "consumer-generated physiological and behavioral measures" collected through connected digital tools [19], and unlike the aforementioned psychological assessments, it offers the benefit of enabling a real-time, continuous and quantitative measurement of an individual's mental state. Many efforts have been made to establish digital biomarkers for mood disorders and affective states, some of which are explored in detail below.

GPS Approach. Studies have shown that GPS data collected from one's mobile phone can act as a powerful predictor for affective disorders including depression and social anxiety [20, 22]. As GPS data captures information about one's range of mobility, home stay and variability in locations visited, signals of mental ill-being were found embedded in the GPS data in multiple occasions. For example, [20] was able to demonstrate the potential of this approach by using fine-grained location data from GPS sensors as a predictor of corresponding, in situ sampling of mental state from 72 study participants. Similarly, in a study conducted with a mobile phone app, Purple Robot [21], higher-level features including circadian movement, normalized entropy and location variance were extracted from raw GPS data of 40 participants for analysis with self-reported depression survey (PHQ-9) [22]. A regression model was trained with the resulting dataset, achieving a cross-validated error of 23.5% in predicting a PHQ-9 score based on the extracted GPS features.

Keystroke Dynamics Approach. Keystroke dynamic refers to the unique characteristics that make up an individual's typing rhythm when using a keyboard or a keypad [23]. Usage of keystroke dynamics in identifying an individual for security applications has been a popular topic for study [24]. Frequently referenced timing features in such studies include time per keystroke, average pause length and pause rate. A variety of keystroke-specific features have been explored as well, including backspace key rate, delete key rate, home key rate and sentence-ending punctuation key rate [23].

Following the promising results in identity authentication applications, keystroke dynamics began to be studied in affective computing. From a field study of participants' keystrokes and their self-reported emotional states, [25] was able to develop classifiers for seven different emotional state, all of which had accuracies above 70%. The study was significant not only in its high achieved accuracy but also in usage of diverse features including those of digraphs (two-letter combinations) and trigraphs (three-letter combinations). Durations between different down keys and up keys of the n-graphs were extracted from participants' keystrokes and were aggregated across participants.

In a separate study exploring the correlations between keystroke dynamics and stress levels, [26] was able to create a KNN-based mode with 75% classification accuracy, further affirming the potential of exploiting continuous monitoring of keyboard interactions for stress detection. On top of keystroke and timing features, the dataset consisted of linguistic features such as language diversity, language complexity and expressivity. Despite the impressive accuracy score, however, it must be noted that introduction of such content-based features may significantly limit the scope of application due to mining of sensitive information.

Mouse Movement Approach. In studies on mouse movements, commonly extracted features are mouse speed, acceleration, direction and number of clicks. Though not as common as studies on keystrokes, a number of studies on mouse movements have demonstrated statistical significance of mouse characteristics in detection of changes in mental states [27, 28].

The authors of [27] designed an experiment that induced emotional states amongst participants by presenting a happy video and a sad counterpart. While the system asked for self-reports on the participants' affective states, it passively gathered mouse movement data without the participants' knowledge. The experiment results showed significant differences in mouse motion characteristics for different levels of arousal. Features that showed particularly high correlation were movement precision, movement smoothness, movement speed and movement acceleration.

Study presented in [28] shared a similar aim of utilizing mouse movement characteristics for development of an empathetic system. More specifically, the paper presented an experiment that collected mouse movements of 136 participants as they were watching an online course. Based on the timing of mouse movement pauses, the system prompted the participants to record their level of boredom. Mouse movement features were extracted from these records, put together with the labels indicating the level of boredom and fed into a statistical classifier implemented with a tree-based algorithm. Though the specificity of the use case and the highly controlled setting of the experiment make the results of the study not widely applicable, the study has its significance in suggesting a novel methodology for using mouse movements to detect changes in emotional state.

Physiological Data Approach. There has been extensive research conducted on physiological signals that mental loads carry. Wealth of novel smartwatches and fitness trackers being released to the market are enabling better understanding of time-dependent physiology of affective disorders, and [25] provides a general overview. In particular, physiological responses studied in correlation with varying stress levels include skin temperature, heart rate, blood pressure and respiration patterns [25].

3   Clara: A System for Passive Sensing of Depression, Stress, and Anxiety in the Workplace

Hereinafter, a system named Clara is proposed with aims to enable unobtrusive measurement and organizational management of workplace mental wellness. The system uses sensing technology that represents and predicts the internal state of one's mental wellness through digital data, and it provides targeted, personalized tools for management. For employers, the system provides an overall report to enable discovery of insights, which can be utilized to strategize effective interventions when necessary.

3.1   Design Principles

Key design principles that drove the development of Clara are presented. The principles described below outline the framework for decision making used in the process of system development.

Unobtrusive Integration. One key strength of Clara lies in its ability to passively and unobtrusively collect the data that it needs to deliver the service. As one of the ultimate aims of the system lies in work productivity enhancement through better management of workplace mental health, conscious decisions were made throughout the development process to ensure that the system minimizes active inputs from the user as much as possible.

Accurate Sensing. In order to optimize the accuracy of depression, anxiety and stress detection, the system collects behavioral data that have previously been reported to contain statistically meaningful signals of an individual's affective state. Until the accuracy of prediction reaches an acceptable threshold, clinical ground truths of users' mental health are collated every week from their responses to DASS-21, a rigorously validated questionnaire for depression, anxiety and stress screening [11].

Protected Confidentiality. As a large portion of the data collected through the system includes what could be viewed as very personal information, careful thoughts have been put into protecting confidentiality. For instance, historical records of both behavioral data and responses to questionnaires are only viewable by the user himself, and when an organization-wide report is generated for the employer, the aggregated data is presented in a way no specific individual is identifiable.

Protected Information Security. When introducing a new software system, information security is a major concern for many employers. To minimize risk, the system gathers the minimum amount of information needed to extract meaningful features for training the behavioral model. For example, in gathering keystroke data, the exact keystroke is not captured. Instead, binary truth values of whether the keystroke is a special character, a number, a backspace or a delete key are delivered to the server with timestamps. The transfer of any collected data is protected through standard MD5 hashing and encryption algorithms [29].

Engaging User Interface. Lack of engaging user interface is one of the most common reasons behind deleting mental health mobile apps [30]. Therefore, throughout development of Clara, design of user-friendly interface was considered a priority. Examples of user interface on the mobile app are given in Fig. 1.

3.2 System Architecture

The high-level architecture of the backend system is presented in Fig. 2. Descriptions of individual components within the architecture follow.

Data Collection. The current version of Clara collects data from two sources: desktop widget and a mobile phone app. Table 1 displays a list of different data collected through the two mediums. For each type of data collected, the table presents its source, raw data sample, collection trigger event and optionality.

Collection trigger event describes a condition that needs to be met for the system to begin collecting corresponding data points. Whereas collection of keystroke and mouse movement simply begins when employees start using their desktops, more complicated sets of rules are applied to trigger collection of data from the mobile phone. For example, GPS-based location is updated to the system only when the system algorithmically determines that the user has traveled more than a certain distance. This threshold acts as a "distance filter", and its value is dynamically determined by the instantaneous speed captured in the reading. The rationale behind dynamically

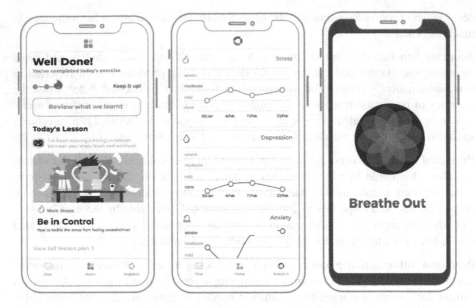

Fig. 1. Clara mobile app user interface

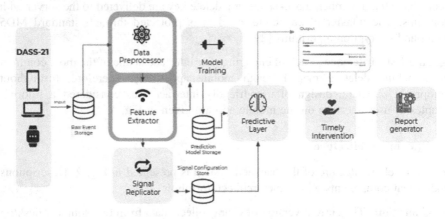

Fig. 2. High-level architecture of the backend system

changing the threshold is to avoid sampling too frequently in the case of high traveling speed. A more detailed description of this implementation can be found in [31], from which the method was taken and adjusted. Likewise, a more detailed description of the trigger methodology for accelerometer implemented in Clara can be found in [32].

Unlike keystroke and mouse movement data that get collected through the desktop widget installed en masse within an organization, the different types of data that get collected on the employee's mobile phone can be selectively opted into the system by each employee. For instance, an employee might choose to provide the system access to his accelerometer data while preventing the system from pulling any data from his

Table 1. Raw data collected by the system

Source	Name	Sample	Trigger event	Optional
Desktop widget	Keystroke dynamic	{timestamp: 1550812094, event_type: KeyUp, is_backspace: True, is_punctuation: False, is_number: False}	Collection triggered when a new key is pressed (event_type = KeyDown) or released (event_type = KeyUp)	No
	Mouse movement	{start_timestamp: 1550812002, end_timestamp: 1550812722, x: 1024, y: 484}	Collection triggered whenever Javascript "onmousemove" event is fired (i.e. when mouse is moved by one or more pixels)	No
Mobile phone app	GPS	{timestamp: 1550989802, latitude: 46.81006, longitude: 92.08174, speed: 18, heading: SW}	Trigger method advanced by [31]. Only collects GPS data when distance travelled exceeds the value of parameter "distance filter", which is dynamically determined by instantaneous speed. Reading is made every 10 min.	Yes
	Accelerometer	{timestamp: 1582091809, a_x: 0.047, a_y: -0.068, a_z: 1.208}	Trigger method advanced in [32]. Accelerometer data collection is initiated when the difference between the magnitude of acceleration in one reading and that of the previous reading is greater than the threshold ($T = 1.1$ m/s2) for 10 consecutive readings. A reading is made every 1 s.	Yes

mobile phone. While higher level of personalization in both screening and delivery of care incentivizes employees to give access to a variety of data points, the degree of flexibility enabled by allowing employees to selectively provide access makes the system capable of catering to a larger group of people with varying levels of comfort in data sharing.

Collection of aforementioned data occurs concurrently with assessment of the employee's mental state through standardized questionnaires. The current version of Clara focuses on measuring employee's depression, anxiety and stress levels, and employees are prompted to fill out the DASS-21 questionnaires every week. The responses to the questionnaires act as clinical ground truth labels for employees' mental state of the week.

Data Preprocessing. Raw data stored in the central database go through series of preprocessing steps before reaching feature extraction. Common high-level preprocessing steps across different data types consist of handling insufficient and erroneous data and de-noising signals.

As keystroke dynamics and mouse movements are captured rather seamlessly with close-to-zero noise via desktop widgets, no particular cleaning or preprocessing strategy specific to these data types is presented. However, in handling GPS and accelerometer data, thorough considerations were made to ensure that the system captures from the data as much meaningful signals as possible. The details of these preprocessing are given below.

GPS Data. Shielding effects and battery exhaustion are some common reasons behind GPS signal losses. To handle missing GPS data in the system, a matrix imputation method based on matrix factorization (MF) [33] is implemented per interval of 7 days. It is worth noting that such MF-based techniques have traditionally been used to provide collaborative recommendations in location-based services [33].

For the purpose of imputing missing spatial values in our system, two separate matrices are constructed using respectively longitudes and latitudes of collected GPS data points. Each element in the matrix represents one GPS data point, and the elements in one row collectively represent data points collected in one day. In each matrix, inferences of missing points are made by factorization, which aims to minimize the errors of the observed points. Using this factorization, both the longitudinal matrix and the latitudinal matrix are reconstructed with missing values imputed.

Accelerometer Data. A particular instance of accelerometer signal is considered insignificant if the motion it captures is not of physical movement of the user. In other words, signals carried by accelerometer when the user simply picks up the phone should not be considered as a valid acceleration input for the model. To correctly identify and remove intervals of such signals, the system calculates the rate of change of acceleration, also known as the jerk. The underlying assumption is that high jerk is associated with physical movement of the individual, whereas low jerk is associated with usage of the phone without the movement. Based on this understanding, a threshold for jerk is defined, and the number of instances of the signal whose jerk is below this threshold is counted in each interval. The ratio of this number to the total number of entries in the interval is used to determine significance of the movement captured in that interval. When this ratio falls under 0.5, the interval is discarded as containing no movement. This approach was previously implemented in [32].

Feature Extraction. A variety of features are extracted from streams of preprocessed data. A comprehensive summary is found in Table 2. A few features require further elaborations, which are provided below.

Table 2. Features extracted from different data streams

Data stream	Feature extracted	Description and comments	Unit
Keystroke	Average pause length	Total pause time/total number of pauses. (Note. threshold of pause T = 500 ms of no keyboard input)	s
	Pause rate	Total number of pauses/total number of keystrokes	–
	Time per keystroke	Total input time/total number of keystrokes	s
	Adjusted time per keystroke	(Total input time - total pause time)/total number of keystrokes	s
	Digraph timing features	Timing between different sets of key down and key up events in digraphs	s
	Trigraph timing features	Timing between different sets of key down and key up events in trigraphs	s
Mouse movement	Average movement speed	Total distance traveled by the cursor during activity/active time during which distance was measured	pixel/s
	Latest average speed before inactivity	Average of movement speed during 120 s before inactivity	pixel/s
	Mouse inactivity occurrences	Number of inactivity occurrences (Note. threshold of inactivity T = 500 ms of 0 change in coordinate)	–
	Average duration of mouse inactivity	Total duration of inactive sessions/mouse inactivity occurrences	s
	Horizontal-to-total movements ratio	Number of horizontal mouse movements/total number of mouse movements	–
	Vertical-to-total movements ratio	Number of vertical mouse movements/total number of mouse movements	–
GPS	Location variance	Logarithm of sum of squared longitudinal variance and squared latitudinal variance	deg^2
	Time spent in moving	(Note. threshold of stationary state T = 1 km/hour for speed)	h
	Total distance traveled	–	km
	Average moving speed	Total distance traveled/time spent in moving	km/h
	Number of unique locations	Number of unique clusters formed by the DBSCAN aclustering	–
	Entropy	$-\sum p_i log\, p_i$ where p_i = percentage of time that a participant spends in location cluster i	–
	Homestay	Time spent at home. Calculated by identifying the location cluster at which most data points are recorded at 0-6am window	h

(continued)

Table 2. (*continued*)

Data stream	Feature extracted	Description and comments	Unit
Accelerometer	Average step duration	Total time for movement recordings/number of steps	s
	Average acceleration magnitude	Root-mean-square sum of accelerations in x, y, and z directions	m/s^2
	Standard deviation of acceleration magnitude	$\sqrt{\frac{1}{M}(\sum\limits_{i=0}^{M-1}(a_i - \bar{a})^2}$ where $\bar{a}$ = average acceleration magnitude	m/s^2
	Average peak acceleration	Average of peak acceleration magnitude in each step	m/s^2

Digraph and Trigraph Features from Keystroke Data. Digraph and trigraph features are extracted by forming two-letter combinations and three-letter combinations in the keystroke data. Digraph features calculated are as follows: difference between timestamps of the first key down and second key down, first key up and second key down, and first key down and last key up. Similarly, trigraph features calculated are as follows: difference between first key down and third key down and first key down and third key up. Also known as duration and latency features, these features are extracted to better capture the rhythm of users' typing on the keyboard.

Directional Features from Mouse Movement. Previous studies have discovered that users frequently make horizontal mouse movements as they gaze through information in paragraphs [34]. In the same studies, vertical mouse movements were more frequently observed when users gazed through dropdowns and menus [34]. These findings suggest coordination between an individual's mouse movements and his reading patterns, which could potentially have indicative signals of his mental state.

For application in our system, mouse movement directions have been categorized into vertical movement and horizontal movement depending on the angle the trajectory of the cursor movement forms with the horizontal axis parallel to the bottom of the laptop screen. Figure 3 illustrates this mapping.

Cluster-Based GPS Features. Cluster-based GPS features refer to features derived from location clusters, created internally in the system by an unsupervised algorithm called DBSCAN [35]. Our implementation of DBSCAN algorithm requires two parameters, epsilon and min_points. These two parameters are used to separate the GPS coordinates into three different categories as one of the following: i) core point if the number of points around the coordinate is greater than min_points within epsilon, ii) border point if the number of points around the coordinate is less than min_points within epsilon and if there's at least one core point within epsilon, and iii) noise point if the coordinate falls under neither of the two aforementioned categories. Upon removal of noise points, the remaining points are iteratively categorized into a cluster until no neighbor, as determined by the reach of epsilon, is found. When this happens, one of the remaining, uncategorized core points is added to a new cluster and its neighbors are again added iteratively. At the end of all iterations, all points end up being labelled with a cluster id.

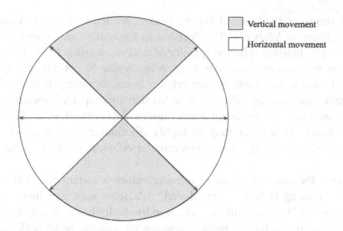

Fig. 3. Directional mapping of mouse movement

The clusters created through this algorithm represent the locations that the user visits, based on the GPS data. The number of unique clusters is therefore indicative of the number of unique locations the user visits, and it is used as a feature in our model. Likewise, for each cluster, a measure of entropy can be calculated using the equation provided in the description box of Table 2. It is worth noting that this implementation has previously been used in [31] to measure the variability of time that an individual spends at different locations.

Step Segmentation from Accelerometer Data. In our system, we consider a single step as the motion that takes place between two consecutive occurrences of the same foot making contact with the ground. A segmentation algorithm advanced in [36] is used to calculate step-based features from the raw accelerometer data. Based on the assumption that the local maxima of the acceleration vector are associated with footfalls, it uses the derivative of the smoothed acceleration, jerk, to identify occurrences of a foot hitting the ground. A low-pass filter, digital Butterworth filter with a critical frequency of 0.05, is used for smoothing purpose before the calculation of jerk.

Once steps are identified within the accelerometer data stream, features such as average step duration and average peak acceleration are calculated.

Model Training and Prediction. Features extracted from the raw data get aggregated into vectors labelled with corresponding ground truth values derived from DASS-21 responses. In such feature aggregation, we consider an interval of 7 days; each interval ends with the day an employee fills in a DASS-21 questionnaire, and the data points collected within the interval are put together with the DASS-21 score calculated from the responses. Per single set of DASS-21 response, three of such feature vectors are constructed, each one labelled with a severity rating for either depression, anxiety or stress. Following the standard DASS-21 scoring scheme, a severity rating that acts as a label for supervised learning can take on one of the following values: normal, mild, moderate, severe and extremely severe.

Upon construction, the labelled feature vectors are fed into a supervised learning algorithm, a variant of Adaboost. The decision to implement an Adaboost variant for model training was motivated by the sparsity of datasets constructed in the system. To better illustrate this concept, consider users who choose to opt-out of accelerometer data collection for concerns ranging from privacy issues to battery drainage. The user's dataset will then have missing values in columns that are properly populated in datasets of other users who did not opt-out of accelerometer data collection. In the latter group of users, accelerometer features may be highly discriminative in predicting affective states, and thus, simply disregarding accelerometer columns would be a poor decision in modeling.

To overcome the problem regarding missing values, a variant of AdaBoost is used. First practical boosting technique introduced, AdaBoost uses weighted ensemble of "weak classifiers" or "base classifiers", which individually has a slightly higher performance than a random classifier, to produce a strong classifier of better performance [37]. The algorithm is also described as a weighted majority-voting scheme because each vote (i.e. classification) from a weak learner is weighted based on its error. For the purpose of binary classification, the traditional AdaBoost algorithm denotes a negative class with -1 and a positive class with +1 [37]. In the variant of Adaboost implemented in Clara, another class, denoted by 0, is added to represent a case in which a base classifier abstains from voting. Advanced in [38], the "Adaboost that abstains" allows a base classifier to "abstain" or output 0 when the particular feature with which it performs learning is missing value. Following this strategy, the model becomes resilient to missing data and is able to handle datasets with large portion of features missing.

With datasets constructed with three labels (depression severity, anxiety severity and stress severity), three models are trained using the aforementioned algorithm. The weights of the learned models are stored in the backend of the system to make real time predictions of corresponding severity levels.

Intervention Delivery and Report Generation. Trigger rules for intervention delivery are as follows: (i) when the predicted severity of at least one affective states out of depression, anxiety and stress reaches "extremely severe" and (ii) when the predicted severity of at least two affective states out of depression, anxiety and stress reach "severe".

A set of interventions are available for users to choose from. One example of an effective intervention built into the system is respiratory biofeedback [39]. In this intervention, the user is given a set of instructions for breathing and relaxation exercises, and the effects of these exercises are captured and made visually available to the user real time. A screenshot of breathing exercise delivered to user as part of this intervention is provided in Fig. 1.

To enable discovery of key insights around the state of workplace mental wellbeing at an organizational level, reports are generated and delivered to employers monthly.

4 Limitations and Future Work

As it currently stands, the system has a few limitations that need modifications through future works. More appraisals around buy-in and trust from different stakeholders are needed to further validate the system.

4.1 Naive Handling of Missing GPS Data

The current method of handling missing GPS data involves usage of MF-based imputation. A brief study on this methodology using a small sample of GPS dataset shows that the approach lacks the robustness needed for a more meaningful usage of the GPS data. Measuring the accuracy of the method involves taking out values from a latitudinal/longitudinal matrix, reconstructing the matrix using imputation and comparing the output with the original values of the matrix. In the preliminary study with a dataset whose missing values were limited to less than 10% of the size of the whole dataset, the MF-based imputation yielded data points, more than 15% of which had greater difference from the ground truth values than the accepted threshold $(T = 500 \text{ m})$.

In order to improve the significance of GPS signals captured, a more effective strategy in handling missing GPS data should be implemented. Some suggestions can be found in [40], where a principled statistical approach is explored based on weighted resampling of the observed data.

4.2 Exclusion of Physiological Signals

As explored in Sect. 2.2.4, physiological signals such as heart rate and skin temperature have been reported as powerful indicators of an individual's affective state. While the current version of Clara only collects behavioral data, integration of physiological signals in the future versions is expected to improve predictive capability of the system. For capturing such signals, however, sensor hardware is required. The upcoming system update will therefore include addition of a pipeline that gathers data from such sensors-equipped wearables and aggregates them to the central storage system before corresponding preprocessing and feature extractions.

5 Conclusion

Clara is an unobtrusive, data-driven monitoring and management solution for workplace mental health. In this paper, we have addressed the limitations of questionnaire-based mental health assessments that Clara overcomes and presented a review of passive sensing technologies that power Clara. We have discussed the overall system architecture of Clara before delving into the details of implementing the smaller components within the system. Last, based on the limitations identified in the first version, we have proposed areas of future work.

With their detrimental effects on productivity, affective disorders at the workplace have an extremely high price tag. Clara, marked by its timely interventions based on passive monitoring technology, has the potential to provide employers of the workplace a solution to effectively manage the mental wellbeing of their employees.

6 Conflict of Interest Disclosure

The co-authors Megan Lam and Caleb Chiu reported holding Board Director positions at Neurum Ltd. No other authors have disclosures to declare.

References

1. Mind the Workplace Report. http://www.mentalhealthamerica.net/tags/mind-workplace-report. Accessed 12 Jan 2019
2. Higginbottom, K.: Poor Mental Health Is Widespread in the Workplace. https://www.forbes.com/sites/karenhigginbottom/2018/09/14/poor-mental-health-widespread-in-the-workplace/#5a67868e72f8. Accessed 12 Jan 2019
3. Creating a mentally healthy workplace - headsup.org.au. https://www.headsup.org.au/docs/default-source/resources/beyondblue_workplaceroi_finalreport_may-2014.pdf?sfvrsn=6. Accessed 12 Jan 2019
4. Dewa, C.S., Thompson, A.H., Jacobs, P.: The association of treatment of depressive episodes and work productivity. Can. J. Psychiatry 56, 743–750 (2011)
5. Work and Well-Being Survey - apaexcellence.org. https://www.apaexcellence.org/assets/general/2016-work-and-wellbeing-survey-results.pdf
6. Headspace Homepage, https://www.headspace.com. Accessed 15 Jan 2019
7. Partnership for Workplace Mental Health. http://www.workplacementalhealth.org/Case-Studies/Delta-Air-Lines. Accessed 16 Jan 2019
8. Graham, A.: Review: brief interventions reduce drinking in patients not seeking treatment. Evid.-Based Ment. Health 5, 116 (2002)
9. Razavi, T.: Self-report measures: an overview of concerns and limitations of questionnaire use in occupational stress research
10. Jones, G., Wright, J., Regele, O., Kourtis, L., Pszenny, S., Sirkar, R., Kovalchick, C.: Evolution of the digital biomarker ecosystem. Digit. Med. 3, 154 (2017)
11. Lovibond, P., Lovibond, S.: The structure of negative emotional states: comparison of the depression anxiety stress scales (DASS) with the beck depression and anxiety inventories. Behav. Res. Ther. 33, 335–343 (1995)
12. Kroenke, K., Spitzer, R.L.: The PHQ-9: a new depression diagnostic and severity measure. Psychiatric Ann. 32, 509–515 (2002)
13. Griffiths, T.C., Myers, D.H., Talbot, A.W.: A study of the validity of the scaled version of the general health questionnaire in paralysed spinally injured out-patients. Psychol. Med. 23, 497 (1993)
14. Pruebas Herramienta de Documentalista. https://www.neps-data.de/Portals/0/Working%20Papers/WP_XLV.pdf. Accessed 20 Jan 2019
15. Cohen, S., Kamarck, T., Mermelstein, R.: A global measure of perceived stress. J. Health Soc. Behav. 24, 385 (1983)
16. Koh, K.B., Park, J.K., Kim, C.H., Cho, S.: Development of the stress response inventory and its application in clinical practice. Psychosom. Med. 63, 668–678 (2001)

17. Sakakibara, B.M., Miller, W.C., Orenczuk, S.G., Wolfe, D.L.: A systematic review of depression and anxiety measures used with individuals with spinal cord injury. Spinal Cord 47, 841–851 (2009)
18. Gross, C.: The standard stress scale (SSS): measuring stress in the life course. In: Blossfeld, H.-P., von Maurice, J., Bayer, M., Skopek, J. (eds.) Methodological Issues of Longitudinal Surveys, pp. 233–249. Springer, Wiesbaden (2016). https://doi.org/10.1007/978-3-658-11994-2_14
19. Rock Health Homepage, https://www.rockhealth.com/reports/. Accessed 02 Feb 2019
20. Chow, P.I., Fua, K., Huang, Y., Bonelli, W., Xiong, H., Barnes, L.E., Teachman, B.A.: Using mobile sensing to test clinical models of depression, social anxiety, state affect, and social isolation among college students. J. Med. Internet Res. 19, e62 (2017)
21. CBITs TECH Website, https://tech.cbits.northwestern.edu/purple-robot/. Accessed 03 Feb 2019
22. Hellhammer, D., Meinlschmidt, G., Kumsta, R.: Mobile Phone Sensor Correlates of Depressive Symptom Severity in Daily-Life Behavior: An Exploratory Study. F1000 - Post-publication peer review of the biomedical literature (2016)
23. Epp, C., Lippold, M., Mandryk, R.L.: Identifying emotional states using keystroke dynamics. In: Proceedings of the 2011 Annual Conference on Human Factors in Computing Systems - CHI 2011 (2011)
24. Maheshwary, S., Pudi, V.: Mining keystroke timing pattern for user authentication. In: Appice, A., Ceci, M., Loglisci, C., Masciari, E., Raś, Zbigniew W. (eds.) NFMCP 2016. LNCS (LNAI), vol. 10312, pp. 213–227. Springer, Cham (2017). https://doi.org/10.1007/978-3-319-61461-8_14
25. Malhi, G.S., Hamilton, A., Morris, G., Mannie, Z., Das, P., Outhred, T.: The promise of digital mood tracking technologies: are we heading on the right track? Evid. Based Ment. Health 20, 102–107 (2017)
26. Solanki, R., Shukla, P.: Estimation of the user's emotional state by keystroke dynamics. Int. J. Comput. Appl. 94, 21–23 (2014)
27. Tsoulouhas, G., Georgiou, D., Karakos, A.: Detection of learner's affective state based on mouse movements. J. Comput. 3, 9–18 (2011)
28. Hibbeln, M., Jenkins, J.L., Schneider, C., Valacich, J.S., Weinmann, M.: How is your user feeling? Inferring emotion through human-computer interaction devices. MIS Q. 41, 1–21 (2017)
29. Heron, S.: Advanced encryption standard (AES). Netw. Secur. 2009, 8–12 (2009)
30. Torous, J., Nicholas, J., Larsen, M.E., Firth, J., Christensen, H.: Clinical review of user engagement with mental health smartphone apps: evidence, theory and improvements. Evid. Based Ment. Health 21, 116–119 (2018)
31. Farhan, Y., Morillo, W., Lu, B., Kamath, R., Bamis, W.: Behavior vs. introspection: refining prediction of clinical depression via smartphone sensing data. In: 2016 IEEE Wireless Health (WH) (2016)
32. A simple method for reliable footstep detection on embedded sensor platforms. http://ozeo.org/lib/exe/fetch.php?media=bodytrack:libby_peak_detection.pdf
33. Zheng, V.W., Zheng, Y., Xie, X., Yang, Q.: Towards mobile intelligence: Learning from GPS history data for collaborative recommendation. Artif. Intell. 184–185, 17–37 (2012)
34. Rodden, K., Fu, X., Aula, A., Spiro, I.: Eye-mouse coordination patterns on web search results pages. In: Proceeding of the Twenty-Sixth Annual CHI Conference Extended Abstracts on Human Factors in Computing Systems - CHI 2008 (2008)
35. Louhichi, S., Gzara, M., Abdallah, H.B.: A density based algorithm for discovering clusters with varied density. In: 2014 World Congress on Computer Applications and Information Systems (WCCAIS) (2014)

36. Pakhomov, A., Sicignano, A., Sandy, M., Goldburt, E.T.: A novel method for footstep detection with extremely low false alarm rate. In: Unattended Ground Sensor Technologies and Applications V. (2003)
37. Freund, Y., Schapire, R.E.: A decision-theoretic generalization of on-line learning and an application to boosting. J. Comput. Syst. Sci. **55**, 119–139 (1997)
38. Conroy, B., Eshelman, L., Potes, C., Xu-Wilson, M.: A dynamic ensemble approach to robust classification in the presence of missing data. Mach. Learn. **102**, 443–463 (2015)
39. Meuret, A.E., Wilhelm, F.H., Roth, W.T.: Respiratory biofeedback-assisted therapy in panic disorder. Behav. Modif. **25**, 584–605 (2001)
40. Barnett, I., Onnela, J.-P.: Inferring mobility measures from GPS traces with missing data. Biostatistics (2018)

System of Nudge Theory-Based ICT Applications for Older Citizens: The SENIOR Project

Giada Pietrabissa[1,2]([⊠]), Italo Zoppis[3], Giancarlo Mauri[3],
Roberta Ghiretti[4], Emanuele Maria Giusti[1,2], Roberto Cattivelli[1,2],
Chiara Spatola[1,2], Gian Mauro Manzoni[1,5],
and Gianluca Castelnuovo[1,2]

[1] Psychology Research Laboratory,
Istituto Auxologico Italiano IRCCS, Milan, Italy
{r.cattivelli, c.spatola, gm.manzoni,
g.castelnuovo}@auxologico.it
[2] Department of Psychology, Catholic University of Milan, Milan, Italy
{giada.pietrabissa, emanuelemaria.giusti}@unicatt.it
[3] Department of Informatics, Systems and Communication, Università Degli
Studi Di Milano-Bicocca, Milan, Italy
{italo.zoppis, giancarlo.mauri}@unimib.it
[4] Auser Regione Lombardia, Milan, Italy
roberta.ghiretti@gmail.com
[5] Faculty of Psychology, eCampus University, Novedrate, Como, Italy

Abstract. *Objective*: Mild Cognitive Impairment (MCI) is rapidly becoming one of the most common clinical manifestation affecting the elderly. The main aim of the SENIOR Project [SystEm of Nudge theory-based Information and Communications Technology (ICT) applications for OldeR citizens] is the development and validation of a new Nudge theory-based ICT coach system for monitoring and empowering persons with MCI. *Methods*: a multi-center randomized controlled clinical trial (RCT) involving 200 senior citizens with MCI will be implemented. Online assessment of demographic, psychological, neuropsychological, and behavioral outcomes will be carried out through the user's device/smartwatch. A machine learning algorithm-based customized profile will elaborate specific nudge-based notifications and suggestions will be provided to the user via SENIOR app. *Expected results and conclusions*: real-time monitoring and tutoring will decelerate the worsening of clinical condition and will improve the general perceived wellbeing of persons with MCI – also empowering care providers through dissemination of knowledge on the condition functioning and therapy. Moreover, the provision of tailored care actions will contribute to a more sustainable national and local healthcare systems.

Keywords: Elderly · Mild cognitive impairment · Nudge theory · Big data · Machine learning

© ICST Institute for Computer Sciences, Social Informatics and Telecommunications Engineering 2019
Published by Springer Nature Switzerland AG 2019. All Rights Reserved
P. Cipresso et al. (Eds.): MindCare 2019, LNICST 288, pp. 29–42, 2019.
https://doi.org/10.1007/978-3-030-25872-6_3

1 Background

1.1 The Importance of Monitoring and Treating Elderly Using a Biopsychosocial Approach

Globally, population aged 60 or over is growing faster than the number of people in younger age groups, and during the next few decades this percentage is likely to rise to historically unprecedented levels. According to the latest estimates, by 2050 population people older than 60 years will nearly double from 12% to 22% [1]. Older people face special challenges. Moreover, the prevalence of physical, social and mental health increases with age, leading a growing number of elderly living in the community to experience multiple health and social care needs that may restrict their social engagement [2] and self-care abilities – with a higher utilization of long-term care and support services [3, 4].

Particularly, mild cognitive impairment (MCI) is rapidly becoming one of the most common clinical manifestations affecting the older citizens. It is characterized by deterioration of memory, attention, and cognitive functioning that is beyond what is expected based on age and educational level [5]. Characteristic of MCI is: (1) a subjective complaint of a memory disturbance (preferably supported by an informant); (2) objective evidence of a memory deficit; (3) generally preserved cognitive functions; (4) ability to perform basic activities of daily living; and (5) the absence of dementia [6]. MCI can also act as a transitional level of evolving dementia with a range of conversion of 10%–15% yearly [7].

Multidisciplinary professional collaboration in primary care is, therefore, required to optimally support older people with MCI in maintaining their independence and functional capacities, in meeting their health and social care needs, as well as in improving their perceived physical, cognitive, personal and social well-being - while minimizing service utilization and expenditure. However, what remains unclear is how collaboration may be undertaken in a multidisciplinary manner in concrete terms [8].

Research demonstrated that risk of further cognitive decline may decrease by the implementation of physical exercises, social engagement and mental activity [9]. For example, a prospective cohort study identified a significant association between engagement in mentally stimulating activities in late life and decreased odds of MCI in a non-clinical population. In 4 years, the risk of MCI decreased by 30% with computer use, 28% with craft activities, 23% with social activities, and 22% by playing games at least 1 to 2 times per week [10].

Still, while the impact of lifestyle, neuropsychological training and their interactions on aging have been frequently studied, no concrete action has yet been implemented to empower and support senior citizens in their everyday life.

The last decade has seen growing popularity and uptake of self-monitoring technology including wireless sensor devices and mobile apps for the long-term treatment of chronic illness [11, 12]. eHealth may help to improve the management of care for elderly and chronically ill patients by facilitating sharing of treatment plans and online health communities – while helping elderly in better managing their chronic conditions and sustaining an active social life.

1.2 From Traditional Mhealth Monitoring to Smart Watches Among Elderly: A New Potential Paradigm

Since 2014, consumer-grade smart watches have penetrated the health research space rapidly and smart watch technical functions, acceptability, and effectiveness in enhancing health outcomes are receiving increasing attention and support in the last years [13]. Rosales et al. (2017) recently suggested wearable technologies as an opportunity to solve problems often related to older people (65+) [14]. Also, Stradolini, Lavalle et al. (2016) proposed an Internet of Things - IoT application to simultaneously and constantly monitor elderly patients and alert healthcare professionals in case of anomalous measured values by using a smart-watch [15].

According to Ehn et al. (2018) devices must be easy to handle – and wearable activity trackers are generally perceived easier to maneuver than tablets or smart-phones, both among elderly and chronic illness patients [16]. However, some of their features - such as tiny screen size, small connectors and reduced power autonomy - can limit the spread of the smartwatches. Also, appropriate user interfaces and dedicated hardware tailored on the potential physical and cognitive impairments experienced by elderly need to be carefully developed.

1.3 The Contribution of Nudge Theory

A *Nudge* is the base element used to define a *Choice architecture,* that is a design of diverse ways in which choices can be presented to the user, also considering the impact of how suggestions are presented on the user process of decision-making [17].

The "Nudge Theory" proposes positive reinforcement and indirect suggestions as ways to influence the behavior and decision making of groups or individuals. This framework has demonstrated to be an effective and viable public tool in encouraging healthier eating choices in adults [18]. By reducing the set of choices, therefore decreasing the cognitive effort associated with processing information, Nudges may challenge the needs of elderly people of remembering or doing things, beside pro-moting healthier behaviours and an active aging lifestyle.

1.4 Big Data Analysis in Elderly

Considering the vast amounts of information clinicians need to take into consideration – i.e. the patients' personal history, familial diseases, genomic sequences, medications, activity on social media, and admissions to hospitals - to guide clinical decision may become an overwhelming task. Analyzing Big Data using a carefully designed statistical model and the machine learning spectrum may improve the knowledge and management of different clinical and sub-clinical conditions in elderly. Gathering all the vital signs of the individuals and detecting any abnormalities, Big Data has a large potential in healthcare and plays major role in monitoring the elderly for earlier diagnosis of health problems [19].

1.5   The Added Value and Step Forward of the SENIOR Project

The SENIOR Project will:

- improve the knowledge of elderly citizens through the collection and examination of large data sets containing a variety of data types
- allow elderly patients to be monitored in a continuous and ubiquitous way (smartwatch) without invasive modalities but using a disappearing and not demanding approach
- tailor the feedbacks, suggestions and indications for MCI patients as suggested by the algorithms improved by big data-machine learning approach
- give "Nudges" to MCI elderly patients to improve their social skills

2   Main Hypotheses and Objectives of the SENIOR Project

The main hypotheses, tested along the SENIOR project, can be summarized as indicated below:

- the creation of a not-invasive, ergonomic, easy-to-use SENIOR platform (smartwatch-based) will serve to continuously monitor selected biological, psychological, social, and environmental data among elderly with MCI;
- smartwatch-based monitoring of elderly with MCI will improve the knowledge of senior citizens' characteristics;
- the collection and analysis of several variables using the big data-machine learning approach will allow the creation of advanced algorithms-based profiles for elderly with MCI;
- the Nudge Theory approach will provide tailored feedbacks and strategies to elderly with MCI according to a given profile – and will enhance the cognitive skills, social interactions, and psychological well-being of the person.

Target objectives of the SENIOR Project are:

Scientific and clinical objectives:

- to define clinical and psychosocial outcomes for elderly with MCI;
- to develop tools to monitor and assist MCI senior citizens with self-management of their conditions;
- to develop a preventive treatment protocol for elderly with MCI;
- to evaluate the clinical efficacy and effectiveness of the new intervention by statistically comparing the SENIOR platform (experimental condition) with standard care (control condition).
- to evaluate costs and resources of the SENIOR approach though impact analysis.

Technological objectives:

- to design a SENIOR virtual coach architecture and platform to manage and record clinical and behavioural parameters of elderly with MCI;
- to develop cooperative architecture and personalized algorithms to support Nudge-based applications for elderly with MCI;

- to identify method(s) to monitor clinical parameters of MCI carriers though a low-cost approach;
- to develop and provide tools and applications for senior citizens with MCI and their caregivers;
- to evaluate the contribution of wearable devices in improving health monitoring in elderly with MCI;
- to create a list of technological specifics for integration with standard software systems.

Integrative objective:

- to implement cognitive-behavioural strategies to modify dysfunctional behaviours and believes and to improve a healthy lifestyle.
- to determine patients' care pathways and integration of health status monitoring within primary care services.

Social objective:

- to improve active socializing to prevent elderly with MCI from a rapid cognitive decline.

3 Methods

The SENIOR Project will provide an innovative, scalable, secure and intelligent system by developing a virtual coach tailored on the individual needs of senior citizens with MCI and by using a smartwatch-based technology in the frame of the Nudge Theory.

The project will involve the collaboration of different partners and will be performed in eight realistic and well-balanced work packages (WP). The Istituto Auxologico Italiano IRCCS[1] will coordinate the consortium (WP8: Consortium Management) and will manage the randomized controlled trial, RCT (WP5: Clinical trial Conduction) by recruiting senior citizens with MCI in their structures as in the Auser Milano Volontariato Onlus (AUSER) centers[2]. The resulting dataset will be sent to WP6 (coordinated by the Catholic University of Milan, UNICATT[3]) for evaluation and data analysis. UNICATT will be also devoted to the study of the interaction between humans and synthetic intelligence (WP4) – results that will be evaluated in WP6. In WP1 – coordinated by the Istituto Auxologico Italiano, IRCCS - enhancement of scientific understanding of the overall smartwatch and health platform functionality and requirements will be conducted.

---

[1] The Istituto Auxologico Italiano IRCCS is one of the main Italian research sites, with four main hospitals and many clinical units located in northern Italy.

[2] AUSER is one of the largest Italian no-profit associations aimed at stimulating active aging through different activities.

[3] The Department of Psychology of the Catholic University of Milan (UNICATT) has a long and notable history of research in the areas of general, developmental, clinical, social and organizational psychology, with extensive expertise in quantitative-qualitative research methodology and statistical analysis.

Results will lead WP2 (coordinated by the University of Milano-Bicocca, UNIMIB[4]) to conduct a market analysis aimed at identifying the adequate equipment of sensors, wearable devices and smartwatches to include in the patients' kit. The software design, development, integration and validation will be carried out in WP3 (UNIMIB) and WP4 (UNICATT). Evaluation and data analysis will be carried out by WP6 (UNICATT). Results will be further discussed and disseminated in WP7 (Dissemination, Demonstration Exploitation and Marketing) led by AUSER.

3.1   Evaluation of Clinical Outcomes

In order to provide evidence for the effectiveness of the SENIOR Project, a multi-center RCT involving 200 senior citizens (100 using the SENIOR virtual coach approach and 100 with standard approach-treatment as usual) will be implemented according to the latest CONSORT statements (Consolidated Standards of Reporting Trials - www. consort-statement.org). The SENIOR protocol will be evaluated by the new model for assessment of telemedicine (MAST- Methodology to assess telemedicine applications - https://ec.europa.eu/digital-single-market/en/news/methotelemed-framework-methodology-assess-effectiveness-telemedicine-applications-europe).

3.2   Participants

Participants will be recruited and screened for admission into the study from the Istituto Auxologico Italiano, IRCCS clinical units and the AUSER units on 3-month basis and monitored for the following 12 months.

Eligibility Criteria
Patients will be included into the study according to the following criteria: (1) age between 65 and 85 years; (2) diagnosis of MCI as measured by the Mini-Mental State Examination (MMSE) questionnaire [20] and an ad hoc Neuropsychological Test Battery [21]; (3) basic knowledge (entry level) of informatics assessed by the CIDA (Centro Informatico di Ateneo - Catholic University of Milan) test of informatics skills; (4) written and informed consent to participate.

Exclusion criteria will be: (1) presence of severe psychiatric disturbance as established by the Diagnostic and Statistical Manual for Mental Disorder [5]th ed. (DSM-5); (2) severe medical conditions that need inpatient treatment and continuous medical surveillance; (3) lack of independence in daily activities; 4) difficulty in sustaining functional movements due to severe medical (orthopedic, neurological, cardiological, etc.) reasons.

---

[4] The Department of Informatics, Systems and Communication (DISCo) of the University Milano Bicocca (UNIMIB) has research experience in software engineering and architectures, databases and information systems, with emphasis on data quality and data integration, ICT in life sciences (bioinformatics, systems biology, medical informatics, telemedicine) data mining, computational models of complex systems, artificial intelligence, Computer Supported Cooperative Work and knowledge management. Specifically, the Biomedical Informatics group (BIMIB) and the Innovative Technologies for Interaction and Services Laboratory (ITIS) groups from UNIMIB will be involved.

A customized version of the Structured Clinical Interview for DSM-5 Disorders (SCID) [22] will be first used to screen for the presence of psychiatric disorders and will be administered by an independent clinical psychologist as part of his work.

3.3 Randomization Procedure

All participants will be randomly assigned to the intervention or control group. The randomization scheme will be generated by using the Web site Randomization.com: http://www.randomization.com. Randomization will take place after the baseline measurement.

3.4 Measures

Paper and pencil as well as online self-report questionnaires, inventories and symptoms checklists will be administered to participants in order to collect relevant periodic data - at baseline and at different follow-up points. Online assessment will be carried out through the SENIOR web-platform. Activity trackers and other smartwatch-based sensors will be used to measure physiological variables.

The following *demographic information* will be considered: (1) age; (2) gender; (3) education; (4) civil status; (5) social support (6) social relationships; (7) socio-economic status (SES).

Physiological-medical outcomes will be: (1) body mass index (BMI); (2) comorbidity indicators, using the Charlson comorbidity index [23]; (3) physical activity and energy expenditure, measured by the biomedical monitoring device (smartwatch).

Beside personality traits [measured by the MMPI-II Personality Inventory [24]], *psychological variables* considered in the study will be: (1) the individuals' perceived quality of the experience, measured using traditional and online Experience Sampling Method-Based questionnaires [25]; (2) the individuals' perceived quality of life (QoL), measured by the SF-26 health survey [26] and the European Quality of Life-5 Dimensions (EQ-5D) [27]; (3) the individuals' psychological status and well-being, as means of the Symptom Checklist-90-R (SCL-90-R) [28], the Outcome questionnaire (OQ 45.2) [29, 30], the Beck anxiety inventory (BAI) and Beck depression Inventory (BDI) [31] (4) self-reported sleep quality, through the Insomnia severity index (ISI) [32], the Pittsburgh sleep Quality index (PSQI) [33], the Sleep Disorder Questionnaire (SDQ); (5) users' satisfaction in managing technological devices and platform, using the Telemedicine Satisfaction Questionnaire (TSQ) [34] and the Quebec User evaluation of Satisfaction with Assistive Technology (QUEST) [35, 36]; (6) patients' engagement and empowerment, using the Patient Activation Measure (PAM) [37] and the Patients Health Engagement (PHE) scale [38]; (7) the patients' motivation to change, as means of the University of Rhode Island Change and Assessment Scale (IT-URICA) [39]; (8) social interactions, through the Pennebaker's method of inferring psychological states via language analysis; 9) stressful life events, using the Paykel Scale of Stressful life events [40].

Also, a *neuropsychological assessment* comprising the MMSE questionnaire [20] and the Neuropsychological Test Battery [21] - which includes measures from five cognitive domains (memory, attention, language, visuospatial functioning, and executive functioning) with at least three measures from each domain (Table 1) - will be undertaken. These tasks will be implemented in both their diagnostic and rehabilitation version to allow the SENIOR virtual coach to identify cognitive difficulties in senior citizens with MCI and to suggest them to undergo an ad hoc training.

Additionally, obese patients will be asked to complete the Weight Efficacy Life Style Questionnaire (WELSQ) and the Impact of Weight in Quality of Life (IWQOL-Lite) [41]. Only to diabetics will be also give the Diabetes Self-Efficacy Scale [42] and Diabetes Empowerment Scale [43].

Table 1. Neuropsychological Tests Administered | Retrieved from *Jak, A.J., et al. (2009). Quantification of Five Neuropsychological Approaches to Defining Mild Cognitive Impairment. The American Journal of Geriatric Psychiatry, 17(5), 368–375.*

Memory	Attention	Language	Visuospatial functioning	Executive functioning
WMS-R logical memory	DRS attention	BNT	WISC-R block design	WCST-48-card version
WMS-R visual reproduction	WAIS-R digit span	Letter fluency	D-KEFS visual scanning	TMT, Part B
CVLT trials 1–5 total, long delay free recall	TMT Part A	Category fluency	>D-KEFS Design Fluency >DRS construction >Clock drawing test	>D-KEFS Color-Word Interference Test >D-KEFS fluency switching (visual and verbal)

Notes: Boston Naming Test (BNT) [44]; California Verbal Learning Test (CVLT) [45]; Dementia Rating Scale (DRS) [46]; Wechsler Memory Scale-Revised (WMS-R) [47]; Wechsler Adult Intelligence Scale-Revised (WAIS-R) [48]; Trail Making Test (TMT) - Part A; Trail Making Test (TMT) - Part B [49]; Wechsler Intelligence Scale for Children-Revised (WISC-R) [50]; Delis-Kaplan Executive Function System (D-KEFS) [51]; modified Wisconsin Card Sorting Test (WCST-48-card version) [52]; Normative data was drawn from Mayo's Older Americans Normative Studies (MOANS) [53] or from other published norms [44, 45, 47–52, 54, 55] except for block design, which used age and education adjusted norms drawn from local unpublished data derived from the UCSD Alzheimer Disease Research Center. DRS: Dementia Rating Scale.

Behavioral outcomes will be: (1) adherence to healthy diet, measured by the Mediterranean Diet Scale (MDS) and using the METADIETA approach (Meteda©); (2) adherence to physical activity, measured by the Recent Physical Activity Questionnaire (RPAQ) [56], the Physical Activity Recall (PAR) interview [57] and the CronoLife SenseWear® armband advance software [58, 59]. Moreover, the Self-Report Habit Index (SRHI) [60] will be used as index of the patients' lifestyle; 3) behavioural and functional indicators - by assessment of the basic instrumental activities of daily living using the Lawton Instrumental Activities of Daily Living (IADL) scale [61] and the WHO Disability Assessment Schedule 2.0 (WH ODAS 2.0) [62] according to the International Classification of Functioning, Disability and Health (ICF) [63].

By integrating target behaviours, a "health score" will be elaborated.

Cost-effectiveness of the SENIOR project will be evaluated considering its direct and indirect cost savings, while its cost-utility will take into consideration each users' needs, abilities, technological skills and psychological profiles reducing costs due to an intelligent algorithm that will increase its performances according to machine learning technique/theory.

3.5 The SENIOR Project Architecture

SENIOR final solution will be represented by:

- a smartwatch dedicated app;
- a set of optional environmental sensors;
- a cloud personalized service.

The customer will install the SENIOR app in his/her smartwatch and will access to SENIOR on-line service. The SENIOR service (user monitoring, personalized nudge advice etc.) will be delivered by a health company/structure and will require an annual fee.

The health company/structure will make revenues based on the number of enabled customers. The SENIOR solution can be proposed, for example, by an insurance company.

The user device (a smartwatch or a smartphone) will use two kind of networks: a local wireless network (Bluetooth LE) to dialogue with local sensors and measuring instruments, and a 3G/4G network to send and receive data from the remote back-end server. The device can be used without depending on wireless or Bluetooth connections due to the presence of a SIM card slot on board.

The security of the communications is guaranteed by the protocols used (Secure Pairing and Connections for BTLE and HTTPS for app-to-backend communications). The data privacy is guaranteed by encrypted communications channels and by using encrypted and obfuscated databases.

3.6 Procedure

In order to help the patient to improve and maintain his/her independence, the personalized virtual coach will elaborate a customized profile (built on the machine learning theory-based algorithm) that will provide the user with specific nudge-based advices-notifications-suggestions.

Different signals will be collected from the user's device and delivered by the SENIOR app to the remote backend server - whose software will analyze the data (physical activity, psychological wellbeing, risk of social exclusion) in order to elaborate a machine learning algorithm that will identify a given pattern.

The remote backend will also help alert the clinicians in presence of negative/dangerous patterns and will also enable caregivers/professionals to deliver personalized treatments plans new personalized pattern rule.

Then the system will transmit a real-time "nudge action" driven by the SENIOR app to the user (Fig. 1). The SENIOR app is self-adaptive to the patient IT skills and level of engagement.

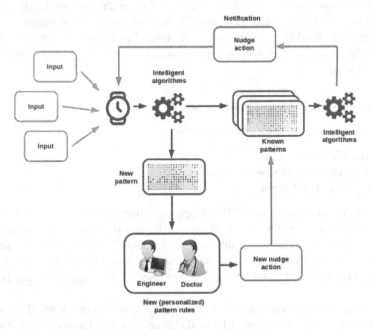

Fig. 1. SENIOR Project IT architecture

3.7 Statistical Analysis

According to a-priori power analysis (G*Power 3.1.3 was used for calculation), 200 participants are required to detect a small interaction effect of treatment × time on outcomes with a 90% statistical power. Two-tailed t-tests for continuous variables and Fisher's exact tests for binary variables will be used for descriptive purposes. Treatment effects (treatment × time interaction effects) as well as moderating and mediating effects will be tested with the General Linear Model [64]. Repeated-measure factorial ANCOVAs will be used for each outcome. Critical alpha for the treatment effects will be set to 0.01 in order to limit the inflation of the type I error rate due to multiple tests, while no adjustment will be applied to alpha = 0.05 for the statistical testing of the other effects. Other further analysis, considering all the collected data, will be performed using advanced informatics approaches - considering the big data and machine learning framework - in order to detect the most useful sorting algorithms to understand the different kinds of elderly patients with MCI.

4 Expected Results and Conclusion

Impact for Older Citizens. Real-time monitoring and tutoring (based on a Nudge theory approach) will decelerate the worsening of mild clinical conditions or the loss of a functional status.

Impact for Care Providers. By combining variable (data integration) through predictive analytic methods, health care providers will better understand the impact of several determinants on the seniors' health – so to readjust their approach based on patient's needs for the delivery of preventive actions.

Scientific and Clinical Impact: home-based ad hoc seniors' assessments and tailored feedbacks with reliable and intelligent tools will be offered to reduce hospitalization rates and to improve disease self-management of seniors with MCI - with consequent strengthening of their QoL. A more active participation of elderly in the care processes (patient engagement and empowerment) will be also facilitated by increased patient-provider interactions. Moreover, the bid data analysis-machine learning approach will improve knowledge of older adults and MCI and allow the identification of more effective treatment strategies.

Societal and Economic Impact: citizens will be directly involved in decision-making processes and follow up procedures, as well as in virtual communities where to share experiences, results, difficulties and successes so to reinforce their motivation and self-efficacy. High-quality and personalized care - with better use of the available healthcare resources – will be then provided, thus contributing to a more sustainable national and local healthcare (clinical and social) systems. The cost-effectiveness of the service will be calculated by means of Effectiveness Indicators and Cost Indicators.

References

1. United Nations Department of Economic and Social Affairs, P.D., World Population Ageing 2015 (ST/ESA/SER.A/390) (2015)
2. Meek, K.P., et al.: Restricted social engagement among adults living with chronic conditions. Int. J. Environ. Res. Public Health **15**, 158 (2018)
3. Lattanzio, F., et al.: Advanced technology care innovation for older people in Italy: necessity and opportunity to promote health and wellbeing. J. Am. Med. Dir Assoc. **15**(7), 457–466 (2014)
4. Littlejohn, H.: Promoting wellbeing in older people with cognitive impairment. Nurs. Older People **12**(10), 37 (2001)
5. Sobral, A., de Araujo, C.M.T., Sobral, M.F.F.: Mild cognitive impairment in the elderly Relationship between communication and functional capacity. Dement. Neuropsychol. **12** (2), 165–172 (2018)
6. Petersen, R.C., et al.: Mild cognitive impairment: clinical characterization and outcome. Arch. Neurol. **56**(3), 303–308 (1999)
7. Eshkoor, S.A., et al.: Mild cognitive impairment and its management in older people. Clin. Interv. Aging **10**, 687–693 (2015)

8. Saint-Pierre, C., Herskovic, V., Sepulveda, M.: Multidisciplinary collaboration in primary care: a systematic review. Fam. Pract. **35**(2), 132–141 (2018)

9. Fang, M.L., et al.: Informing understandings of mild cognitive impairment for older adults: implications from a scoping review. J. Appl. Gerontol. **36**(7), 808–839 (2017)

10. Krell-Roesch, J., et al.: Association between mentally stimulating activities in late life and the outcome of incident mild cognitive impairment, with an analysis of the APOE ε4 Genotype. JAMA Neurol. **74**(3), 332–338 (2017)

11. Choi, Y.K., et al.: Smartphone applications to support sleep self-management: review and evaluation. J. Clin. Sleep Med. **14**(10), 1783–1790 (2018)

12. Pellegrini, C.A., et al.: Smartphone applications to support weight loss: current perspectives. Adv. Health Care Technol. **1**, 13–22 (2015)

13. Reeder, B., David, A.: Health at hand: a systematic review of smart watch uses for health and wellness. J. Biomed. Inf. **63**, 269–276 (2016)

14. Rosales, A., et al.: Older people and smartwatches, initial experiences. El Profesional de la Informacion **26**(3), 457 (2017)

15. Stradolini, F., Lavalle, E., De Micheli, G., Motto Ros, P., Demarchi, D., Carrara, S.: Paradigm-shifting players for iot: smart-watches for intensive care monitoring. In: Perego, P., Andreoni, G., Rizzo, G. (eds.) MobiHealth 2016. LNICST, vol. 192, pp. 71–78. Springer, Cham (2017). https://doi.org/10.1007/978-3-319-58877-3_9

16. Ehn, M., et al.: Activity monitors as support for older persons' physical activity in daily life: qualitative study of the users' experiences. JMIR Mhealth Uhealth **6**, e34 (2018)

17. Thaler, R.H., Sunstein, C.R.: Nudge: Improving Decisions about Health, Wealth, and Happiness. Yale University Press, New Haven and London (2009)

18. Arno, A., Thomas, S.: The efficacy of nudge theory strategies in influencing adult dietary behaviour: a systematic review and meta-analysis. BMC Public Health **16**, 676 (2016)

19. Tao, J., Shuijing, H.: The elderly and the big data how older adults deal with digital privacy. In: International Conference on Intelligent Transportation, Big Data and Smart City (ICITBS), Changsha, China (2016)

20. Folstein, M.E., Folstein, S.E., PR, M.: Mini-mental state. A practical method for grading the cognitive state of patients for the clinician. J. Psychiatry Res. **12**(3), 189–198 (1975)

21. Jak, A.J., et al.: Quantification of five neuropsychological approaches to defining mild cognitive impairment. Am. J. Geriatr. Psychiatry **17**(5), 368–375 (2009)

22. First, M.B., et al.: Structured Clinical Interview for DSM-5-Research Version (SCID-5 for DSM-5, Research Version; SCID-5-RV). American Psychiatric Association, Arlington (2015)

23. Frenkel, W.J., et al.: Validation of the Charlson comorbidity index in acutely hospitalized elderly adults: a prospective cohort study. J. Am. Geriatr. Soc. **62**(2), 342–346 (2014)

24. Ben-Porath, Y.S., Sherwood, N.E.: The MMPI-2 Content Component Scales: Development, Psychometric Characteristics, and Clinical Application. University of Minnesota Press, Minneapolis (1993)

25. Verhagen, S.J.W., et al.: Use of the experience sampling method in the context of clinical trials. Evid. Based Ment Health **19**(3), 86–89 (2016)

26. Apolone, G., Mosconi, P.: The Italian SF-36 Health Survey: translation, validation and norming. J. Clin. Epidemiol. **51**(11), 1025–1036 (1998)

27. Savoia, E., et al.: Assessing the construct validity of the Italian version of the EQ-5D: preliminary results from a cross-sectional study in North Italy. Health Qual. Life Outcomes **4**, 47 (2006)

28. Sarno, I., et al.: SCL-90-R Symptom Checklist-90-R Adattamento italiano Firenze Giunti, Organizzazioni Speciali (2011)

29. Lo Coco, G., et al.: The factorial structure of the outcome questionnaire-45: a study with an Italian sample. Clin. Psychol. Psychother. **15**(6), 418–423 (2008)
30. Chiappelli, M., et al.: The outcome questionnaire 45.2. Italian validation of an instrument for the assessment of psychological treatments. Epidemiol. Psichiatr. Soc. **17**(2), 152–161 (2008)
31. Sica, C., Ghisi, M.: The Italian versions of the beck anxiety inventory and the beck depression Inventory-II: psychometric properties and discriminant power. In: Lange, M.A. (ed.) Leading-Edge Psychological Tests and Testing Research, NOVA Science Publishers (2007)
32. Castronovo, V., et al.: Validation study of the Italian version of the Insomnia Severity Index (ISI). Neurol Sci **37**(9), 1517–1524 (2016)
33. Curcio, G., et al.: Validity of the Italian version of the Pittsburgh Sleep Quality Index (PSQI). Neurol. Sci. **34**(4), 511–519 (2013)
34. Yip, M.P., et al.: Development of the telemedicine satisfaction questionnaire to evaluate patient satisfaction with telemedicine: a preliminary study. J. Telemed. Telecare **9**(1), 46–50 (2003)
35. Mao, H.F., et al.: Cross-cultural adaptation and validation of the Quebec User Evaluation of Satisfaction with Assistive Technology (QUEST 2.0): the development of the Taiwanese version. J. Telemed Telecare **24**(5), 412–421 (2010)
36. Demers, L., Weiss-Lambrou, R., Ska, B.: Development of the Quebec User Evaluation of Satisfaction with Assistive Technology (QUEST). Assist. Technol. **8**(1), 3–13 (1996)
37. Graffigna, G., et al.: Measuring patient activation in Italy: Translation, adaptation and validation of the Italian version of the patient activation measure 13 (PAM13-I). BMC Med. Inf. Decis. Mak. **15**, 109 (2015)
38. Graffigna, G., et al.: Measuring patient engagement: development and psychometric properties of the Patient Health Engagement (PHE) scale. Front. Psychol. **6**, 274 (2015)
39. Pietrabissa, G., et al.: Stages of change in obesity and weight management: factorial structure of the Italian version of the university of Rhode island change assessment scale. Eat Weight Disord. **22**(2), 361–367 (2017)
40. Baratta, S., Colorio, C., Zimmermann-Tansella, C.: Inter-rater reliability of the Italian version of the Paykel Scale of stressful life events. J. Affect. Disord. **8**(3), 279–282 (1985)
41. Kolotkin, R.L., Head, S., Brookhart, A.: Construct validity of the impact of weight on quality of life questionnaire. Obes. Res. **5**(5), 434–441 (1997)
42. Messina, R., et al.: Assessing self-efficacy in type 2 diabetes management: validation of the Italian version of the Diabetes Management Self-Efficacy Scale (IT-DMSES). Health Qual. Life Outcomes **16**(1), 71 (2018)
43. Anderson, R.M., et al.: The Diabetes Empowerment Scale-Short Form (DES-SF). Diab. Care **26**(5), 1641–1642 (2003)
44. Kaplan, E.F., Goodglass, H., Weintraub, S.: The Boston Naming Test Philadelphia. Lea & Febiger, Philadelphia (1983)
45. Delis, D.C., et al.: The California Verbal Learning Test New York. Psychological Corporation (1987)
46. Springate, B.A., et al.: Screening for mild cognitive impairment using the dementia rating scale-2. J. Geriatr. Psychiatry Neurol. **27**(2), 139–144 (2014)
47. Wechsler, D.: Wechsler Memory Scale-Revised New York. Psychological Corporation (1987)
48. Wechsler, D.: Wechsler Adult Intelligence Scale-Revised Manual San Antonio. The Psychological Corporation (1981)
49. Reitan, R.M., Wolfson, D.: The Halstead-Reitan Neuropsychological Test Battery. Neuropsychology Press, Tucson (1985)

50. Wechsler, D.: Wechsler Intelligence Scale for Children-Revised New York. Psychological Corporation (1974)
51. Delis, D.C., Kaplan, E., Kramer, J.H.: Delis-Kaplan Executive Function System (D-KEFS). The Psychological Corporation, San Antonio (2001)
52. Lineweaver, T.T., et al.: A normative study of Nelson's: (1976) modified version of the Wisconsin card sorting test in healthy older adults. Clin. Neuropsychol. **13**, 328–347 (1999)
53. Ivnik, R.J., et al.: Mayo's older Americans normative studies: WMS-R norms for ages 56–94. Clin. Neuropsychol. **6**, 49–82 (1992)
54. Norman, M.A., et al.: Demographically corrected norms for the California verbal learning test. J. Clin. Exp. Neuropsychol. **22**(1), 80–94 (2000)
55. Gladsjo, J.A., et al.: Norms for letter and category fluency: demographic corrections for age, education, and ethnicity. Assessment **6**(2), 147–178 (1999)
56. Golubic, R., et al.: Validity of electronically administered recent physical activity questionnaire (RPAQ) in ten European countries. PLoS One **9**(3), e92829 (2014)
57. Baxter, S.D., et al.: A validation study concerning the effects of interview content, retention interval, and grade on children's recall accuracy for dietary intake and/or physical activity. J. Acad. Nutr. Diet. **114**(12), 1902–1914 (2014)
58. Martien, S., et al.: Energy expenditure in institutionalized older adults: validation of sensewear mini. Med. Sci. Sports Exerc. **47**(6), 1265–1271 (2015)
59. Machac, S., et al.: Validation of physical activity monitors in individuals with diabetes: energy expenditure estimation by the multisensor sensewear Armband Pro3 and the step counter Omron HJ-720 against indirect calorimetry during walking. Diab. Technol. Ther. **15**(5), 413–418 (2013)
60. Gardner, B., de Bruijn, G.J., Lally, P.: A systematic review and meta-analysis of applications of the self-report habit index to nutrition and physical activity behaviours. Ann. Behav. Med. **42**(2), 174–187 (2011)
61. Graf, C.: The Lawton instrumental activities of daily living (IADL) scale. Medsurg Nurs. **18**(5), 315–316 (2009)
62. Janca, A., et al.: The World Health Organization Short Disability Assessment Schedule (WHO DAS-S): a tool for the assessment of difficulties in selected areas of functioning of patients with mental disorders. Soc. Psychiatry Psychiatr. Epidemiol. **31**(6), 349–354 (1996)
63. World Health Organization, International classification of functioning, disability and health: ICF Geneva World Health Organization. http://www.who.int/iris/handle/10665/42407(2001)
64. Kraemer, H.C., et al.: Mediators and moderators of treatment effects in randomized clinical trials. Arch. Gen. Psychiatry **59**(10), 877–883 (2002)

Virtual Reality for Anxiety and Stress-Related Disorders: A SWOT Analysis

Javier Fernández-Alvarez[1](✉), Desirée Colombo[2], Cristina Botella[2,3],
Azucena García-Palacios[2,3], and Giuseppe Riva[1,4]

[1] Department of Psychology of the Catholic University,
Largo Gemelli 1, 20100 Milan, Italy
{javier.fernandezkirszman,giuseppe.riva}@unicatt.it

[2] Department of Basic Psychology, Clinic and Psychobiology,
Universitat Jaume I, Castellón, Spain
{dcolombo,botella,azucena}@uji.es

[3] CIBER Fisiopatología Obesidad y Nutrición, Instituto Salud Carlos III,
Madrid, Spain

[4] Applied Technology for Neuro-Psychology Lab at IRCCS Istituto
Auxologico Italiano, Milan, Italy
{p.cipresso,g.riva}@auxologico.it

Abstract. Virtual Reality (VR) Therapy has emerged in the 90s as an appealing way of delivering exposure treatment. Throughout these years, ample evidence has been published. Although there is an agreed consensus regarding its efficacy, currently a quick shift in the field is being experienced, especially due to the advent of off-the-shelf technology that is greatly facilitating its dissemination. In this context, theoretical discussions of the field appear as an important action in order to take stock of the mounting evidence that has been produced and the main challenges for the coming future. To stimulate the discussion in a burgeoning field, a SWOT analysis is proposed, which may help to map the field of VR therapy for anxiety and stress-related disorders. Overall, it is undoubted that VR appears as a well-established technology for the treatment of ASRD and the main challenges are in line with the possibility of hurdling the same obstacles that the whole field of clinical psychology and psychotherapy has to deal with: How to bridge the gap between research and clinical practice.

Keywords: Virtual reality therapy · Anxiety disorders · SWOT analysis

1 Introduction

Anxiety and stress-related disorders (ASRD) are among the most prevalent mental disorders [1]. Having an ASRD is sometimes perceived as a minor psychopathological manifestation. However, not only suffering from an ASRD can be devastating by itself, but also it may constitute the correlate of a chronic, serious and disabling mental or physical dysfunction. A clear indicator in this regard is the high comorbidity of ASRD with a vast array of other disorders [2].

Despite the well-established efficacy of a range of psychological treatments [3], a large amount of people does not receive adequate treatment or remains untreated [4, 5]. In this context, the development of new therapeutic strategies can be part of the

© ICST Institute for Computer Sciences, Social Informatics and Telecommunications Engineering 2019
Published by Springer Nature Switzerland AG 2019. All Rights Reserved
P. Cipresso et al. (Eds.): MindCare 2019, LNICST 288, pp. 43–54, 2019.
https://doi.org/10.1007/978-3-030-25872-6_4

solution [6]. Particularly, Information and Communication Technologies (ICTs) may hurdle some of the existing obstacles, such as the dissemination and implementation of the already existing treatments [7].

Virtual Reality (VR) is one of the technological advancements that has been developed more than two decades ago and since then has shown a spark of interest in the scientific community. Initially, it emerged as an alternative for the delivery of in vivo exposure. Although applying exposure to anxiety disorders is one of the few undisputable procedures in clinical psychology research [8], a number of studies have shown that both therapists [9–11] and patients [12, 13] are reluctant to undergoing in vivo exposure. In that sense, the possibility of creating virtual environments capable of provoking analogue emotional reactions to real stimuli arouse as an appealing strategy for the whole spectrum of ASRD. Therefore, the term coined for applying exposure by means of VR has been Virtual Reality Exposure Therapy (VRET).

In these 25 years, the field of VR for ASRD has experienced profound changes, in line with the logical evolution of clinical psychology as a field and VR as a technology in the society in general. With the goal of describing the salient aspects of the present and future of the field, this study aims to conduct a SWOT analysis. Although this is not the first study of this kind for VR, more than 15 years have gone by since that article and the state-of-the-art and future challenges are very different. Besides, it is interesting to compare that study with the current one in order to establish the extent to which the field of VR has changed.

2 Methods

For previous studies, we had carried out several systematic searches of the literature [14, 15], so a direct contact with the current literature in the field was already performed. An update of the literature search was conducted in order to include the latest studies that have been published recently. This study involves people from two of the main laboratories working with VR, as recently stated in a bibliometric analysis of research on VR [16].

The decision of doing a SWOT analysis was based on the fact that this approach has shown to be effective at mapping the general picture of a particular field. Usually used in organizational settings, it has also been sometimes implemented for clinical research, for example for describing the field of negative effects in clinical psychology [17]. This type of study may promote new unexplored avenues of future research as well as alerting the scientific community with regard to the aspects that need to be carefully addressed.

Despite this paper is focused on ASRD, general aspects of virtual reality therapy, regardless of the specificity for these clinical conditions, will be taken into consideration.

3 Strengths and Weaknesses of VR for Anxiety Disorders

The therapeutic strengths of VR are extensively agreed in the literature. On the one hand, the controllability of the stimuli can be of paramount importance for the delivery of exposure. Although the presupposed mechanism of exposure was initially thought to be habituation, nowadays evidence supports that the operating principle is the inhibitory learning [18]. Thus, the necessity to violate confirming biases associated with the feared stimuli rather than exposing the individual to the feared stimuli in a hierarchical way. In any case, VR offers a secure modality that in vivo exposure does not guarantee. The most illustrative example is constituted by the extensive research to treat PTSD in veterans of war given the possibility of recreating the same contextual information [19].

In this sense, the strongest aspect of VR for ASRD revolves around the fact that in these 25 years dozens of clinical trials have been carried out and nowadays there is a large body of evidence that supports its equal efficacy to in vivo exposure. Interestingly, improvements are observed not only in self-report measures [20], but also in behavioural [21] and physiological measures [22, 23]. Besides, evidence suggests that VR is more accepted than in vivo exposure [12], and its attrition and deterioration rates are comparable to face-to-face interventions [15, 24].

One aspect of paramount importance is that increasing attention is being paid to the quality, standards and guidelines to carry out VR clinical trials [25, 26]. However, this is part of a weakness detected by experts in VR for healthcare, who identified that most of the clinical trials until 2013 were of dubious quality. Throughout these years, indeed, the weaknesses of research on VR have consistently been identified, including the aforementioned problems in clinical trials' designs (e.g. small sample sizes [27] or problems with the randomization of participants [26]), the scarcity of process-focused research studies [28] or the lack of implementation of VR in naturalistic settings.

From the three described problems, it could be stated that research quality has considerably improved, including publications in the best clinical journals with powered samples [29–33]; the research on process-focused research has seen a slow but still important progress; and the implementation of VR in clinical settings is definitely the most serious shortcoming.

With regard to process-focused research, some signs of progress have been achieved in therapeutic alliance (TA). Although none clinical study had the primary aim of exploring TA, there are some theoretical discussion on the topic [34–37]. Besides, three RCTs [38–40] and one pilot study [41] included TA as a secondary outcome measure. Currently, the results indicate that TA in VR treatments is similar to face-to-face approaches. That is, there is a consistent positive association between TA and outcome. A spark of interest was also shown in the predictors of outcome. In total, four studies explored the role of expectations as a predictor of outcome in VRET [42–45], indicating that it constitutes a relevant non technical aspect that plays a relevant role in VRET. Likewise, some studies were conducted to look into the levels of engagement as a key process in VR outcomes, with mixed findings [46, 47].

Last but not least, the first studies to shed light upon the mechanisms of change in VR are starting to appear, in line with the advent of the process-based CBT movement that Stefan Hofmann and Steven Hayes have recently promoted [48]. As an example,

Norr and colleagues [49] performed moderator analyses to explore the characteristics of the patients who improved the most for prolonged exposure versus VR exposure. Their results indicate that being young, not to take antidepressants and having greater PTSD hyperarousal symptoms predicted a greater reduction in PTSD symptoms undergoing VR exposure. In another study, mediational analyses revealed that the reduction of posttraumatic symptoms leads to the change of depressive symptoms and not the other way around [50]. Likewise, Maples-Keller and colleagues [44] investigated the role of reexperiencing symptoms in VRET for PTSD, showing its importance in line with Emotional Processing Theory. Finally, a further research line explored the role of cognitive mechanisms in spider phobia VRET. In line with the conceptualization of exposure in cognitive behaviour models, both the phobic stimuli and self-efficacy have proven to be predictors of change in two different studies [51, 52].

Apart from cutting edge research, another well-established advantage of VR as a clinical tool revolves around the possibility of providing patients with contextually relevant stimuli. This feature is gaining more importance with the proliferation of personalized systems [53] as well as user-friendly software that allow to create virtual environment with almost none programming skills. In terms of hardware, head-mounted displays are significantly decreasing their price, which permits to acquire VR devices for very affordable prices [54].

Precisely in terms of hardware, it is interesting the results of a recent systematic review which synthesized the VR equipment used by all the existing trials in the field [55]. The authors found that among the 82 included studies, a great proportion utilized the eMagin z800 and then many different devices were only rarely implemented. The most salient aspect shared by all these devices share is that all are stationary. Among the commonly sold HMDs sold on the market, none was used in these studies. It must be stated, however, that in the latest studies published during the last couple of years, researchers are starting to use off-the-shelf devices in line with the abovementioned decrease of the prices [56].

As previously stated, the lack of implementation of VR in clinical settings is the most critical aspect that should be mentioned. On the one hand this can be explained by the overall problems that literature has detected in order to bridge the gap between research and practice [57], and the difficulties to translate basic science to applied contexts [58]. Besides, in the case of VR, even when prices are significantly decreasing, therapists might not see the reason to justify a still high expenditure [54].

4   Opportunities and Threats that Foresee the Future Challenges in the Field

As described before, VR has mainly been studied as a replacement of exposure. However, we consider that there are numerous opportunities for the future of VR in the field of ASRD given the capabilities of this interactive and immersive technology. Four potential ways in which VR can really go beyond exposure:

(a) VR as an embodied tool. Such an approach considers that the body plays an instrumental role in the processing of cognition. Apart from merely reproducing certain stimuli of the real world, VR can interact with the real world modifying it [59]. In particular, VR has shown to be effective at fooling the body matrix, which in turn is essential in the regulation of the psychological and physiological processes of individuals. Specifically, a technique called "body swapping", which permits to promote changes in the body memory, may be useful in order to work on body image distortions that sometimes are present in individuals suffering from ASRD [60]. Likewise, this technique can be helpful for social anxiety disorder, in which body image plays an important role [60] and bodily aspects may be relevant targets to deactivate safety behaviours. Furthermore, an interventional study, based on this paradigm, has shown that assigning a dissimilar avatar to social anxiety individuals helped them to reduce the levels of anxiety, which highlights the relevance of self-representation in this condition [61].

(b) Integration of VR with psychophysiology is opening new avenues, in particular, to intervene in the self-regulation of specific processes that have shown to be predictive of a range of disorders, including anxiety. Specifically, a physiological process that is impaired in ASRD is Heart Rate Variability (HRV) [62]. Although HRV biofeedback has shown to be effective for ASRD [63], the integration of VR environments may enhance the engagement and thus the effectiveness of biofeedback training. Existing examples are already available. For example, Repetto tested a virtual reality mobile based biofeedback [64] or Lorenzetti and colleagues implemented a real-time functional magnetic resonance imaging neurofeedback protocol with the aim of enhancing emotional states in healthy subjects [65]. Another technology that may be integrated with VR and is gaining interest is eye-tracking. Extensive research has shown the presence of perceptual and attentional biases in anxiety disorders, and preliminary research using VR suggests that it is an effective way of delivering attentional bias modification [66].

(c) VR for the training of psychological strategies of affect and emotion regulation. For example, autobiographical memory training could be achieved through VR environments that permit to stimulate the evocation of specific memories. Some initial evidence in this regard was achieved by Baños and colleagues [67] who used a system that used symbolic information for the re-elaboration of traumatic events in PTSD patients. The utilization of non-symbolic information (i.e. bringing the person to real place where the events took place) has not been researched yet but constitutes a promising avenue to explore. Likewise, 360 degrees videos may be utilized for the training of specific situations that are dysfunctional. For example, in the case of social anxiety disorders, training how to interact with people in stressful situations may be important to train assertiveness. Besides, certain emotion regulation strategies that are causing problems may be also trained, such as cognitive reappraisal in order to decrease rumination or fostering acceptance instead of dealing with experiential avoidance.

(d) One of the weaknesses of VR that could be transformed into strength in the near future is the utilization of VR as an assessment tool. Clinically, the possibility of providing a patient with multiple scenarios can be of tremendous help in order to make accurate diagnoses. Especially, in order to determine the extent to which personality is compromised in the context of an anxiety disorder [68]. In this line the existing associations between multisensory integration (process that has extensively been research in VR), attachment and personality (disorders) constitutes a very promising line to further explore. Although there are some existing examples in the literature, this is a research line that can be greatly expanded.

Among the threats, in line with all ICTs, it must be mentioned the time that research needs to demonstrate efficacious procedures. Currently, the classic validation design of any treatment supposes a series of steps that culminate in conducting a randomized controlled trial as the gold standard criteria of quality [69]. Should all the recommended steps be taken; the whole process is a matter of years until the final results are available. Given that technological developments, including VR, are ever changing, much faster testing procedures are required. Two highly recommended approaches are qualitative research and single case experimental design, which luckily is re-emerging as a very powerful research design, especially when testing new treatment approaches [70].

Another aspect that needs particular attention in order to not become a weakness is how embodied conversational agents (ECA) are incorporated in therapeutic interventions, practices that are defined by human interaction. There is no doubt that ECAs will grow exponentially in the next years, in line with the overall explosion of artificial intelligence. Indeed, there are already examples of development and pilot studies starting to implement ECAs in the context of anxiety disorders [71]. The first examples of self-led interventions are showing very promising results, and if personalized the possibility of increasing the personalization of the virtual stimuli depending on the individual necessity and preference, would greatly strengthen VR as a clinical tool.

First and foremost, there is an ethical concern regarding the extent to which the interventions will be open for the massive public and how regulation and monitoring of users will be done. In this sense, works like the one conducted by Freeman and colleagues [31] are promising examples given the high quality of the clinical trial. Besides, it is of utmost relevance to establish when people do need human support [72] given that in many cases it should be needed additional therapeutic content in order to achieve full recovery. However, in terms of regulation and ethical concerns, it is not only important to ensure the effectiveness but also the privacy of the users' data, including nonverbal data that current virtual systems can record [73].

On a similar but different note, the potential threat of ECAs is also anchored in the perceptions that clinical psychologists and psychotherapists may have. Many clinical psychologists may perceive ECAs as their substitutes. Indeed, different studies show that therapists are not only concerned about the difficulties that incorporating VR may entail (lack of training, technical and financial obstacles), but also that they are unfamiliar with VR as a clinical tool and thus they have concerns about its efficacy, the potential negative effects or the potential way VR may affect the therapist-client relationship [74–76]. With the advent of consumer VR platforms, Lindner and colleagues [77] revealed that attitudes towards VRET are overall positive and that familiarity with VR was higher in comparison to previous studies, although no direct comparison can be established for being completely different populations.

Finally, it is also very relevant the opinions of the community regarding the use of VR for health purposes. The first study exploring public perceptions of VR in health care suggests that overall there are positive attitudes towards VR for health care, including ASRD. Despite the predominance of positive comments, there are also concerns, such as the dependency of technology. Indeed, in a society in which technology-mediated experiences are starting to be omnipresent, there is increasing evidence showing that there is an overuse of virtual engagement, which far from helping contributes to unhealthy lifestyles that may lead in adjunction to other factors to the development of mental disorders. In this context, it is rather logical that the general public may perceive VR treatments with some extent of skepticism.

Weaknesses can be transformed into opportunities if correctly addressed or into threats if not. In that sense, one of the most challenging aspects is to achieve a real scale of VR. Every 10 years, a Delphi study of the field of psychotherapy is conducted. The last two versions carried out seven and seventeen years ago respectively, predicted that the use of VR was going to sprout out [78, 79]. While in the span of time between the first and second Delphi study the prediction clearly did not become true, a well and truly regrowth of VR emerged in the last years, which might lead to believe that the implementation of VR in clinical settings will finally flourish. The main reason to believe so is that costs have dramatically decreased and thus hardware and software costs are much more accessible if compared to a few years ago.

All in all, we do not have to forget that VR, like any other technology, is only a tool, which can be used properly or improperly. Besides, and most important, the core of our interest as clinical psychologists, either researchers or clinicians, is to understand the clinical phenomena and not be led by the usually mistaken idea of thinking that cutting-edge technologies will necessarily entail solutions for the problems we have to face with.

Acknowledgement. This work was supported by the Marie Skłodowska-Curie Innovative Training Network AffecTech (project ID: 722022) funded by the European Commission H2020.

References

1. Bandelow, B., Michaelis, S.: Epidemiology of anxiety disorders in the 21st century. Dialogues Clin. Neurosci. **17**(3), 327 (2015)
2. Watson, D.: Differentiating the mood and anxiety disorders: a quadripartite model. Ann. Rev. Clin. Psychol. **5**, 221–247 (2009). https://doi.org/10.1146/annurev.clinpsy.032408. 153510
3. Olatunji, B.O., Cisler, J.M., Deacon, B.J.: Efficacy of cognitive behavioral therapy for anxiety disorders: a review of meta-analytic findings (2010). https://doi.org/10.1016/j.psc. 2010.04.002
4. Alonso, J., et al.: Treatment gap for anxiety disorders is global: results of the world mental health surveys in 21 countries. Depress. Anxiety (2018). https://doi.org/10.1002/da.22711
5. WHO: Prevalence, severity, and unmet need for treatment of mental disorders in the world health organization world mental health surveys. J. Am. Med. Assoc. 2581–2590 (2004). https://doi.org/10.1001/jama.291.21.2581
6. Wagner, R., Silove, D., Marnane, C., Rouen, D.: Delays in referral of patients with social phobia, panic disorder and generalized anxiety disorder attending a specialist anxiety clinic. J. Anxiety Disord. (2006). https://doi.org/10.1016/j.janxdis.2005.02.003

7. Kazdin, A.E., Blase, S.L.: Rebooting psychotherapy research and practice to reduce the burden of mental illness. Perspect. Psychol. Sci. (2011). https://doi.org/10.1177/1745691610393527
8. Hoyer, J., Beesdo, K., Gloster, A.T., Runge, J., Höfler, M., Becker, E.S.: Worry exposure versus applied relaxation in the treatment of generalized anxiety disorder. Psychother. Psychosom. (2009). https://doi.org/10.1159/000201936
9. Pittig, A., Kotter, R., Hoyer, J.: The struggle of behavioral therapists with exposure: self-reported practicability, negative beliefs, and therapist distress about exposure-based interventions. Behav. Ther. (2019). https://doi.org/10.1016/j.beth.2018.07.003
10. Cook, J.M., Biyanova, T., Elhai, J., Schnurr, P.P., Coyne, J.C.: What do psychotherapists really do in practice? An internet study of over 2,000 practitioners. Psychotherapy (2010). https://doi.org/10.1037/a0019788
11. Schumacher, S., Weiss, D., Knaevelsrud, C.: Dissemination of exposure in the treatment of anxiety disorders and post-traumatic stress disorder among German cognitive behavioural therapists. Clin. Psychol. Psychother. (2018). https://doi.org/10.1002/cpp.2320
12. Garcia-Palacios, A., Botella, C., Hoffman, H., Fabregat, S.: Comparing acceptance and refusal rates of virtual reality exposure vs. in vivo exposure by patients with specific phobias. CyberPsychol. Behav **10**, 722–724 (2007). https://doi.org/10.1089/cpb.2007.9962
13. Garcia-Palacios, A., Hoffman, H.G., Kwong See, S., Tsai, A., Botella, C.: Redefining therapeutic success with virtual reality exposure therapy. CyberPsychol. Behav. **4**, 341–348 (2002). https://doi.org/10.1089/109493101300210231
14. Botella, C., Fernández-Álvarez, J., Guillén, V., García-Palacios, A., Baños, R.: Recent progress in virtual reality exposure therapy for phobias: a systematic review. Curr. Psychiatry Rep. **19** (2017). https://doi.org/10.1007/s11920-017-0788-4
15. Fernández-Álvarez, J., et al.: Deterioration rates in virtual reality therapy: an individual patient data level meta-analysis. J. Anxiety Disord. **61**, 3–17 (2019). https://doi.org/10.1016/j.janxdis.2018.06.005
16. Cipresso, P., Giglioli, I.A.C., Raya, M.A., Riva, G.: The past, present, and future of virtual and augmented reality research: a network and cluster analysis of the literature. Front. Psychol. (2018). https://doi.org/10.3389/fpsyg.2018.02086
17. Rozental, A., et al.: Negative effects in psychotherapy: commentary and recommendations for future research and clinical practice. BJPsych Open (2018). https://doi.org/10.1192/bjo.2018.42
18. Craske, M.G., Treanor, M., Conway, C.C., Zbozinek, T., Vervliet, B.: Maximizing exposure therapy: an inhibitory learning approach. Behav. Res. Ther. **58**, 10–23 (2014). https://doi.org/10.1016/j.brat.2014.04.006
19. Botella, C., Serrano, B., Baños, R.M., Garcia-Palacios, A.: Virtual reality exposure-based therapy for the treatment of post-traumatic stress disorder: a review of its efficacy, the adequacy of the treatment protocol, and its acceptability (2015). https://doi.org/10.2147/NDT.S89542
20. Carl, E., et al.: Virtual reality exposure therapy for anxiety and related disorders: a meta-analysis of randomized controlled trials (2018)
21. Morina, N., Ijntema, H., Meyerbröker, K., Emmelkamp, P.M.G.: Can virtual reality exposure therapy gains be generalized to real-life? A meta-analysis of studies applying behavioral assessments. Behav. Res. Ther. **74**, 18–24 (2015). https://doi.org/10.1016/j.brat.2015.08.010
22. Loucks, L., et al.: You can do that?!: Feasibility of virtual reality exposure therapy in the treatment of PTSD due to military sexual trauma. J. Anxiety Disord. **61**, 55–63 (2019). https://doi.org/10.1016/j.janxdis.2018.06.004

23. Côté, S., Bouchard, S.: Documenting the efficacy of virtual reality exposure with psychophysiological and information processing measures. Appl. Psychophysiol. Biofeedback **30**, 217–232 (2005). https://doi.org/10.1007/s10484-005-6379-x
24. Benbow, A.A., Anderson, P.L.: A meta-analytic examination of attrition in virtual reality exposure therapy for anxiety disorders. J. Anxiety Disord. **61**, 18–27 (2019). https://doi.org/10.1016/j.janxdis.2018.06.006
25. Birckhead, B., et al.: Recommendations for methodology of virtual reality clinical trials in health care by an international working group: iterative study. JMIR Ment. Health **6**, e11973 (2018). https://doi.org/10.2196/11973
26. McCann, R.A., et al.: Virtual reality exposure therapy for the treatment of anxiety disorders: an evaluation of research quality. J. Anxiety Disord. **28**, 625–631 (2014). https://doi.org/10.1016/j.janxdis.2014.05.010
27. Page, S., Coxon, M.: Virtual reality exposure therapy for anxiety disorders: small samples and no controls? Front. Psychol. **7**, 1–4 (2016). https://doi.org/10.3389/fpsyg.2016.00326
28. Meyerbröker, K., Emmelkamp, P.M.G.: Therapeutic processes in virtual reality exposure therapy: the role of cognitions and the therapeutic alliance. J. CyberTher. Rehabil. **1** (2008)
29. Reger, G.M., et al.: Randomized controlled trial of prolonged exposure using imaginal exposure vs. virtual reality exposure in active stress disorder (PTSD). J. Consult. Clin. Psychol. **84**, 946–959 (2016). https://doi.org/10.1037/ccp0000134
30. Donker, T., et al.: Effectiveness of self-guided app-based virtual reality cognitive behavior therapy for acrophobia. JAMA Psychiatry (2019). https://doi.org/10.1001/jamapsychiatry.2019.0219
31. Freeman, D., et al.: Automated psychological therapy using immersive virtual reality for treatment of fear of heights: a single-blind, parallel-group, randomised controlled trial. Lancet Psychiatry **5**, 625–632 (2018). https://doi.org/10.1016/S2215-0366(18)30226-8
32. Minns, S., et al.: Immersive 3D exposure-based treatment for spider fear: a randomized controlled trial. J. Anxiety Disord. **61**, 37–44 (2019). https://doi.org/10.1016/j.janxdis.2018.12.003
33. Lindner, P., et al.: Therapist-led and self-led one-session virtual reality exposure therapy for public speaking anxiety with consumer hardware and software: a randomized controlled trial. J. Anxiety Disord. **61**, 45–54 (2019). https://doi.org/10.1016/j.janxdis.2018.07.003
34. Miragall, M., Baños, R.M., Cebolla, A., Botella, C.: Working alliance inventory applied to virtual and augmented reality (WAI-VAR): psychometrics and therapeutic outcomes. Front. Psychol. **6**, 1–10 (2015). https://doi.org/10.3389/fpsyg.2015.01531
35. Ngai, I., Tully, E.C., Anderson, P.L.: The course of the working alliance during virtual reality and exposure group therapy for social anxiety disorder. Behav. Cogn. Psychother. **43**, 167–181 (2015). https://doi.org/10.1017/S135246581300088X
36. Wrzesien, M., Burkhardt, J.M., Botella, C., Alcañiz, M.: Towards a virtual reality- and augmented reality-mediated therapeutic process model: a theoretical revision of clinical issues and HCI issues. **16**, 124–153 (2015). https://doi.org/10.1080/1463922X.2014.903307
37. Wrzesien, M., et al.: How technology influences the therapeutic process: evaluation of the patient-therapist relationship in augmented reality exposure therapy and in vivo exposure therapy. Behav. Cogn. Psychother. **41**, 505–509 (2013). https://doi.org/10.1017/S1352465813000088
38. Anderson, P.L., et al.: Virtual reality exposure therapy for social anxiety disorder: a randomized controlled trial. J. Consult. Clin. Psychol. **81**, 751–760 (2013). https://doi.org/10.1037/a0033559
39. Moldovan, R., David, D.: One session treatment of cognitive and behavioral therapy and virtual reality for social and specific phobias. Preliminary results from a randomized clinical trial. J. Evid.-Based Psychother. **14**, 67–83 (2014)

40. Bouchard, S., et al.: Virtual reality compared with in vivo exposure in the treatment of social anxiety disorder: a three-arm randomised controlled trial. Br. J. Psychiatry. 1–9 (2016). https://doi.org/10.1192/bjp.bp.116.184234

41. Levy, F., Leboucher, P., Rautureau, G., Komano, O., Millet, B., Jouvent, R.: Fear of falling: efficacy of virtual reality associated with serious games in elderly people. Neuropsychiatr. Dis. Treat. 12, 877–881 (2016). https://doi.org/10.2147/NDT.S97809

42. Price, M., Anderson, P., Henrich, C.C., Rothbaum, B.O.: Greater expectations: using hierarchical linear modeling to examine expectancy for treatment outcome as a predictor of treatment response. Behav. Ther. 39, 398–405 (2008). https://doi.org/10.1016/j.beth.2007.12.002

43. Price, M., Anderson, P.L.: Outcome expectancy as a predictor of treatment response in cognitive behavioral therapy for public speaking fears within social anxiety disorder. Psychotherapy 49, 173–179 (2012). https://doi.org/10.1037/a0024734

44. Price, M., Maples, J.L., Jovanovic, T., Norrholm, S.D., Heekin, M., Rothbaum, B.O.: An investigation of outcome expectancies as a predictor of treatment response for combat veterans with PTSD: comparison of clinician, self-report, and biological measures. Depress. Anxiety 32, 392–399 (2015). https://doi.org/10.1002/da.22354

45. Norrholm, S.D., et al.: Fear load: The psychophysiological over-expression of fear as an intermediate phenotype associated with trauma reactions. Int. J. Psychophysiol. 98, 270–275 (2014). https://doi.org/10.1016/j.ijpsycho.2014.11.005

46. Price, M., Mehta, N., Tone, E.B., Anderson, P.L.: Does engagement with exposure yield better outcomes? Components of presence as a predictor of treatment response for virtual reality exposure therapy for social phobia. J. Anxiety Disord. 25, 763–770 (2011). https://doi.org/10.1016/j.janxdis.2011.03.004

47. Reger, G.M., Smolenski, D., Norr, A., Katz, A., Buck, B., Rothbaum, B.O.: Does virtual reality increase emotional engagement during exposure for PTSD? Subjective distress during prolonged and virtual reality exposure therapy. J. Anxiety Disord. 61, 75–81 (2019). https://doi.org/10.1016/j.janxdis.2018.06.001

48. Hofmann, S.G., Hayes, S.C.: The future of intervention science: process-based therapy. Clin. Psychol. Sci. 7, 37–50 (2019). https://doi.org/10.1177/2167702618772296

49. Norr, A.M., et al.: Virtual reality exposure versus prolonged exposure for PTSD: which treatment for whom? Depress. Anxiety (2018). https://doi.org/10.1002/da.22751

50. Peskin, M., et al.: The relationship between posttraumatic and depressive symptoms during virtual reality exposure therapy with a cognitive enhancer. J. Anxiety Disord. (2019). https://doi.org/10.1016/j.janxdis.2018.03.001

51. Côté, S., Bouchard, S.: Cognitive mechanisms underlying virtual reality exposure. CyberPsychol. Behav. 12, 121–129 (2009). https://doi.org/10.1089/cpb.2008.0008

52. Tardif, N., Therrie, C., Bouchard, S.: Re-examining psychological mechanisms underlying virtual reality-based exposure for spider phobia. Cyberpsychol. Behav. Soc. Netw. 22, 39–45 (2019). https://doi.org/10.1089/cyber.2017.0711

53. Pizzoli, S.F.M., Mazzocco, K., Triberti, S., Monzani, D., Alcañiz Raya, M.L., Pravettoni, G.: User-centered virtual reality for promoting relaxation: an innovative approach. Front. Psychol. 10, 1–8 (2019). https://doi.org/10.3389/fpsyg.2019.00479

54. Lindner, P., et al.: Creating state of the art, next-generation virtual reality exposure therapies for anxiety disorders using consumer hardware platforms: design considerations and future direction. Cogn. Behav. Ther. (in press). https://doi.org/10.1080/16506073.2017.1280843

55. Jerdan, S.W., Grindle, M., Van Woerden, H.C., Kamel Boulos, M.N.: Head-mounted virtual reality and mental health: critical review of current research. J. Med. Internet Res. 20, 1–16 (2018). https://doi.org/10.2196/games.9226

56. Carlbring, P., et al.: Therapist-led and self-led one-session virtual reality exposure therapy for public speaking anxiety with consumer hardware and software: a randomized controlled trial. J. Anxiety Disord. **61**, 45–54 (2018). https://doi.org/10.1016/j.janxdis.2018.07.003

57. Fernández-Álvarez, J., Fernández-Álvarez, H., Castonguay, L.G.: Resumiendo los nuevos esfuerzos para integrar la práctica y la investigación desde la perspectiva de la investigación orientada por la práctica. Rev. Argent. Clin. Psicol. (2018). https://doi.org/10.24205/03276716.2018.1070

58. Maples-Keller, J.L., et al.: When translational neuroscience fails in the clinic: dexamethasone prior to virtual reality exposure therapy increases drop-out rates. J. Anxiety Disord. **61**, 89–97 (2019). https://doi.org/10.1016/j.janxdis.2018.10.006

59. Repetto, C., Riva, G.: From virtual reality to interreality in the treatment of anxiety disorders. Neuropsychiatry (London) (2011). https://doi.org/10.2217/npy.11.5

60. Aderka, I.M., Gutner, C.A., Lazarov, A., Hermesh, H., Hofmann, S.G., Marom, S.: Body image in social anxiety disorder, obsessive-compulsive disorder, and panic disorder. Body Image (2014). https://doi.org/10.1016/j.bodyim.2013.09.002

61. Aymerich-Franch, L., Kizilcec, R.F., Bailenson, J.N.: The relationship between virtual self similarity and social anxiety. Front. Hum. Neurosci. **8**, 944 (2014). https://doi.org/10.3389/fnhum.2014.00944

62. Chalmers, J.A., Quintana, D.S., Abbott, M.J.A., Kemp, A.H.: Anxiety disorders are associated with reduced heart rate variability: a meta-analysis. Front. Psychiatry. **5** (2014). https://doi.org/10.3389/fpsyt.2014.00080

63. Goessl, V.C., Curtiss, J.E., Hofmann, S.G.: The effect of heart rate variability biofeedback training on stress and anxiety: a meta-analysis. Psychol. Med. **47**, 2578–2586 (2017). https://doi.org/10.1017/S0033291717001003

64. Repetto, C., Gaggioli, A., Pallavicini, F., Cipresso, P., Raspelli, S., Riva, G.: Virtual reality and mobile phones in the treatment of generalized anxiety disorders: a phase-2 clinical trial. Pers. Ubiquitous Comput. (2013). https://doi.org/10.1007/s00779-011-0467-0

65. Lorenzetti, V., et al.: Emotion regulation using virtual environments and real-time fMRI neurofeedback. Front. Neurol. **9**, 390 (2018). https://doi.org/10.3389/FNEUR.2018.00390

66. Urech, A., Krieger, T., Chesham, A., Mast, F.W., Berger, T.: Virtual reality-based attention bias modification training for social anxiety: a feasibility and proof of concept study. Front. Psychiatry **6**, 1–5 (2015). https://doi.org/10.3389/fpsyt.2015.00154

67. Baños, R.M., Guillen, V., Quero, S., García-Palacios, A., Alcaniz, M., Botella, C.: A virtual reality system for the treatment of stress-related disorders: a preliminary analysis of efficacy compared to a standard cognitive behavioral program. Int. J. Hum Comput Stud. **69**, 602–613 (2011). https://doi.org/10.1016/j.ijhcs.2011.06.002

68. Cipresso, P., Riva, G.: Personality assessment in ecological settings by means of virtual reality. In: The Wiley Handbook of Personality Assessment, pp. 240–248 (2016)

69. Fleming, T.M., et al.: Maximizing the impact of e-therapy and serious gaming: time for a paradigm shift. Front. Psychiatry **7**, 65 (2016)

70. Kazdin, A.E.: Single-case experimental designs. Evaluating interventions in research and clinical practice (2018). https://doi.org/10.1016/j.brat.2018.11.015

71. Provoost, S., Lau, H.M., Ruwaard, J., Riper, H.: Embodied conversational agents in clinical psychology: a scoping review (2017). https://doi.org/10.2196/jmir.6553

72. Schueller, S.M., Tomasino, K.N., Mohr, D.C.: Integrating human support into behavioral intervention technologies: the efficiency model of support (2017). https://doi.org/10.1111/cpsp.12173

73. Bailenson, J.: Protecting nonverbal data tracked in virtual reality. JAMA Pediatr. (2018). https://doi.org/10.1001/jamapediatrics.2018.1909

74. Schwartzman, D., Segal, R., Drapeau, M.: Perceptions of virtual reality among therapists who do not apply this technology in clinical practice. Psychol. Serv. **9**, 310–315 (2012). https://doi.org/10.1037/a0026801
75. Segal, R., Bhatia, M., Drapeau, M.: Therapists' perception of benefits and costs of using virtual reality treatments. Cyberpsychol. Behav. Soc. Netw. **14**, 29–34 (2010). https://doi.org/10.1089/cyber.2009.0398
76. Kramer, T.L., Pyne, J.M., Kimbrell, T.A., Savary, P.E., Smith, J.L., Jegley, S.M.: Clinician perceptions of virtual reality to assess and treat returning veterans. Psychiatr. Serv. **61**, 1153–1156 (2014). https://doi.org/10.1176/ps.2010.61.11.1153
77. Lindner, P., Miloff, A., Zetterlund, E., Reuterskiöld, L., Andersson, G., Carlbring, P.: Attitudes toward and familiarity with virtual reality therapy among practicing cognitive behavior therapists: a cross-sectional survey study in the era of consumer VR platforms. Front. Psychol. **10**, 1–10 (2019). https://doi.org/10.3389/fpsyg.2019.00176
78. Norcross, J.C., Hedges, M., Prochaska, J.O.: The face of 2010: a delphi poll on the future of psychotherapy. Prof. Psychol. Res. Pract. (2002). https://doi.org/10.1037/0735-7028.33.3.316
79. Norcross, J.C., Pfund, R.A., Prochaska, J.O.: Psychotherapy in 2022 : a delphi poll on its future. **44**, 363–370 (2013). https://doi.org/10.1037/a0034633

Experiencing Dementia from Inside: The Expediency of Immersive Presence

Francesca Morganti[(✉)] [iD]

University of Bergamo, Bergamo, Italy
francesca.morganti@unibg.it

Abstract. The lengthening of life expectancy has shown a positive trend of neurodegenerative diseases and, among these, dementia seems to have a large incidence in the world population. Unfortunately, in their individual, social and institutional contexts people with dementia are very often stripped of their "being a person" and, finding themselves in a condition of particular frailty, they become the object of exclusion. More recently the idea of being aware about pathological cognitive decline linked to neurodegenerative diseases is growing worldwide through the Dementia Friendly Community movement. It is asking to general population to perform inclusive behaviors towards people living with different forms of dementia (including Alzheimer's disease) by maintaining their personal and professional role within the urban community. Despite the large amount of Dementia Friendly initiatives, if a member of the community doesn't have the opportunity to personally observe this living condition among her/his close relationships she/he probably tend to consider the dementia population as largely needful and highly usefulness, without exactly understand how they can contribute in this inclusive process. In order to support the urban community members in their broadly availability to adequately play their social role towards people living with dementia, the present research introduces ViveDe: examples of immersive experiences possible trough virtual reality. With the aim of pushing the general population in understanding how living with dementia could be like, different daily situation where proposed and social perspective change was analyzed.

ViveDe experience revealed how "being present" in the daily challenges an urban space proposes (e.g. exploiting her/his duty at home, going around in a unknown city, having some leisure time with friends) sheds new light on the role each community's member can play towards people with dementia.

Keywords: Cognitive frailty · Alzheimer · Dementia Friendly · ViveDe · 360° video · Virtual reality

1 Living with Dementia

1.1 The Cognitive Frailty Increasing

An urge amount of research in cognitive neuropsychology developed during the last 10 years was focused on dementia and cognitive decline. This research mainstream is addressable to the urgency data about aging population and to the exponential increase

© ICST Institute for Computer Sciences, Social Informatics and Telecommunications Engineering 2019
Published by Springer Nature Switzerland AG 2019. All Rights Reserved
P. Cipresso et al. (Eds.): MindCare 2019, LNICST 288, pp. 55–70, 2019.
https://doi.org/10.1007/978-3-030-25872-6_5

in neurodegenerative diseases [1]. The most recent report available about the spread of dementia in Italy, in fact, showed there are at least 1 million people with dementia in 2017 (of which about 600,000 with Alzheimer's dementia) and about 3 million people taking care of them. These numbers are estimated to tripling for 2050. Considering also that up to now about 50% of dementia diagnoses worldwide do not seem to detect mild cognitive decline in the elderly population, one can easily imagine the repercussions of these data on the economic and social landscape of the coming decades. At present it's a largely shared opinion that in the next 20 years' people suffering from dementia will increase and formal caregiving (such as health institutions and governmental welfare) will be insufficient for facing the wide amount of assistance request [2].

Dementia is specifically defined as a cognitive impairment (a decline in performance prior to the known or presumed beginning of the disease), global (involving all cognitive functions) and chronic (which is prolonged continuously over time). The cognitive performance required to face the external environment challenges becomes unsuccessful in dementia. Nowadays, to outline the nosographic boundaries of an intermediate situation between brain aging and dementia is still a difficult task, especially because the relationships between these two conditions are not yet clear. For some scholars, brain aging and dementia represent the extremes of a continuum in which dementia is the terminal phase of an inexorable process and an expression of functional exhaustion of the brain [3]. For others, dementia is a pure pathology, distinct from aging that represents a risk factor but not the cause of the disease [4]. However, a perspective that is not only biological, but embraces also the social dimension, shows how the term dementia should be used in a largely descriptive way to draw a clinically identified condition that refers to the person in its entirety and not exclusively to his or her brain [5]. Accordingly, "being a person in dementia" is a condition given to an individual by the others that constitute her/his relational and social context. Similarly, the definition of dementia in this case is referring to a multiple-cause clinical syndrome. In addition to cognitive decline, there are symptoms that affect the sphere of personality, of affectivity, of conception and perception, as well as of vegetative functions and of behavior. Thus, it is possible to define dementia as a progressive and irreversible disease of organic origin, prevalently found in elderly people, which presents a compromise of memory functions, with communicative difficulties in its forms of expression and understanding consequent to disturbance of language, with the inability to perform daily activities in spite of the integrity of motor skills, and with the consequent inability to perform goal oriented gestures and actions, such as taking care of personal hygiene or organizing domestic activities [6]. Therefore, the manifestations of dementia here described tend to have a strong impact on the functional status of the subject (both in the individual and social sphere) significantly interfering with her/his quality of life.

Luckily in the misfortune dementia course is not always so sudden but, in most cases, allows people to continue to live in partial autonomy especially in the early stages of the disease. Accordingly, it become necessary to value the person in order to warrantee her/him a good quality of life. It means to value also her/his temperament and her/his personality (built in the experience of life), on which depends, in large part, the way in which the individual faces both old age and eventually dementia. Hilman [7] in this regard claims that it is necessary:

- to last those parts of the character last that allow the person to always positively overcome the challenges of life in a creative and functional way according to her/his own well-being;
- to leave those parts of the character that hinder an optimal path in old age and dementia;
- to keep those parts of the character that allow the person to be considered by all those who surround it as unique, peculiar and special.

However, this autonomy is subordinated to the change in inclusiveness, that the contexts in which the person finds her/himself living daily, may have developed. We'll discuss about it later in the manuscript, after better understood what living with dementia could mean.

1.2 How Living with Dementia Is like?

The way a person with cognitive frailty experience everyday space plays a significant role in the ways she/he can face the contextual challenges and gain autonomy in daily activity. Moreover, the way the context is represented will become even more crucial in the ways the individual perceive the possibilities for building social relations.

Some aspects of how living with dementia can be like emerges from the experience reported by the patients themselves [8]. The personal experience of living with dementia is influenced by social elements (e.g. the modality in which member s of the community talk and behave toward them), and to have the opportunity of being considered with the full possibility of being a valued member of the society they live in, seems to have a great impact upon the emotional and psychological well-being of people with dementia [9]. Moreover, considering how people with dementia experience their surrounding space (both owns home and long term-care settings), showed that lived space continually decreases due to the progression of dementia but individuals continues to experience the spatial dimensions of life through lived space even in the illness [10].

Unfortunately, even the literature in the field can provide us with a detailed picture about the challenges/skill balance people with dementia do about living every day, it doesn't be able to give us an idea about how experiencing dementia daily can be. Generally, "from the outside" we observe people living with dementia without understanding why they are presenting some behaviors (such as agitation, wandering, irritation, memory fault and inability to conclude some easy tasks) during a daily situation (such as having a family lunch or going to bed). This inability to detect which cognitive difficulties can lead the person to not have socially adequate behaviors, often leads us to confuse these behaviors with evidence of a "personality change" and not as a symptom of an in progress cognitive impairment in the person who is living with dementia. Moreover, living with a cognitive frailty inevitably contains in itself suffering, fear, anguish and, often, a double difficulty of recognition. There is a difficulty in recognizing oneself, on the part of those who carry cognitive impairments and in integrating the new image of oneself with the past (especially when awareness in the pathology is preserved). Furthermore, there is a difficulty in recognizing the person with cognitive frailty on the part of the community members. Difficulty that often results in distancing oneself from those who start to be considered primarily as a burden. This double difficulty results in a mutual isolation, in which the community tends to exasperate the behavior of protection against the person with cognitive frailty, often limiting their daily autonomy. While the latter, in an attempt to silence the anxiety related to the progress of cognitive decline, will start towards an isolation that will lead it to live with the daily limitations to which the cognitive compromise binds she/he irreversibly.

Determining how every day social life could be for people with dementia might contribute to overcome this situation. This can be possible starting from the point of view of people with dementia who live in an urban community and at the same time by providing the community with insight about the role and actions to be taken in supporting all the members in identifying the cognitive and relational possibilities that can be brought at play including the person with dementia within the same community [11]. If this situation is kept and interwoven in a strongly interconnected social network that welcomes people living with dementia, supports them, enhances them, and gives them back competence, a good quality of social life can still be possible. For this to happen, however, there is a need to enhance "best practices" in education based on the idea that people with dementia require relational and emotional paths that unfold around the person to continue living an everyday life that is as autonomous as possible. Above all, in the cohabitation with the pathology, a more inclusive community have to be planned.

2 How to Implement a Dementia Friendly Community "Revolution"

By supporting the idea of inclusiveness for people living with dementia described above, Dementia Friendly communities (DFC) were developed worldwide [11]. DFC are urban realities in which each member, in her/his personal and professional role, learns to understand what to do and what the other person expects to be done in living with people who no longer have full control of their cognitive faculties and will continue being part of the same urban community. Accordingly, a DFC is not made up exclusively of health professionals and family members of people with dementia, but it is a community where each member finds its role in combining their possible life-paths with people with cognitive decline whether they are their customers, neighbors or simple acquaintances. Specifically, a Dementia Friendly Community has as its basis the relationship constituted by the various focal points of the community. Therefore, not only those who take daily-care of people with dementia are involved in this network and constitute its important node. Contrarywise, all the representative sectors of an urban community (such as the neighborhood, the transport services, the educational institutions, the legal and financial services, the sales companies, the religious communities, etc.) are involved in a DFC.

All-over the world many Dementia Friendly communities are growing with both private and governmental contribution, such for example the Alzheimer's Disease International in UK [12], the Dementia Friendly America, in USA [13] and the Alzheimer's Australia Dementia Friendly, in Australia [14]. Even if at present they can show several different perspectives on how to improve a DFC growth, their contribution appears to focus more on the institutional level (such as the local welfare services) than on the entire urban community. Moreover, their efforts seem overcome being focused on an educational intervention that can raise citizens' awareness about dementia and on the exercise of a responsible and inclusive citizenship. The neighborhoods, the public and the businesses services that the person with dementia face with every day, in fact, have to be supported in understanding what role they can have in order to create a friendly ground on which to allow the rooting of a full inclusiveness of the person himself. It is therefore necessary to learn how a "friendly" community can be formed around the person [5].

2.1 How to Become Dementia Friendly?

If the stated mission is to turn any urban community as an inclusive one toward people suffering from this kind of illness, any community member has to turn aware about "what living with dementia means". Thus, by this way the individual will be not excluded but will be fully understood and, above all, will be supported in continuing her/his individuality in spite of, and together with, her/his cognitive frailty.

Consistent with DFC this perspective, the bio-ecological theory of Urie Bronfenbrenner [15] illustrates the importance of experience in conveying an inclusive change towards people. It highlights the active role that have to be recognized to individuals who "inhabit" the environment, and, at the same time, it underlines the effects that their action has with respect to the determination of the surrounding environment. The behavior of the individuals belonging to a community is determined not only by the individuals-environment "per sè", but it is co-determined by the individual-environment coupling experienced at that peculiar moment. Accordingly, to find ways to start an inclusive change suitable for all the elements of the community network, it appears to be necessary studying the positioning people with dementia have in the community during their daily living. Thus, it is desirable to understand the perception people living with dementia have of the activity, of the roles and of the relationships that can be identified in the situations they live in. It will be, in fact, the active role that is recognized to the person with dementia, and the effects that their action has with respect to the determination of the surrounding environment, that can build an inclusive network of people. Maintaining people with dementia within it.

The rising question is still there: How to implement a DFC "cultural revolution" within community members? It is from this operationality question the present research starts. If the context itself is defining the idea of inclusion, it is exactly in the light of supporting a situation awareness that the DFC change will deem. Accordingly, the understanding of the context in which the person with dementia is living every day and of the situations within which she/he is building a close and mutual relationship with the member of the community can provide the possibility to identify the correct DFC educational approach. In our hypothesis, it is by negotiating meanings within the community, and by avoiding a prescriptive approach that imposes an "institutional" Dementia Friendly change, without understanding the points of view of all the elements involved in the community itself, that this essential revolution could be done.

2.2   Towards an Experiential Dementia Friendly Education Approach

At present the DFC programs worldwide doesn't seem to have individuated the experiential approach as one of the main expediencies for its educational mission. Instead to think about the opportunity provided from first-person perspective as one of the elective educative playgrounds in encouraging the performance of inclusive behaviors towards people living with dementia, several second- third-person actions were planned in urban situations requiring a large amount of efforts to organize it [11]. The main aim of this contribution is to show how, by providing people with appropriate contents to fully subjectively experience how living with dementia could be, we support them to understand which community role they can have in a Dementia Friendly perspective.

This first- person approach can be considered to be not an easy challenge for a double motivation. First, the wide experiential gap between the general population and people living with dementia introduces several emotional, cognitive and behavioral differences that convey the experience of living with dementia difficult to understand from the outside (especially if a member of the community doesn't have the opportunity to personally have closeness with this living condition in their family or among their daily relationships). Second, the dementia population is generally considered as largely needful and highly usefulness from the general public and this stereotyped representation appears to be stronger when addressed to severe cognitively impaired people (such as in Alzheimer disease). Thus, even if broadly available to adequately play their social role, urban community members don't exactly understand how they can contribute in a Dementia Friendly Community.

The recent wide diffusion of low-cost interactive technologies, such as 360° videos explorable through virtual reality eyeglasses, can provide new opportunities for creating experiences able to vehiculate a changing perspective on dementia. Moreover, such experiential technology, if accompanied with an educational program, will be able to support the adequate positioning of community members towards people living with this neurodegenerative disease.

2.3   The Role of Virtual Presence for Inclusiveness Change

The more recent development of virtual reality applications, due to its interactive nature, was made for pushing out storytelling [16]. At present, storytelling is considered as an effective pivot for emotions arousal that kick off correspondent actions. When user experience is warranted by optimal levels of virtual presence [17], some perspective changing is made possible by feeling of being "part of the story" while watching a meaningful content by interacting with it.

From the literature in the field we know that the sense of presence will be strong inasmuch as the virtual system enables an inclusive, extensive, surrounding and vivid illusion. The immersive quality of virtual experience would be enhanced by the perceptive features and by the proprioceptive feedback provided by the virtual technology and/or, as in the last years the research on presence has emphasized, by being exposed to interactive meaningful situations [18]. The sense of agency ownership, in fact, seems to be today the key presence element. It is provided not only by the visual reference of the agent body in the virtual environment, but also from the dynamic a virtual reality is able to support through a continuous coupling between perception and action. Thus, not only highly immersive technological solutions are needed to experience presence, but also subjective involvement plays an important role. Accordingly, some new generation researches are investigating how the virtual presence, the user flow-experience, and the storytelling identification, were significantly linked to empathetic disposal for actors and situations. Especially if empathetic situations are depicted in the proposed experience [19]. The results are highlighting how, like in the serious game for example, the same contextual and individual dimensions are related with an interest in learning different possibilities to face a situation considered as meaningful from the user. The "lived" virtual experience, in fact, appears to enhance interest in learning more about the game-specific topic, and on the specific skills the serious game would like to teach. Unfortunately, for how concerns the acquisition of socially valuable actions (e.g. inclusiveness) data suggests only that empathetic contents lead to moti-vation in increasing another's welfare, but only predicting this commitment without measuring it.

In order to overcome this gap and starting from the idea that presence is not a propriety of the immersive and interactive technology "per sè", but is a domain of human cognition that interplays with such kind of technological devices, the contri-bution proposed here aimed in understand how, when exposed by virtual reality to the perspective people with dementia have in exploring daily environments, users not only engage with the provided stories, but also construct and develop a perspective changing in their social role by actively adopting, consuming, and experiencing these immer-sively experienced stories. According to this, the ViveDe project was developed and introduced here.

In the next paragraphs different daily situations were described as presented to the general public by the use of immersive virtual reality in order to support a Dementia Friendly changing on them.

3   ViveDe: The Virtual Dementia Daily Experiences

The following paragraph will describe the ViveDe project developed from the Dementia Friendly Italia research group at the University of Bergamo (http://www.vivede.it). ViveDe introduces everyday situations that people can experience through the use of 360° videos explorable one the x/y axis by Virtual Reality eyeglasses. These daily experiences are provided from the point of view of a person living with dementia in order to give at the general public a first-person perspective on how living with dementia could be. ViveDe experiences take into account the different situations of dementia people ordinary everyday life.

3.1   ViveDe Scenario Developments

More than to tailor the scenarios on the well-known characteristics of cognitive impair-ment in dementia, derived from the neuropsychological expertise and from the wide symptoms description provided by the scientific literature in the field, in developing

ViveDe three different researches were conducted. Considering the main roles individual could have within a DFC community we had:

1. Early-dementia people (10 individuals) from different urban contexts (e.g. a big city, a smaller one, a seaside village, etc.) were involved in providing their perspective about how is difficult to face with everyday challenges without asking caregivers, relative, friends to support them daily. By introducing the Cultural Probe qualitative method [20] the daily dimension of aging-in-place with dementia was investigated. The 'capture artifacts' returned by people with dementia after a 2-months period were mainly small narratives, photographs, diagrams, calendar notes. They provide image-rich responses from the participant and constitutes useful elements in determining what could be the appropriate scenario to develop in ViveDe project.
2. Semi-structured interviews were conducted with caregivers, relatives, close friends about the daily habits people with dementia they live nearby have. These interviews were conducted in order to detect which could be the more frequent situations in which their support is required. In particular, focus was on the pattern of everyday activity the patient could still have faced with independently, if a collaborative context had been found.
3. A participatory ethnography was conducted by observing people with dementia and their caregivers in exploring the urban context they live within. From this perspective data were collected about activities proposed by neighbors, shopkeepers, desk clerks, bar and restaurant waiters to people with dementia. Main focus of this analysis, conducted following Bronfenbrenner's theoretical approach, was to determine the stereotypes and inappropriate behaviors usually presented from micro- to meso-situations that have to include individuals with dementia.

From the qualitative and quantitative data collected during this project phase the scripts proposed here were developed. The main ViveDe scenarios developed are:

Come Back Home
Day interior. The subjective of a panting person climbing the stairs of a building. One perceives the difficulty of returning home after a hypothetical outdoor walk. The person appears confused: there is no certainty about where the person is, nor about the exactness of the floor of the building in which the apartment he/she wants to reach is located. There is no one around, there are no distinctive elements to recognize the doors of the apartments. The person rings the house bell at one of the two doors on the floor and waits. No reply. She/he has keys in hand, but he does not use them. She/he waits. After a few moments the person, recognizing the doormat as a known element that can be placed in the sphere of the most remote memories, tries several times to use the bunch of keys he has in hand to ascertain the type of key with that of the lock on the door.

Entry into the apartment. Moment of emotional agitation due to not being sure to be on the right assessment. The apartment is perceived as definitely belonged to someone else. Running out of the apartment with the fear of being mistaken for thieves. The front door remains open. The person hesitates on the landing, he turns his gaze to the entrance and enters again recognizing him as his own.

Search for known elements in the living room and bedroom. Each "recognized" element decreases the state of agitation of the person. Confabulations on some of the elements encountered (e.g. basic necessities on the dining table, clothes in the closet) that obviously denote a confusion of space and time.

Search for a comfortable place in the apartment (e.g. a chair, a sofa). Waiting "watchful" of the arrival of a hypothetical landlord. Clear evidence of the impossibility of someone else arriving. Waiting with crescendo of anxiety and agitated thoughts. Dissolution.

Neighbors and Friends

Day interior. The subjective of a person sitting in an armchair inside an apartment. The person waits. The ambient conditions of the room are becoming unpleasant (e.g. too much noise coming in through the open window, the sun that overheats the living room and the seated person). Someone is ringing the doorbell. No reaction of the person in subjective. Noise of keys turned into the lock. The entrance door opens.

A person appears happily greets and enters carrying a shopping bag. It is understood that there is confidence between the two people but not full familiarity. The newly entered person, however, presents herself/himself making sure that she/he is recognized as the next-door neighbor. Show the keys and "justifies" for having used so it was agreed between them earlier. Once confirmed to agreement, closes the window and makes sure that the sun is not unpleasant for the person sitting in the chair.

The neighbor goes to the kitchen and finds in the fridge and in the pantry inappropriate objects (a hairdryer between the dishes and a book in the ice department). There is no negative reaction or judgment to the unusual findings. She shows objects to the person in the chair, appoints them, explains their main function and puts them in the right place while continues to show them to his interlocutor. Continuing to talk with the person sitting in the armchair, the neighbor begins to arrange the house and prepare lunch. Scene dissolution.

Having Lunch

Opening the scene with the subjective of being seated with the table set in a singular manner (e.g. soup in the citrus squeezer, fork instead of a dish and chopping board instead of a placemat).

The neighbor enters the dining room after finishing to work in the adjoining room. She is surprised about this arrangement of the table and, without judgement, shows to the person the inadequacy of this situation. The person in subjective gives a confused motivation about this and the neighbor understands how the person has no awareness of the difficulty in eating a soup with a fork. Scene dissolution.

Reopening of the scene with a table perfectly set for two. The tablecloth is well cleaned and ironed, the soup is steaming on the plate and the tablespoon is clearly visible on the napkin on the right. The neighbor puts a background music asking the person in subjective if this is her/his favorite song, which seems to be a song from many years ago. She sits in front of the person and asks to explain why she/he likes this song so much. As she begins to listen to the song together with the person in subjective, the scene ends.

Daily Shopping

At the Bakery

Day interior. Subjective of a person who enters alone in a bakery. There are some people waiting. The face of the waiting person reveals the belief that the person should not go around alone. There is a nod of agreement with the person at the desk.

The person's turn has arrived, while in the meantime the shop counts to fill people with evident haste. General consensus of people waiting to declare each one with different motivations (e.g. work, tiredness, reservations already made in advance, small amount of purchase to be made, etc.) to not have much time to waste. The evidence of the next loss of time is clearly attributable to the person who is about to be served.

The subjective of the person is focused on sheet of paper held in hand nervously. The perception of an "hostile" atmosphere does the person tend to hide the paper in his pocket, trying not to reveal the difficulties in making the purchase without the use of a memorandum. Some bystanders share an ill-considered moment of laughter. The atmosphere, however, is of nervous haste and little inclination to patience. As if this kind of episode was renewed every day.

The person is invited to make his order. Keeping the ticket hidden in the pocket, the person tries hesitantly to remember the written sequence, confusing types and quantities, omitting some things that are replaced with others in an attempt not to make others aware of the difficulty of memory. The order even if not quite, however, seems plausible to the person and bystanders. Even if, the bread seller kindly explains to him that they do not sell olive oil in this store but can find it in the fruit and vegetable shop across the street. The person says he has already planned to go to the greengrocer soon after.

The person prepares to pay by clumsily looking for the wallet in his pockets and dropping some things (scattered banknotes, small coins, some cards, including one with his own name and surname with emergency phone number written on it, that the person hides quickly from the view of the bystanders) while the bag is already ready its shopping bag.

While the person is about to pay something confuses the person who gives salesmen a 50 cents coin, solicits the rest and tries to quickly "take away" the bag with the goods purchased in an attempt to get out from that situation as soon as possible because it is developing anxiety on him. It is pointed out by the sales clerk that the amount is not sufficient to purchase, so the person replaces the 50 cents coin with 50 euro. While the salesman goes into the back of the shop to get the change, the person takes his bag and leaves, without realizing that he has not taken the change.

At the Greengrocer

Day interior. The person is greeted with a kind indifference. The other customer now in the shop does not seem to know the person at all. Both have a basket in hand to be filled between the boxes of fruit and vegetables present in the store. Items are placed in an order that only the merchant seems to understand. Everything is very confusing. Furthermore, the shopkeeper does not seem willing to help customers as he is distracted by the continuous ringing of cell phones for home orders.

The person therefore consults his shopping list and prepares to fill the basket where he replaces ginger in enormous quantities, mistaking it for potatoes and mixing zucchini and cucumbers thinking that they are the same vegetable. She/he delivers the basket to the shopkeeper to be weighed. While this operation is carried out with a small conversation the baker enters breathlessly in the shop waving the forgotten change just before.

The person at the beginning refuses this money and then thanks him surprised almost this money was a gift that someone is doing to him. The baker also reminds him that he was just looking for olive oil in the bakery that is available for sale right here. The person purchases it without much conviction.

Meanwhile, the other customer has placed his basket on the counter to wait for it to be weighed. The person observes it and potatoes contained in the basket are "taken furtively" and placed in their bag without the greengrocer nor the customer noticing, while the rest of the basket is clumsily thrown to the ground. The other customer is irritated, she would like to leave the store quickly. The person appears to be mortified and tries to convince the shopkeeper to accept a sum of money which seems to him to be suitable for the compensation of the damage but is not. The shopkeeper does not accept the money and urges him to go home.

After having noticed the loss of the person on this point, the shopkeeper proposes to the person to have the shopping at home and ask about any address she/he can have written in the pocket. In that way the phone number for emergencies was found. Thus, he calls the family member and agreeing with the latter the exact address where to meet.

Wandering in an Unknown Place

Exterior late night/early morning. Subjective of a person who is waking up approximately at 5 AM. The person exit home without being accompanied by a caregiver and she/he takes a bicycle. She/he is wandering while the city starts the daily activity (e.g. garbage truck working, people going by car). Time passes and becomes full day. The person reaches an isolated place and sits near the sea water edge as she/he is waiting for something.

After some time, a couple of adults is reaching the same place. They look at the person with some interest and, after a small discussion, the woman is approaching the seated person asking her/him if any help is eventually needed.

The person answers everything is ok and to be only waiting for a boat that will take her/him back to Milano. Considering the person as confused and disoriented the couple decided to friendly engage with the person a small conversation in order to understand if they could be helpful in accompanying the person at home. After a few exchanges the man ask to the person if she/he had some ticket in the pocket to catch the boat and if he can check it. Luckily the person shows a ticket with a name and a telephone number written on, thus the couple can reach the person's relatives providing them with the exact place in which they find the person waiting for a boat. After the phone call the couple goes away, leaving the person alone. The person continues to dangerously approach the seawater. Time is passing, the evening is arriving, no one is coming to take the person home.

At the Restaurant

Exterior night. Subjective of a person entering a restaurant accompanied by someone who could be a spouse. The restaurant is full of people, there is a lot of confusion:

chatter, background music, waiters who go fast between the tables, children playing at the entrance. The person hesitates, the spouse solicits entry.

They enter the room in search of known faces. They seem to arouse the curiosity of many. The person does not recognize any known face even if some greeted them as embarrassed or hastily. Having to untangle in such confusion causes in the person the desire to leave the restaurant immediately, also because the table is not positioned in the manner in which the person expected it to be. All this is immediately communicated to the spouse in an obsessive manner.

Meanwhile, the guests (all of the same age, therefore supposedly friends) are positioning themselves at the table (some undecided moving several times, even leaving occupied more places with bags and jackets that are constantly repositioned) and some of them get up to give the welcome to the person and his spouse who are coming. In "shuffling" the seats at the table the only disagreeing diner is sitting in front of the person. The dislike is overtly expressed by the person. Someone laughs, someone fears the worst.

Finally, everyone sits, and the waiter arrives. He speaks very quickly, often interrupting himself to respond to the jokes of the guests. The person grabs the menu, but the list of dishes graphically appears illegible and the noise continually distracts her/him from reading. She/he order quickly to not show its difficulty, repeating two different main courses and a dessert. This kind of uncommon request irritates the spouse and once again urges the sarcasm of the unsympathetic.

Everything proceeds quite well (even if for the person the music seems to have variations of volume and the conversation at times appears as non-sense) until the ordered dishes arrive. The person starts to eat spaghetti trying to roll them with a knife. Being unable in doing that, she/he reduces spaghetti into small pieces in order to take them with the dessert spoon. The spouse realizes the embarrassment arousing in diners and can't hold back a frustration reaction that make her radically rethink the possibility of having an adequate social life that includes also the person with dementia (e.g. "You were right: it had been better to stay home!").

3.2 Changing Social Perspective on Dementia: Preliminary Results

As explained before, the experiences proposed by ViveDe are easily experimented through a new generation smartphone by using a virtual reality cardboard. For this reason, following a series of public interventions aimed at discussing about Dementia Friendly behaviors with the population of the Lombardy area (in northern Italy) the scenarios described below were proposed to the general public during the last year. According with the end user target we had to work with in supporting the creation of a Dementia Friendly community, not all the scenarios were proposed every time. Instead, different scenarios were selected according to the social role and the activity perspective each group of community members can have on dementia and people living with it. Thus, for general public and high-school students, who were supposed to be people with dementia neighbors or family members, the "at home" scenario and/or the "going out" ones were proposed, while for people involved in commercial activities the "restaurant" and/or the "have shopping" were considered as more appropriate.

Within the several different supervision request on how to become Dementia Friendly requested to our research group from different urban communities a specific research on the effectiveness of ViveDe was planned in a II degree secondary school. As the main goal was to use the first-person experience provided by ViveDe 360° scenarios in supporting the understanding of perspective people living with dementia have in daily activity, perspective changes in end users after the ViveDe experience have to be measurable. Thus, before and after the immersive sessions, a questionnaire about the social perspective participants have on people living with dementia was proposed. The questionnaire is composed by 6 items through which every participant can answer on a five-point Likert's scale. Items are about the need for people with dementia to always be supported in everyday life, to be exclusively helped by family members, to have the urge in reaching health-care facilities and so on. Moreover, participants were asked about the awareness of having a key role as community member (both in their individual and professional roles) in supporting people with dementia autonomous living. At last, on the basis of the questionnaire answers provided, participants were involved in a 1-h debriefing session for discussing their opinion, comments, feelings, suggestion about how to be like a dementia person have created a better Dementia Friendly behavior in their personal and professional daily activity.

Data were collected on 74 participants (Female 38/Male 36) aged from 14 to 17 years old (Mean 15,31; Sd 0,97) attending a secondary school in northern Italy. The scenario proposed were the "Daily shopping" and "Wandering in a unknown place" ones. A paired-samples t-test was conducted to compare questionnaire answers. As summarized in Table 1 and depicted in Fig. 1, there were significant differences in answers provided pre and post ViveDe experiences.

Table 1. Means (standard deviation) and significance values for paired sample t Test on agreement/disagreement answers provided by participants before and after ViveDe experiences.

Item	Student's T	Significance	Mean (sd) Pre ViveDe	Mean (sd) Post ViveDe
Q1	T (73) = 7.1	P = .001	3.88 (0.92)	2.85 (0.97)
Q2	T (73) = 10.20	P = .001	2.09 (0.88)	3.39 (0.90)
Q3	T (73) = 3.70	P = .001	2.86 (0.73)	2.36 (0.97)
Q4	T (73) = 6.20	P = .001	3.78 (1.06)	2.73 (0.94)
Q5	T (73) = 12.40	P = .001	4.01 (0.96)	2.09 (0.86)
Q6	T (73) = 12.20	P = .001	2.16 (0.83)	3.96 (1.05)

These results show that ViveDe experience really does have an influence in changing social perspective about dementia people rights/needs and also on the role that each member of the community can have in creating a more inclusive behavior. Specifically, results suggest that when individuals were exposed to a first-person perspective on how could be living with dementia and having to face everyday challenges the idea of not being engaged in a possible relationship with them if not personally involved in a personal or professional way dramatically changes.

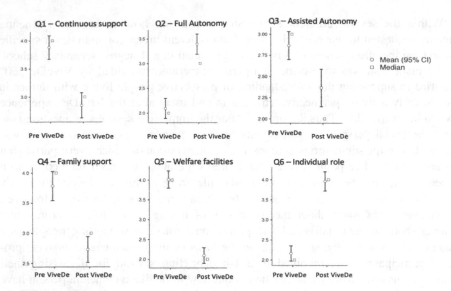

Fig. 1. Differences between pre and post ViveDe experiences for each questionnarire items

4 Conclusions

After the ViveDe experience many individuals have had the opportunity to discuss what it means to live daily with dementia. The reactions were multiple. It immediately emerged that it is difficult to define a person in dementia. What remains of the person when the rationality is intermittent? When the reasoning is fallacious, and exposes us to risks in the management of our assets or relationships? When the form of abstract and evolved reasoning is externally defined as a delirium or a hallucination? All these questions began to be answered after the experience in ViveDe.

Moreover, the question the pathology poses to the individuals has therefore become a question for the whole community: How to remains loving children, good neighbors or competent managers of a commercial exercise, even in front of a person with dementia who wants to continue living his daily life autonomously? Mainly because continuing to be people in dementia has risked the "ability to assemble and maintain relationships". Therefore, trying to create relationships for individuals meant to understand and identify, not only with the disease, but also with the interests, desires and needs of the person with dementia.

The debriefings conducted with the people who have benefited from the experiences proposed by ViveDe have finally shown many surprising elements. First of all, the feeling of being unexpectedly involved in some uncomfortable experience, that the individuals may not think is concerning to them. The surprise of understanding how to be able to include the other, who had always been perceived as totally incapable or different before the ViveDe experience. The surprise of being able to play a fundamental role in including the unexpected in our daily practices. Finally, the surprise of having discovered potentially a little more Dementia Friendly or the surprise of willing to be in the next future.

The most radically surprising change, however, was the one made on mistrust. The fear of the other person who is different from us, but who has something that could concern us closely is, at the beginning of the experience, very present in individuals who had the ViveDe experience. In particular there were a mistrust in having to manage a situation that individuals know they could never have full government on. In addition, there were a mistrust in matching themselves with the ability to truly be able to do own's part in making the community really inclusive for people with dementia. Both these mistrusts were surprisingly won after experiencing ViveDe. Some behaviors, that were not considered useful, become essential. They appear to distrust the falls and people find themselves as Dementia Friendly.

Finally, community members generally experienced indifference regarding dementia that allowed them to say: "it's not me having to deal with this!". It leads individuals to delegating and to feel safe from any implication with the disease, if the latter does not really concern us closely. The possibility of experiencing the role of a person with dementia provided by ViveDe scenarios appeared also to modify this attitude. Accordingly, in the next future ViveDe will want to push on the possibility to reduce indifference and therefore it intends to continue to invite all members of the community to win the initial surprising mistrust even when this is persistently present. Only in this way will it be possible to create small Dementia Friendly communities even in contexts that can be defined as uninterested in inclusive culture.

In conclusion, the idea of using 360° videos regarding the daily life of people with dementia provided by ViveDe, has never had the ambition to provide universally repeatable solutions in order to build Dementia Friendly communities starting from effective action plans in any specific context. On the contrary, it plans to present experiential paths that led to choose a first-person privileged perspective for the observation of what it means to live with dementia in specific contexts. For every member of an urban community this will mean to have an opportunity to reflect on how to weigh up own's action choices, in order to choose the most practicable ones for the introduction of inclusive behaviors.

It will certainly not be possible to monitor the path that members of a future Dementia Friendly community have begun to undertake after the ViveDe experience, but this experience can be considered as warranting a smoother step towards the goal. It was started by allowing community members to have a moment of reflexivity on their experience, in order to have the possibility to understand the necessary change and to make it last in time. These were the first seeds of Dementia Friendly culture to be planted, and only the time passing will tell us if they have really paid off. For how concerns the present time, the wish is to have been able to give an example of how to convey more inclusive perspective change in a field in which a social perspective changing is, not only possible, but also strongly necessary.

Acknowledgement. I would fully thank, once again, Giuseppe Riva who, without imposing me a rework, always stimulates new challenges in my research pathways.

References

1. Prince, M., Comas-Herrera, A., Knapp, M., Guerchet, M., Karagiannidou, M.: World Alzheimer Report 2016. Alzheimer Disease International, London (2016)
2. Lucca, et al.: Prevalence of dementia in the oldest old: the monzino 80-plus population based study. Alzheimer Dement. **11**, 258–270 (2015)
3. Drachman, D.A.: If we live long enough, will we all be demented? Neurology **44**, 1563–1565 (1994)
4. Khachaturian, Z.: Toward a comprehensive theory of Alzheimer's disease: challenges, caveats, and parameters. Ann. N. Y. Acad. Sci. **924**, 184–194 (2000)
5. Kitwood, T.: Dementia Reconsidered: The person comes First. Open University Press, Buckingham and Philadelphia (1997)
6. American Psychiatric Association.: Diagnostic and statistical manual of mental disoders (5ª ed.), Author, Washington, DC (2013)
7. Hilman, J.: La forza del carattere. Adelphi, Milano (2000)
8. Wolverson, E.L., Clarke, C., Moniz-Cook, E.D.: Living positively with dementia: a systematic review and synthesis of the qualitative literature. Aging Ment. Health **20**(7), 676–699 (2016)
9. Patterson, K., Clarke, C., Wolverson, E., Moniz-Cook, E.: Through the eyes of others – the social experiences of people with dementia: a systematic literature review and synthesis. Int. Psychogeriatr. **30**, 791–805 (2018)
10. Førsund, L.H., Grov, E.K., Helvik, A.S., Juvet, L.K., Skovdah, K., Eriksen, S.: The experience of lived space in persons with dementia: a systematic meta-synthesis. BMC Geriatr. **18**, 33 (2018)
11. Morganti, F.: Le comunità Dementia Friendly: Verso l'inclusione delle persone con demenza. Franco Angeli, Milano (2018)
12. Alzheimer's Disease International.: Dementia Friendly Communities (DFCs): New domains and global examples (2015). www.alz.co.uk/adi/pdf/dementia-friendly-communities.pdf
13. Dementia Friendly America.: Dementia Friendly America (2016). www.dfamerica.org/sector-guides-1
14. Alzheimer's Australia Dementia Friendly.: Creating Dementia-Friendly a Communities: Community toolkit (2016). https://act.fightdementia.org.au/files/Community_toolkit.pdf
15. Bronfenbrenner, U.: Rendere umani gli esseri umani. Bioecologia dello sviluppo. Erickson, Trento (2010)
16. Shin, D.: Empathy and embodied experience in virtual environment: to what extent can virtual reality stimulate empathy and embodied experience? Comput. Hum. Behav. **78**, 64–73 (2017)
17. Riva, G., Mantovani, F., Capideville, C.S., Preziosa, A., Morganti, F., Villani, D.: Affective interactions using virtual reality: the link between presence and emotions. Cyberpsychol. Behav. **10**, 45–56 (2007)
18. Morganti, F.: Embodied space in natural and virtual environments: implications for cognitive neuroscience research. Commun. Comput. Inf. Sci. **604**, 110–119 (2016)
19. Bachen, C.M., Hernández-Ramos, P.F., Raphael, C., Waldron, A.: How do presence, flow, and character identification affect players' empathy and interest in learning from a serious computer game? Comput. Hum. Behav. **64**, 77–87 (2016)
20. Graham, C., Rouncefield, M., Gibbs, M., Vetere, F., Cheverst, K.: How probes work. In: OZCHI 2007 Proceedings of the 19th Australasian Conference on Computer-Human Interaction: Entertaining User Interfaces, pp. 29–37 (2007)

Psychological Correlates of Interoceptive Perception in Healthy Population

Daniele Di Lernia[1(✉)], Silvia Serino[2], and Giuseppe Riva[1,3]

[1] Department of Psychology, Università Cattolica del Sacro Cuore,
Largo Gemelli, 1, 20100 Milan, Italy
{daniele.dilernia, giuseppe.riva}@unicatt.it
[2] MySpace Lab, Department of Clinical Neurosciences University Hospital
Lausanne (CHUV), Lausanne, Switzerland
[3] Applied Technology for Neuro-Psychology Lab,
IRCCS Istituto Auxologico Italiano, Via Magnasco, 2, 20149 Milan, Italy
g.riva@auxologico.it

Abstract. Investigating awareness of internal state of the body (i.e. interoception) is a promising field in the neuroscience domain. Evidence indicated interoceptive alterations in a wide variety of conditions. However, among literature, there is a consistent lack of information regarding the psychological correlates of interoceptive awareness (IA) in healthy population.
Methods: 54 subjects performed a complete interoceptive assessment for accuracy (IAc), metacognitive awareness (IAw), and sensibility (IAs) measured through M.A.I.A questionnaire. Subjects also performed psychological assessment for depression (BDI), anxiety (BAI), state and trait anxiety (STAI), and eating disorders (EDI-3) risks. **Results**: IAc and IAw positively correlated across the whole sample and IAw strongly positively correlated with several MAIA subscales. Significant negative correlations were also found with state anxiety and depressive symptoms. Female subjects exhibited a different interoceptive pattern with a negative relationship between IAc and BMI, and IAw and state anxiety. Conversely, male subjects exhibited a positive relationship between IAw and BMI, and IAc and Age, while IAw showed a negative relationship with state anxiety and depression. **Conclusions**: Perception of internal state of the body and relative metacognitive awareness appeared only partially connected. Different interoceptive patterns between male and female subjects appeared primarily related to specific body perceptions rather than gender differences. Considering the relationship between interoception and wellbeing, knowledge regarding how interoceptive processes work could help develop tailored technological interventions that utilize interoceptive treatments and multisensory stimulation to enhance human well-been through technology.

Keywords: Interoception · Interoceptive awareness · Emotions ·
Interoceptive technology · Interoceptive stimulation · Interoceptive treatments

© ICST Institute for Computer Sciences, Social Informatics and Telecommunications Engineering 2019
Published by Springer Nature Switzerland AG 2019. All Rights Reserved
P. Cipresso et al. (Eds.): MindCare 2019, LNICST 288, pp. 71–82, 2019.
https://doi.org/10.1007/978-3-030-25872-6_6

1 Introduction

Our body represents the focal lens that allows us to perceive the world. We live, explore, and relate to others through our body and its perceptions. Furthermore, the way we process and integrate perceptions coming from the body defines who we are, our self, and – ultimately – our wellbeing [1–4]. Several authors explored the relationship between the perception of the body and the human well-being, and these efforts resonated with different scientific solutions aimed at enhancing healthy bodily processing through the new field of embodied technology. From this perspective, embodied technology represents a new outlook focused upon the possibility to use technology to stimulate bodily perceptions with the ultimate goal of promoting a balanced autonomic functioning both in healthy both in clinical populations [2, 5, 6].

Traditionally, the study of body perception has always been related to proprioceptive signals, nonetheless in the last two decades neuro-scientific evidence brought light to a brand new concept of interoceptive perceptions. Interoception, defined as the psychological sense of the entire organism [7], reshaped several domains of science bringing a new perspective to several fields from psychology to cognitive sciences to neuroscience. Nonetheless, to properly explore technological solutions applied to the interoceptive domain, more data need to be collected especially regarding behavioural interoceptive functioning in healthy population.

Interoception can be explored on different axes. The most accepted framework has been proposed by Garfinkel, Seth, Barrett, Suzuki and Critchley [8] and described three interoceptive axes: interoceptive accuracy (IAc) i.e. subject's ability to correctly perceive his own body, metacognitive awareness (IAw) i.e. subject's confidence in the accuracy evaluation, and sensibility (IAs) i.e. subject's cognitive evaluation of his bodily perceptions. These axes have been explored in different contexts, with a main focus upon accuracy alterations in different clinical [9] and non-clinical conditions, nonetheless across literature there is a consistent lack of information regarding psychological correlates (e.g. mood both in trait both in state conditions, body-related psychological processes and beliefs) of interoception in healthy samples. This gap not only creates an area of unidentified knowledge but it also interferes with the ability to correctly elaborate interoceptive information in other contexts. Beginning to address this issue and moving toward a more complex knowledge about interoceptive processes, the study explored psychological correlates of interoception in healthy population.

In healthy subjects, we hypothesize a positive correlation between IAc and IAw. According to literature [10], we also hypothesize a positive relationship between anxiety and IAc and a negative relationship between depressive symptoms and IAc [11]. Considering evidence related to eating disorder [12] we also hypothesize a negative relationship between interoceptive accuracy and EDI-3 risk subscales.

2 Methods

2.1 Participants

Sample size calculation based on previous studies [8, 10, 13] indicate a total sample size of fifty-six subjects [$\rho^2 = 0.3$, α err prob. = 0.05, power = .95]. Fifty-six subjects were recruited at the Catholic University of the Sacred Heart of Milan, campus of Psychology. Data for two subjects were not collected due to ECG technical issues. Fifty-four subjects [18.5% male] were included into the study. Exclusion criteria were the presence of current psychological or physical diagnoses. Subjects received instruction to avoid medications in the 12 h before the meeting. Similar instruction was given for nicotine and caffeine, and subjects were asked to avoid them in the 2 h before the experiment. All subjects gave written informed consent in accordance with the Declaration of Helsinki (2008). The protocol was approved by the Ethics Committee of Catholic University of Sacred Heart of Milan.

2.2 Procedure

Subjects were accommodated in a comfortable room and received information about the experiment. After information was given, they proceeded to sign written consent and took part to a brief anamnestic interview with a psychologist specialized in psychopathological and personality assessment. Following the interview they proceeded to compile a series of psychological questionnaires. After the questionnaires, subjects were connected to a portable ECG device with Ag/AgCl electrodes to perform the interoceptive tasks. At the end of the tasks, electrodes were removed and subjects were debriefed.

2.3 Psychological Assessment

Depressive mood alterations were assessed through the Beck Depression Inventory (BDI-II) [14] that is a 21 self-reported questionnaire able to discriminate different levels of depression. The instrument is among the most diffused and well validated whereas scores under 13 indicate normal mood variations, while scores above 14 are able to differentiate from mild, to moderate, to severe depressive status [15, 16].

Anxiety was assessed both in state and trait dimensions through the 40-items State Trait Anxiety Inventory (STAI) [17], whereas scores above 40 indicate clinical anxiety both in trait and status conditions. Due to known correlations between STAI and BDI [18] measures, anxiety was also assessed through the BAI [19], a specific scale that provides a trait-like measure of anxiety without overlapping constructs with the BDI. Risks for eating disorders were assessed through EDI-3 [20] risk subscales [21]. The EDI-3 questionnaire [20–22] is a specific instrument able to assess different eating related subclinical risks, through three specific subscales: Drive for Thinness (DT) is a subscale connected to behavioural and cognitive drives linked to anorexia nervosa tendencies. Bulimia (B) is a subscale that assess for bulimic tendencies, and Body Dissatisfaction (BD) is a scale that explores a generalized construct related to a diffuse dissatisfaction towards the body. The sum of the scores from these subscales composes a Global Risk Index (EDRC).

2.4   Interoceptive Measures

Interoception has been recently operationalized in three separate constructs: interoceptive accuracy, interoceptive metacognitive awareness, interoceptive sensibility [8]. Interoceptive Accuracy (IAc) was assessed through a well validated and wide utilized heart beat perception task, originally designed by Schandry [23]. Subjects were connected to a portable ECG unit sampling at 250 Hz [24–28] with Ag/AgCl electrodes and they were instructed to count their own heartbeats in specific intervals time intervals (25, 35, 45, and 100 s). Accuracy index was calculated according to: $1/4\sum$ $(1 - (|\text{recorded heartbeats} - \text{counted heartbeats}|)/\text{recorded heartbeats})$.

Interoceptive metacognitive awareness (IAw) is a response of confidence that assesses how much subjects considered their answers to the accuracy tasks correct. IAw is evaluated with a Visual Analogue Scale that ranges from "not confident at all" to "fully confident" according to Garfinkel, Seth, Barrett, Suzuki and Critchley [8].

Interoceptive sensibility was assessed through The Multidimensional Assessment of Interoceptive Awareness (MAIA) questionnaire [29]. The M.A.I.A. is a multidimensional 32 items questionnaire with 8 subscales. The M.A.I.A. is a multidimensional 32 items questionnaire with 8 subscales. The Noticing (NO) subscale expresses subject's awareness of uncomfortable, comfortable, and neutral body sensations. The Not-Distracting (ND) subscale expresses subject's tendency not to ignore or distract oneself from sensations of pain or discomfort. The Not-Worrying (NW) subscale expresses subject's tendency not to worry or experience emotional distress with sensations of pain or discomfort. The Attention Regulation (AR) subscale expresses subject's ability to sustain and control attention to body sensations. The Emotional Awareness (EA) subscale expresses subject's awareness of the connection between body sensations and emotional states. The Self-Regulation (SR) subscale expresses subject's ability to regulate distress by attention to body sensations. The Body Listening (BL) subscale expresses subject's ability to active listening to the body for insight. The Trusting (TR) subscale expresses subject's experience of one's body as safe and trustworthy. Responses are given on a 6 points likert scale, from 0 to 5. Each subscale score ranges from 0 to 5.

2.5   Statistical Analyses

Linear and non-linear correlational analyses were run for variables of main interest in the whole sample and across the different gender subsamples. Following literature suggestions [18] and results from previous studies [13] we also implemented different factors structures for BDI [15, 16], to identify cognitive and somatic (body related) depressive symptoms.

3   Results

3.1   Sample Psychological Characteristics and Psychological Measures

Total sample of N = 54 was comparable for age [mean = 25.74 years; SD = 6.38] and BMI [mean = 21.01; SD = 2.24] with other healthy sample in literature [8]. Sample showed moderate levels of anxiety [STAI_T mean = 42.63, SD = 9.81; STAI_S mean = 34.18, SD = 7.77; BAI mean = 10.88, SD = 7.55] and depressive symptoms [mean = 8.72; SD = 6.72]. EDI-3 subscales indicated a generalized high Global risk index [EDRC mean = 22.5; SD = 7.9] and Body Dissatisfaction [BD mean = 11.70; SD = 8.84], a moderate Drive for thinness [DT mean = 7.66; SD = 7.89] and a low Bulimia risks [B mean = 3.09; SD = 3.37]. Results are summarized in Table 1.

Table 1. Psychological assessment scores

	N	Min	Max	Mean	SD
Age	54	19.0	48.0	25.74	6.38
BMI	54	17.26	28.71	21.012	2.24
BDI_tot	54	.0	37.0	8.72	6.72
BDI_cogn	54	.0	25.0	5.25	4.91
BDI_som	54	.0	12.0	3.46	2.42
STAI_T	54	25.0	64.0	42.63	9.81
STAI_S	54	21.0	62.0	34.18	7.77
BAI	54	.0	34.0	10.88	7.55
EDI_DT	54	.0	27.0	7.66	7.89
EDI_B	54	.0	13.0	3.09	3.37
EDI_BD	54	.0	32.0	11.70	8.84
EDI_EDRC	54	.0	67.0	22.46	17.13

BMI: body mass index, BDI_tot: BDI total score, BDI_cogn: BDI cognitive factors, BDI_som: BDI somatic factors, STAI_T: STAI trait anxiety, STAI_s: STAI state anxiety, BAI: Beck Anxiety Inventory, EDI_DT: EDI Drive for thinness subscale, EDI_B: Bulimia subscale, EDI_BD: Body Dissatisfaction subscale. EDI_EDRC: EDI Global Risk Index (EDRC).

Several significant correlations were found between psychometric variables. Results are summarized in Table 2.

Table 2. Correlation analyses for psychometric variables

	Age	BMI	BDI_tot	BDI_cogn	BDI_som	STAI_T	STAI_S	BAI	EDI_DT	EDI_B	EDI_BD
Age	1										
BMI	.463**	1									
BDI_tot	−.013	.083	1								
BDI_cogn	−.027	.074	.961**	1							
BDI_som	.019	.079	.828**	.641**	1						
STAI_T	−.167	.137	.495**	.486**	.390**	1					
STAI_S	.185	.303*	.375**	.385**	.260	.337*	1				
BAI	−.312*	−.032	.360**	.343*	.306*	.361**	.084	1			
EDI_DT	−.122	.141	.165	.172	.109	.295*	−.037	.193	1		
EDI_B	.057	.353**	.497**	.435**	.497**	.553**	.339*	.249	.387**	1	
EDI_BD	−.069	.164	.341*	.347*	.244	.483**	.214	.289*	.615**	.589**	1
EDI_EDRC	−.081	.219	.350**	.344*	.274*	.494**	.160	.287*	.855**	.680**	.916**

**Correlation is significant at level 0.01 (two tails). *Correlation is significant at level 0.05 (two tails). BMI: body mass index, BDI_tot: BDI total score, BDI_cogn: BDI cognitive factors, BDI_som: BDI somatic factors, STAI_T: STAI trait anxiety, STAI_s: STAI state anxiety, BAI: Beck Anxiety Inventory, EDI_DT: EDI Drive for thinness subscale, EDI_B: Bulimia subscale, EDI_BD: Body Dissatisfaction subscale. EDI_EDRC: EDI Global Risk Index (EDRC).

3.2 Interoceptive Accuracy, Metacognitive Awareness, Sensibility

Total sample interoceptive accuracy mean score was 0.54 [SD = 0.22] while interoceptive metacognitive awareness mean score was 43.68 [SD = 20.88]. M.A.I.A. scores are reported in Table 3 and correlations in Table 4.

Table 3. MAIA subscales scores

Scale	Min	Max	Mean	SD
NO	1.00	4.75	3.07	.91
ND	1.33	4.00	2.39	.66
NW	.00	5.0	2.50	1.25
AR	.43	4.57	2.69	.97
EA	1.0	4.8	3.17	.88
SR	.00	5.00	2.37	1.18
BL	.00	4.66	2.49	1.17
TR	.33	5.00	3.16	1.16

NO: Noticing subscale, ND: Not Distracting subscale, NW: Not Worrying subscale, AR: Attention Regulation subscale, EA: Emotional Awareness subscale, SR: Self-Regulation subscale, BL: Body Listening subscale, TR: Trusting subscale.

Table 4. Correlation analyses for interoceptive variables

	IAc	IAw	MAIA_NO	MAIA_ND	MAIA_NW	MAIA_AR	MAIA_EA	MAIA_SR	MAIA_BL
IAc	1								
IAw	.406**	1							
MAIA_NO	.152	.371**	1						
MAIA_ND	.202	.272*	.186	1					
MAIA_NW	−.137	.176	.154	−.240	1				
MAIA_AR	.248	.453**	.579**	.137	.348**	1			
MAIA_EA	.165	.591**	.534**	.252	.280*	.426**	1		
MAIA_SR	.225	.463**	.550**	.086	.382**	.580**	.583**	1	
MAIA_BL	.134	.563**	.501**	.133	.214	.674**	.575**	.641**	1
MAIA_TR	.244	.372**	.419**	.163	.385**	.527**	.500**	.600**	.555**

**Correlation is significant at level 0.01 (two tails). *Correlation is significant at level 0.05 (two tails). IAc: interoceptive accuracy, IAw: interoceptive metacognitive awareness, MAIA_NO: Noticing subscale, MAIA_ND: Not Distracting subscale, MAIA_NW: Not Worrying subscale, MAIA_AR: Attention Regulation subscale, MAIA_EA: Emotional Awareness subscale, MAIA_SR: Self-Regulation subscale, MAIA_BL: Body Listening subscale, MAIA_TR: Trusting subscale.

IAc positively correlated with IAw [r = .406; p = .002], and IAw positively correlated with several MAIA subscales including Noticing [r = .371; p = .006], Not Distracting [r = .272; p = .046], Attention Regulation [r = .453; p = .001], Emotional Awareness [r = .591; p < .001], Self-Regulation [r = .463; p < .001], Body Listening [r = .563; p < .001], and Trusting [r = .372; p = .006].

3.3 Relationship Between Measures and Gender

Several significant correlations were found between MAIA subscales and different psychometric variables [Table 5].

Table 5. Correlation analyses between MAIA subscales and psychometric variables

	BDI_tot	BDI_cogn	BDI_som	STAI_T	STAI_S	BAI	EDI_DT	EDI_B	EDI_BD	EDI_EDRC
MAIA_NO	−.077	−.082	−.049	−.106	−.236	.257	−.170	−.237	−.292*	−.276*
MAIA_ND	−.237	−.218	−.216	−.228	−.167	−.098	−.009	−.195	−.095	−.092
MAIA_NW	−.086	−.125	.016	−.187	−.116	−.173	−.139	.011	−.182	−.156
MAIA_AR	−.015	−.049	.058	−.123	−.267	.095	−.191	−.173	−.492**	−.376**
MAIA_EA	−.058	−.030	−.100	−.241	−.281*	.149	.053	−.231	−.255	−.153
MAIA_SR	−.290*	−.302*	−.193	−.496**	−.447**	−.072	−.161	−.448**	−.421**	−.380**
MAIA_BL	−.075	−.047	−.114	−.278*	−.312*	.054	−.155	−.188	−.368**	−.298*
MAIA_TR	−.050	−.076	.016	−.550**	−.230	−.019	−.405**	−.279*	−.603**	−.552**

**Correlation is significant at level 0.01 (two tails). *Correlation is significant at level 0.05 (two tails). MAIA_NO: Noticing subscale, MAIA_ND: Not Distracting subscale, MAIA_NW: Not Worrying subscale, MAIA_AR: Attention Regulation subscale, MAIA_EA: Emotional Awareness subscale, MAIA_SR: Self-Regulation subscale, MAIA_BL: Body Listening subscale, MAIA_TR: Trusting subscale. BMI: body mass index, BDI_tot: BDI total score, BDI_cogn: BDI cognitive factors, BDI_som: BDI somatic factors, STAI_T: STAI trait anxiety, STAI_s: STAI state anxiety, BAI: Beck Anxiety Inventory, EDI_DT: EDI Drive for thinness subscale, EDI_B: Bulimia subscale, EDI_BD: Body Dissatisfaction subscale. EDI_EDRC: EDI Global Risk Index (EDRC).

Correlations between interoceptive variables remained significant when splitting for gender, nonetheless some interesting results emerged in the female group [Fig. 1] that showed a negative correlation between IAw and BMI [r = −.297; p = .050] and a negative correlation between IAc and state anxiety (STAI) [r = −.319; p = .035].

	Age	BMI	IAc	IAw	BDI_tot	BDI_cogn	BDI_som	STAI_T	STAI_S	BAI	EDI_DT	EDI_B	EDI_BD	EDI_EDRC
Age		0,45	X	X	X	X	X	X	0,34	X	X	X	X	X
BMI	0,45		X	-0,29	X	X	X	0,35	0,45	X	0,30	0,49	0,37	0,43
IAc	X	X		0,43	X	X	X	X	-0,32	X	X	X	X	X
IAw	X	-0,29	0,43		X	X	X	X	X	X	X	X	X	X
BDI_tot	X	X	X	X		0,94	0,77	0,68	X	0,45	X	0,60	0,37	0,40
BDI_cogn	X	X	X	X	0,94		0,51	0,65	X	0,43	X	0,49	0,36	0,36
BDI_som	X	X	X	X	0,77	0,51		0,50	X	0,33	X	0,60	X	0,33
STAI_T	X	0,35	X	X	0,68	0,65	0,50		0,41	0,33	X	0,57	0,51	0,49
STAI_S	0,34	0,45	-0,32	X	X	X	X	0,41		X	X	X	X	X
BAI	X	X	X	X	0,45	0,43	0,33	0,33	X		X	0,30	X	X
EDI_DT	X	0,30	X	X	X	X	X	X	X	X		0,39	0,58	0,84
EDI_B	X	0,49	X	X	0,60	0,49	0,60	0,57	X	0,30	0,39		0,63	0,71
EDI_BD	X	0,37	X	X	0,37	0,36	X	0,51	X	X	0,58	0,63		0,91
EDI_EDRC	X	0,43	X	X	0,40	0,36	0,33	0,49	X	X	0,84	0,71	0,91	

Fig. 1. Correlation table for the female subsample. If r value is present, correlation is significant at level 0.05 (two tails). BMI: body mass index, IAc: interoceptive accuracy, IAw: interoceptive metacognitive awareness, BDI_tot: BDI total score, BDI_cogn: BDI cognitive factors, BDI_som: BDI somatic factors, STAI_T: STAI trait anxiety, STAI_s: STAI state anxiety, BAI: Beck Anxiety Inventory, EDI_DT: EDI Drive for thinness subscale, EDI_B: Bulimia subscale, EDI_BD: Body Dissatisfaction subscale. EDI_EDRC: EDI Global Risk Index (EDRC).

Correlation between IAc and IAw remained strong [r = .433; p = .003]. Conversely, male subjects exhibited different interoceptive patterns whereas strong significant positive correlations were found between IAw and BMI [r = .680; p = .030] and IAw and Age [r = .712; p = .021] in an opposite direction than female subjects. Moreover, in male sample no significant correlation was found between IAc and IAw [r = .478; p = .162] while significant negative correlations were found for IAw and somatic symptoms of depression [r = −.678; p = .031] and IAw and trait anxiety on both STAI [r = −.739; p = .015] and BAI [r = −.716; p = .020] (Fig. 2).

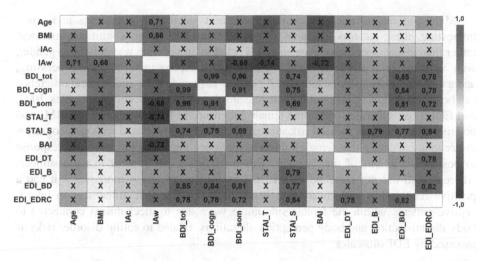

Fig. 2. Correlation table for the male subsample. If r value is present, correlation is significant at level 0.05 (two tails). BMI: body mass index, IAc: interoceptive accuracy, IAw: interoceptive metacognitive awareness, BDI_tot: BDI total score, BDI_cogn: BDI cognitive factors, BDI_som: BDI somatic factors, STAI_T: STAI trait anxiety, STAI_s: STAI state anxiety, BAI: Beck Anxiety Inventory, EDI_DT: EDI Drive for thinness subscale, EDI_B: Bulimia subscale, EDI_BD: Body Dissatisfaction subscale. EDI_EDRC: EDI Global Risk Index (EDRC).

4 Discussion

The study analyzed psychological correlates of interoceptive perception in healthy sample population. As hypothesized a significant positive relationship was found between interoceptive accuracy and metacognitive awareness. Nonetheless, it is worth noticing that this relationship was weak, suggesting that the two constructs have a high degree of separation. Across the whole sample, interoceptive accuracy acted as a partially independent factor with weak connections with psychological correlates measured through self-reported instruments.

Albeit interoceptive accuracy showed weak connections with psychological correlates, metacognitive awareness appeared to be strongly related to psychological factors and to MAIA subscales. As a matter of fact, interoceptive sensibility subscales showed strong positive relationships with metacognitive awareness, suggesting a possible congruency of constructs, especially for MAIA Emotional Awareness subscale. From this perspective, metacognitive awareness showed a high sensitivity to psychological correlates of emotions. Negative relationships were found with anxiety and depressive symptoms, confirming respectively previous results for accuracy and supporting previous evidence from literature [10, 11, 18].

Interoceptive sensitivity measured via MAIA subscales appeared strongly connected to psychological correlates of emotions. Specifically, Self-Regulation (SR) scale, whose score indicates subject's ability to regulate distress by attention to body sensations, was the most sensitive to emotion and mood alterations due to strong negative relationships with all anxiety and depression measures.

Male and female subjects exhibited different interoceptive patterns and, quite interesting, these patterns appeared related to body perception cognitive processes, rather than gender specificity. Age and BMI acted in an opposite way related to gender, with a positive relationship in males regarding interoceptive metacognitive processing, and a negative relationship in females. A possible explanation for such radical difference can be found analyzing in detail the relationships between interoceptive variables, BMI, and EDI-3 risk subscales within the female subgroup. In female subjects, the BMI was positive related with all the EDI risk subscales and negatively related with metacognitive awareness, indicating that female subjects experience negative perceptions in response to positive variations of their weight. This pattern was not present in male subjects whereas BMI did not correlate with EDI-3 risk subscales and – moreover – it had a positive relationship with awareness. It therefore possible that differences in interoceptive patterns within the female subsample were due to mechanisms connected to body dissatisfaction and body perception alterations, related to eating disorder risks as assessed by EDI subscales.

5 Conclusion and Technological Applications

Interoception represents an emerging field of study in the consciousness domain and understand how perception of bodily inputs works can lead to a brand new perspective regarding several pathological and non-pathological conditions. From this point of view, interoceptive technological devices able to stimulate and manipulate the perception of inner bodily sensations may provide new innovative solutions with several applications in clinical and non-clinical fields. Such interoceptive technological devices have already been developed [30, 31] and used for assessment purposes [13, 32]; nonetheless they can also be used to achieve different goals beyond psychological and psychopathological assessment. This kind of technology can be used in non-pathological contests to improve embodiment and body ownership [33], and it also can be used to enhance human well-being through manipulation of the parasympathetic and sympathetic autonomic system [30, 31]. Merging interoceptive stimulation devices with other technologies such as virtual reality (VR), vibration multisensory systems, and "positive technologies" [2, 3, 34, 35] can therefore offer new forms of treatment for clinical and subclinical conditions [9, 36, 37]. As a matter of fact,, considering the relation between interoceptive perception and well-being [2], the understanding of interoceptive integration processes can lead to new form of interventions that can show effectiveness in a broad range of clinical and non-clinical alterations.

6 Conflict of Interest Statement

The authors had no conflict of interest.

Acknowledgments. GR was funded by the MIUR PRIN research project "Unlocking the memory of the body: Virtual Reality in Anorexia Nervosa" (201597WTTM).

References

1. Riva, G.: The neuroscience of body memory: from the self through the space to the others. Cortex **104**, 241–260 (2017)
2. Riva, G., et al.: Embodied medicine: mens sana in corpore virtuale sano. Front. Hum. Neurosci. **11**, 120 (2017). https://doi.org/10.3389/fnhum.2017.00120
3. Riva, G., et al.: Positive and transformative technologies for active ageing. Stud. Health Technol. Inform. **220**, 308–315 (2016)
4. Riva, G.: The neuroscience of body memory: from the self through the space to the others. Cortex **104**, 241–260 (2018). https://doi.org/10.1016/j.cortex.2017.07.013
5. Critchley, H.D., Garfinkel, S.N.: Interactions between visceral afferent signaling and stimulus processing. Front. Neurosci. **9**, 286 (2015). https://doi.org/10.3389/fnins.2015.00286
6. Watson, D.R., et al.: Computerized exposure therapy for Spider Phobia: effects of cardiac timing and interoceptive ability on subjective and behavioral outcomes. Psychosom. Med. **81**, 90–99 (2018)
7. Craig, A.D.: Interoception: the sense of the physiological condition of the body. Curr. Opin. Neurobiol. **13**(4), 500–505 (2003). https://doi.org/10.1016/s0959-4388(03)00090-4
8. Garfinkel, S.N., et al.: Knowing your own heart: distinguishing interoceptive accuracy from interoceptive awareness. Biol. Psychol. **104**, 65–74 (2015). https://doi.org/10.1016/j.biopsycho.2014.11.004
9. Di Lernia, D., et al.: Pain in the body. Altered interoception in chronic pain conditions: a systematic review. Neurosci. Biobehav. Rev. 71, 328–341 (2016). https://doi.org/10.1016/j.neubiorev.2016.09.015
10. Pollatos, O., et al.: Differential effects of anxiety and depression on interoceptive accuracy. Depress. Anxiety **26**(2), 167–173 (2009). https://doi.org/10.1002/da.20504
11. Dunn, B.D., et al.: Heartbeat perception in depression. Behav. Res. Ther. **45**(8), 1921–1930 (2007). https://doi.org/10.1016/j.brat.2006.09.008
12. Pollatos, O., et al.: Reduced perception of bodily signals in anorexia nervosa. Eat. Behav. **9**(4), 381–388 (2008). https://doi.org/10.1016/j.eatbeh.2008.02.001
13. Di Lernia, D., et al.: Feel the time. Time perception as a function of interoceptive processing. Front. Hum, Neurosci. **12**(74) (2018). https://doi.org/10.3389/fnhum.2018.00074
14. Beck, A.T., et al.: An inventory for measuring depression. Arch. Gen. Psychiatry 4, 561–571 (1961)
15. Steer, R.A., et al.: Dimensions of the Beck Depression Inventory-II in clinically depressed outpatients. J. Clin. Psychol. **55**(1), 117–128 (1999)
16. Storch, E.A., et al.: Factor structure, concurrent validity, and internal consistency of the Beck Depression Inventory-Second Edition in a sample of college students. Depress. Anxiety **19**(3), 187–189 (2004). https://doi.org/10.1002/da.20002
17. Spielberger, C.D., et al.: Manual for the state-trait anxiety inventory (1970)
18. Dunn, B.D., et al.: Can you feel the beat? Interoceptive awareness is an interactive function of anxiety- and depression-specific symptom dimensions. Behav. Res. Ther. **48**(11), 1133–1138 (2010). https://doi.org/10.1016/j.brat.2010.07.006
19. Beck, A.T., et al.: An inventory for measuring clinical anxiety: psychometric properties. J. Consult. Clin. Psychol. **56**(6), 893 (1988)
20. Garner, D.M., et al.: Development and validation of a multidimensional eating disorder inventory for anorexia nervosa and bulimia. Int. J. Eat. Disord. **2**(2), 15–34 (1983)
21. Eshkevari, E., et al.: Increased plasticity of the bodily self in eating disorders. Psychol. Med. **42**(4), 819–828 (2012). https://doi.org/10.1017/S0033291711002091

22. Clausen, L., et al.: Validating the eating disorder inventory-3 (EDI-3): a comparison between 561 female eating disorders patients and 878 females from the general population. J. Psychopathol. Behav. Assess. **33**(1), 101–110 (2011). https://doi.org/10.1007/s10862-010-9207-4

23. Schandry, R.: Heart beat perception and emotional experience. Psychophysiology **18**(4), 483–488 (1981). https://doi.org/10.1111/j.1469-8986.1981.tb02486.x

24. Hugeng, H., Kurniawan, R.: Development of the 'healthcor'system as a cardiac disorders symptoms detector using an expert system based on Arduino UNO". Int. J. Technol. **7**(1), 78 (2016)

25. Ševčík, J., et al.: System for EKG monitoring. Int. J. Adv. Res. Artif. Intell. **4**(9) (2015)

26. Stojanović, R., et al.: Alternative approach to addressing infrastructure needs in biomedical engineering programs (case of emerging economies). Folia Medica Facultatis Medicinae Universitatis Saraeviensis **50**(1) (2015)

27. Villarrubia, G., et al.: EKG mobile. Adv. Sci. Technol. Lett. **49**, 95–100 (2014)

28. Villarrubia, G., De Paz, Juan F., Corchado, Juan M., Bajo, J.: EKG intelligent mobile system for home users. In: Bazzan, Ana L.C., Pichara, K. (eds.) IBERAMIA 2014. LNCS (LNAI), vol. 8864, pp. 767–778. Springer, Cham (2014). https://doi.org/10.1007/978-3-319-12027-0_62

29. Mehling, W.E., et al.: The multidimensional assessment of interoceptive awareness (MAIA). PLoS ONE **7**(11), e48230 (2012). https://doi.org/10.1371/journal.pone.0048230

30. Di Lernia, D., et al.: Toward an embodied medicine: a portable device with programmable interoceptive stimulation for heart rate variability enhancement. Sensors **18**(8) (2018). https://doi.org/10.3390/s18082469

31. Di Lernia, D., Riva, G., Cipresso, P.: iStim. A new portable device for interoceptive stimulation. In: Cipresso, P., Serino, S., Ostrovsky, Y., Baker, Justin T. (eds.) MindCare 2018. LNICST, vol. 253, pp. 42–49. Springer, Cham (2018). https://doi.org/10.1007/978-3-030-01093-5_6

32. Di Lernia, D., et al.: Interoceptive axes dissociation in anorexia nervosa: a single case study with follow up post-recovery assessment. Front. Psychol. **9**(2488) (2019). https://doi.org/10.3389/fpsyg.2018.02488

33. Crucianelli, L., et al.: Bodily pleasure matters: velocity of touch modulates body ownership during the rubber hand illusion. Front. Psychol. **4**, 703 (2013). https://doi.org/10.3389/fpsyg.2013.00703

34. Serino, S., et al.: The role of age on multisensory bodily experience: an experimental study with a virtual reality full-body illusion. Cyberpsychol. Behav. Soc. Netw. **21**(5), 304–310 (2018). https://doi.org/10.1089/cyber.2017.0674

35. Zanier, E.R., et al.: Virtual reality for traumatic brain injury. Front. Neurol. **9**(345) (2018). https://doi.org/10.3389/fneur.2018.00345

36. Castelnuovo, G., et al.: What is the role of the placebo effect for pain relief in neurorehabilitation? Clinical implications from the Italian Consensus Conference on pain in neurorehabilitation. Front. Neurol. **9**, 310 (2018)

37. Di Lernia, D., et al.: Ghosts in the machine. Interoceptive modeling for chronic pain treatment. Front. Neurosci. **10**, 314 (2016). https://doi.org/10.3389/fnins.2016.00314

Development of a Computational Platform to Support the Screening, Surveillance, Prevention and Detection of Suicidal Behaviours

Juan Martínez-Miranda[1,2]($\boxtimes$) (iD), Antonio Palacios-Isaac[3],
Fernando López-Flores[3], Ariadna Martínez[3], Héctor Aguilar[3],
Liliana Jiménez[3], Roberto Ramos[1], Giovanni Rosales[1], and Luis Altamirano[3]

[1] Centro de Investigación Científica y de Educación Superior de Ensenada,
Unidad de Transferencia Tecnológica Tepic - CICESE-UT3, Tepic, Nay., Mexico
{jmiranda,lramos,grosales}@cicese.mx
[2] Consejo Nacional de Ciencia y Tecnología - CONACyT, Mexico City, Mexico
[3] Servicios de Salud de Nayarit, Tepic, Nay., Mexico
clinicausame@hotmail.com, jferlf@hotmail.com, ariadna44@hotmail.com,
licnolilijima@hotmail.com

Abstract. The use of new technologies in the prevention and detection of suicidal behaviours have a strong potential to reach and offer immediate support to individuals at risk, their caregivers and in the long run to health care policymakers. In this paper, we describe the development of a computational platform to support suicide prevention activities through two main components. The first one is a Clinical Decision Support System developed to help specialists with the screening, treatment management, and the collection and analysis of suicide-related data for surveillance purposes. The second component of the platform is HelPath, a mobile-based application, addressed to individuals identified with suicidal behaviour (ideation, planning or attempt). HelPath offers support for the remote and continuous collection of data for the assessment of risk factors and offers suggestions and activities based on Cognitive Behaviour Therapy that can prevent to commit suicide. The main functionalities of each component are described emphasising how each of these functionalities impacts in the different key actions required to get an integral strategy for suicide prevention.

Keywords: Suicide prevention · Suicidal behaviours ·
Clinical decision support system · Embodied Conversational Agents

1 Introduction

According to some estimations of the World Health Organisation (WHO), over 800,000 people die every year around the world due to suicide [44]. The same

P. Cipresso et al. (Eds.): MindCare 2019, LNICST 288, pp. 83–101, 2019.
https://doi.org/10.1007/978-3-030-25872-6_7

WHO's report highlights that suicide is the second leading cause of death in the 15–29 years old population; it represents the 1.4% of all deaths worldwide, and it was the 17th leading cause of death during 2015. Moreover, there is also evidence that for each individual who commits suicide, there could be 20 others attempting it [35]. These facts reveal how important is to consider the prevention of suicide as a higher priority on the global public health agenda. Nevertheless, an effective prevention of suicide is a not easy task considering that this phenomenon results from a complex interaction of biological, genetic, psychological, sociological, cultural and environmental factors [41]. Although complex, suicide is preventable but it should include an integral strategy involving not only the health sector but also others such as education, employment, social welfare, and the judiciary, to name a few. Important resources are necessary to achieve both short-to-medium and long-term objectives, there should be an effective planning, and the applied strategy should be regularly evaluated to assess its results and identify improvements for the future [42].

In order to facilitate the implementation of different preventive strategies and the involvement of various sectors, there is necessary that national governments adopt a clear commitment to deal with this phenomenon. Currently, some countries have already implemented national prevention strategies such as surveillance, means restriction, media guidelines, stigma reduction and raising of public awareness, crisis intervention services, as well as training for health workers, educators, police and other gatekeepers [42]. Each strategy should be implemented through specific actions allowing the assessment of their effectiveness. In a recent systematic review, seven interventions were assessed to get an updated evidence for the effectiveness of suicide prevention: *(i)* public and *(ii)* physician education; *(iii)* media strategies; *(iv)* screening; *(v)* restricting access to suicide means; *(vi)* treatments; and *(vii)* internet or hot-line support [46]. The obtained results indicate that no single strategy clearly stands above the others, and the efficacy of some of them depends on the groups of population addressed.

The development of ICT-based applications can facilitate the implementation and follow-up of different strategies and interventions at different stages. The potential beneficiaries of these applications are not only suicidal people and their caregivers, but also other key actors such as their relatives, teachers and bereaved survivors [21]. Internet and mobile-based applications can increase the availability, accessibility, and acceptability of different suicidal prevention actions, ranging from the screening of people in risk, the support of psychotherapeutic treatment, the collection and analysis of data for surveillance purposes, to the provision of guided or unguided "self-help" interventions.

Much of these technology-based interventions are relatively new and there is not yet strong evidence about their effectiveness on suicide prevention, but they have the potential to reach and help a larger population of vulnerable people. Moreover, stakeholders of different countries including policy and public management professionals, specialists of the mental health area, and professionals related to the social area and non-governmental organisations, recognised the usefulness and advantages of new technologies as resources that should be incorporated into suicide prevention programs [23].

In this paper, we present the design and development of a computational platform with the aim to support the identification and prevention of suicidal behaviours. The platform is composed of two main components: **(i) a clinical decision support system** to help specialists with the screening, treatment management, and the collection and analysis of suicide-related data for surveillance purposes; and **(ii) a mobile-based application** addressed to people identified with suicidal behaviours (ideation, planning or attempt) to support the detection of risk factors and offer activities that can prevent the occurrence of these behaviours.

The platform was developed in the context of a collaborative research project with specialists (psychiatrists, psychologists, epidemiologists and public health managers) from the public health sector to facilitate its adoption in different primary care and specialised health services. The rest of the paper is organised as follows: Sect. 2 summarises some related work in the use of new technologies for suicide prevention. Section 3 presents in detail the design and main functionalities of the developed computational platform. Finally, Sect. 4 presents some conclusions and the ongoing and future work to evaluate the proposed platform.

2 Related Work

In the last years, several ICT-based solutions have been developed to support the prevention of suicide including informative websites, online self-help interventions, electronic therapy (e-therapy) interventions, interactive websites (chats), Internet forums, social networks, apps and video-games. Some of these applications are addressed to help health-care professionals with different activities during patients' suicide risk identification and intervention; some others are addressed to provide direct guided or unguided self-help to individuals in risk; and some others are addressed to involve relatives, family, gatekeepers and general public to increase the level of awareness of the suicide phenomenon [21].

Due to the evidence that a correct and early identification of individuals in risk contributes to enhancing treatment referrals and intervention [9,25,27], there are some current efforts in the development of computer-based systems for the screening of suicide risk and provider follow-up actions. For example, in [8] the authors describe the implementation of a computerised screening of suicidal ideation for youths in a paediatric primary care. A total of 1,547 youths responded to the system and 209 were identified with suicidal thoughts in the previous month. After a deeper mental health evaluation, 71 received a mental health service within 6 months. These results proved the feasibility of ICT-based screening in paediatric primary care, and the youth willingness to disclose suicidal ideation on a computerised screen.

More recently, the study presented in [6] describes the implementation of adolescents suicide screening and follow-up recommendations to providers into an existent clinical decision support system (CDSS) in primary care. In a sample of 2,134 patients, the system screened positive in suicidality over the 6% of them, and providers documented follow-up actions for 83% of patients screened positive. A similar ongoing study is presented in [15], where the authors describe a protocol for the development of an electronic CDSS to support general practitioners in the identification, assessment and management of suicidality in primary care.

Another key aspect for the design of improved suicide prevention strategies is the collection and analysis of all the data that helps to better understand this phenomenon. Surveillance systems should be used to register not only suicide cases but also suicide attempts and self-harm situations. The analysis and dissemination of these data can help public health professionals and policymakers in the implementation of preventive actions [43]. Most of the current efforts in the collection and analysis of suicides, attempts and self-harms for surveillance purposes involves the integration of the electronic records obtained from independent ICT health systems, usually form the emergency department. Examples of these surveillance systems include the data repositories implemented at regional [12,39], national [28] and international [16] level containing the anonymised and merged collected records.

In addition to the development of ICT-based solutions addressed to directly support health-care professionals and policymakers, the new technologies also offer opportunities to provide *digital interventions* to individuals at risk through online programs and mobile applications. This kind of interventions helps to reach a larger population that currently cannot or does not get as much access to mental health services as required due to costs, logistical issues, stigma or convenience. Moreover, such interventions have the potential to improve the scalability of effective treatments for self-harm and suicidal ideation [2].

Examples of these digital interventions include an internet-based program to reduce suicidal ideation, depression and hopelessness among students of secondary school [31]; a mobile app for suicide prevention in Australian indigenous youth [38]; a web-based cognitive behaviour therapy intervention for the prevention of suicidal behaviour in medical interns [10]; an online preventive suicide intervention for adolescents [14]; and a mobile app for the reduction of suicidal self-injury [7], to name a few. A deeper review of these and other similar digital interventions can be seen in [45]. In general, the use of these tools for the decreasing of suicidal ideation and self-harm may be more effective than waitlist control, though it remains unclear whether these reductions would be clinically meaningful. Nevertheless, the effectiveness of these technological solutions seems to be the next field to explore in the coming decade [46].

In the next section we describe a computational platform that implements three of the features described in the above described technological solutions: *(i)* a web-based application to support with the **screening** of individuals with suicidal behaviour and **follow-up actions**; *(ii)* a component for the analysis and visualisation of the collected data for the **surveillance** of suicidality; and *(iii)* a mobile application based on cognitive behaviour therapy to provide **self-help interventions** to prevent and detect suicidal behaviours.

3 The Computational Platform to Support Suicide Prevention

The proposed computational platform aims to contribute at different stages of the suicide prevention process, from the identification and screening of individuals with a suicidal behaviour to the support in the management of the provided treatment and follow-up actions. Two main modules were designed as the basis of the platform:

- A web-based **clinical decision support system (CDSS)** to help health-care professionals with:
  - The implementation of a standardised screening protocol.
  - The decision support in primary care for referring the patient to specialised services according to the results from the screening.
  - The implementation of a patient electronic psychological record to support with the management of the provided treatment.
  - The analysis and visualisation of the collected information for surveillance purposes.
- A **mobile-based (HelPath)** application to support patients with:
  - The collection and recording of relevant data that can be used to better assess their evolution.
  - The offering of suggestions and activities based on cognitive-behaviour therapy that can help to manage their current state.
  - The detection of factors that can be associated with a risk of suicidality.
  - Facilitate direct contact with the health-care providers and/or relatives in case of risk.

The CDSS can be deployed in both, primary care centres and in centres with specialised (psychological and psychiatric) health-care services. According to the role of the user (general practitioner, mental health specialist, epidemiologist or public health specialist), different functionalities are provided. All the information collected in each health-care centre, as well as some of the data collected through the patient's mobile application are stored in the central offices of the public health-care services. Figure 1 presents the main components of the platform. In the following sub-sections, each of the main features provided by the CDSS and the mobile application is explained.

3.1 The Clinical Decision Support System

Screening. When an individual seeks for help at the first time due to symptoms associated with some affective disorder, many times this first contact is with a general practitioner in a primary care centre. The patient usually does not identify what is the origin of the problem and is the clinician who has to identify whether the patient would need the provision of the mental health services. In the cases when the general practitioner identifies thoughts or ideas related to

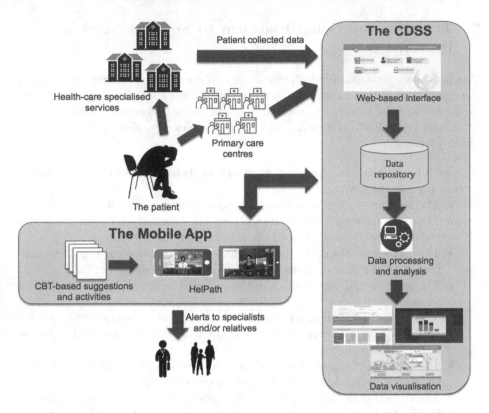

Fig. 1. The main components of the ICT-based platform to support suicide prevention.

suicidality, many times the patient is referred with "depression" to the mental health specialist. Nevertheless, in most of the cases, this assessment is not the result of applying a standardised instrument to diagnose a specific affective disorder leaving this task to the mental health specialist. In order to support a better assessment of the individuals that attend to primary care with this kind of problems, our CDSS implements an electronic version of three validated instruments used to identify different mental health disorders. The selection of these instruments was agreed with the clinicians of the project taking into account that are straightforward to apply by general practitioners in the primary care centres, and that most of the mental health professionals from the specialised centres are familiarised with these questionnaires.

The first instrument is the Calderon Depressive Syndrome Scale [4] which has been validated in the Mexican population [22]. The questionnaire consists of 20 items measured with a Likert type scale and depending on the responses, the individual can be diagnosed as non-depressive/with incipient depression/with middle depression/with severe depression. The second questionnaire implemented as part of the screening process is the Spanish validated version [33] of the Plutchik Suicide Risk Scale [29]. This scale contains 15 self-report items that should be answered with "yes" or "no" describing the degree to which an individual reveals characteristics similar to those of a suicide prototype. The obtained total score range of 0–15 indicates no suicide risk (0–5); suicide risk (6–9); and high suicide risk (>10). The third questionnaire is the Hamilton Anxiety Rating Scale [11] implemented in its Spanish validated version [17]. The scale consists of 14 items, each defined by a series of symptoms, and measures both psychic and somatic anxiety. Each item is scored on a scale of 0 (not present) to 4 (very severe), with a total score range of 0–56, where <17 indicates mild severity, 18–24 mild to moderate severity, 25–30 moderate to severe, and >30 severe to very severe. These three questionnaires are administered to the patients after the requesting of some personal and sociodemographic data.

In addition to the results obtained from each questionnaire, it is important the assessment of whether the individual is presenting a specific suicidal behaviour such as ideation or planning. Thus, following the clinicians' advice, when the patient answer affirmatively any of the questions related with suicidality (i.e. question number 19 from the Calderon Depressive Syndrome Scale "Do you feel a desire to be dead?"; questions number 13 "Have you ever thought about committing suicide?" or 14 "Have you ever told anyone you would commit suicide?" from Plutchik Suicide Risk Scale), then the system asks the question "Have you think how to do it?". If the patient responds "no", then the patient is assessed as an individual with *suicidal ideation*. On the other hand, if the response is affirmative, the system asks for an input describing how the patient has thought to do it. In this latter case, the patient is assessed as an individual with *suicidal planning*.

Depending on the obtained results from the three questionnaires, the CDSS implements a rule-based inference system to suggest the referral of the patient to the mental health services either to receive psychological or psychiatric attention. When an individual is admitted in the emergency department of a hospital due to a suicidal attempt, once the patient is stabilised and out of danger, the clinician performs the interview to enter into the system the patient's data and the results of the questionnaires. Moreover, the *suicidal attempt* behaviour is recorded jointly with the used self-harm method according to the WHO's International Classification of Diseases, ICD-11. All this information collected during the screening stage is then available to the mental health specialists to decide the specific actions during the follow-up process.

Follow-Up and Treatment Management. Once the patient is referred to the mental health services, the psychologists or psychiatrists responsible for the follow-up actions can easily access the patient's data collected in primary care. At this point, the specialist can complete all the information required in the electronic psychological record. The required data include the patient's family background, his/her school and occupational history, information about family and friends networks of support, among others. During this stage, the specialist can take the decision whether the patient is suitable for the use of the HelPath App as a complement of the treatment. If HelPath is recommended, some of the data stored in the patient's psychological record are then used by the mobile application as indicators to better assess further risks of suicidality (see Sect. 3.2). Moreover, all the information collected by the mobile application is also stored in the electronic psychological record for the specialist can observe the evolution of the patient's condition according to some factors such as the self-reported mood, negative thoughts or irrational beliefs, and physical or social activities.

As a complement to the patient's continuous self-reported information collected in the HelPath App, there is also the option that the specialists can apply again any of the validated instruments to get more data about the evolution of the patient's condition. Thus, through the CDSS's treatment management module the specialists can administer to the patient any of the three selected questionnaires used during the screening stage. This will allow the generation of plots to easily visualise the scores obtained at different times from each scale. Also, the system was designed to smoothly add other validated instruments for those specialists that want to use additional scales during the treatment of the patient.

Surveillance. As defined in [43], the registration not only of suicides but also of suicide attempts can add valuable information for the design of suicide prevention strategies. Having the records about suicide attempts and self-harm available to perform data analyses, e.g. on demographic and clinical risk groups is fundamental for the development, implementation, and evaluation of suicide prevention programmes [5]. Thus, our CDSS implements a surveillance module where all the information collected during the screening stage can be analysed and visualised in terms of different sociodemographic variables that each health professional can define in the user interface. As previously explained, all the suicide attempts received by the emergency departments can be registered including the used self-harm method. This information is also complemented with the recordings of all the individuals identified with suicidal ideation and planning.

Our CDSS's suicidality surveillance module implements the processing and visualisation of the data collected in all the primary care and specialised services according to the different filtering parameters that can be defined in the user interface. Moreover, all the cases related to the different suicidal behaviours are georeferenced according to the location of the health care centres where those cases were detected. Using a city map (or state or the whole country maps) the visualisation of the number of cases can be easily identified through a heat map layer representing with different colours the quantity of detected cases related to suicide attempts, ideation and planning at each health care centre during a specific period of time (see Fig. 2(a)). Additionally, through the surveillance user interface different plots can be generated to identify incidence rates during specific time periods according to the gender, age, occupation, marital status among some others (see an example in Fig. 2(b)).

3.2   The HelPath App

There are currently several apps and web-based interventions with the potential to prevent suicidal behaviours through the provision of educational and support information; assessment of risk; facilitating the access to safety plans and the offering of crisis support [18]. A critical point of these applications is their ability to engage and motivate the users to promote their continuous and long-term use facilitating the effective provision of the information and support. One strategy to catch and keep the interest of the users is the use of Embodied Conversational Agents (ECAs) that act as virtual peers of the users to get information about the user's condition and to provide immediate feedback. The main characteristic of an ECA is the ability to emulate a person to person conversation through a combination of dialogue interaction represented in a human-like appearance with a set of body movements and facial expressions. In recent years the development and use of ECAs for suicide prevention have emerged acting as virtual counsellors to support individuals in risk, or as virtual patients for learning purposes where medical students, college or university teachers, or formal and informal caregivers are trained in the identification of clues associated with suicidal behaviours [19].

In our HelPath App, we developed an ECA as the main interface with the users. We have developed a set of four ECAs (two males and two females) for the users to choose -at the beginning of each session- their preferred ECA's appearance and clothes. The inputs from the user to the ECA are constrained to the selection of different options and values through the controls in the graphical user interface (see Fig. 3). We selected this solution to ensure data validity and accuracy, and to minimise errors in automatic speech recognition and natural language understanding, which is particularly important when designing health counselling interactive systems [3]. All the verbal responses from the ECA to the user are communicated via voice using the text-to-speech of the mobile device. The main functionality of the ECA is the collection of relevant data from the patient and the provision of suggestions and activities, based on Cognitive Behaviour Therapy (CBT), during short daily sessions. Another important functionality of HelPath is the identification of risk factors associated with a suicidal behaviour inferred from the patient's reported data and validated with a suicidal scale. In these cases, the app sends an SMS alert to the specialists or patient's relatives promoting a direct face-to-face contact.

CBT for Suicide Prevention. Different studies have shown the evidence about the use of CBT in the reduction and prevention of suicidal cognitions and suicidal behaviours, and that better patient outcomes arise when this type of therapy is focused on these suicidal cognitions and behaviours as dysfunctional individual factors rather than symptoms of mental illness [20,37]. Thus, we have implemented five modules based on principles of the CBT in our HelPath App where the ECA is responsible for offering most of the content and motivating to the user in the execution of the recommended activities. The five modules are the following:

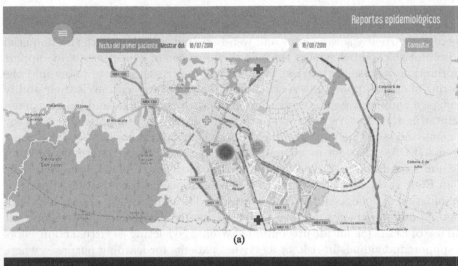

(a)

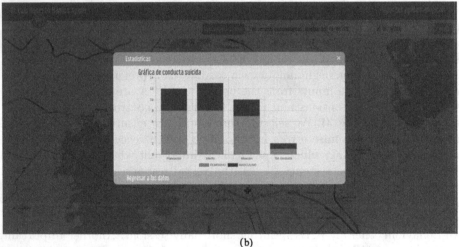

(b)

Fig. 2. (a) A heat map for the visualisation of suicidal behaviour (ideation, planning and attempt) cases detected in the different health care centres from a city. (b) Generation of plots with the information of suicidal behaviour cases divided by gender.

1. An initial psychoeducation activity.
2. The emotions and mood monitoring.
3. Cognitive modification.
4. Behavioural activation.
5. Relaxation techniques.

Psychoeducation. An important initial phase of a CBT-based intervention is to dedicate some time to explain the patients about their symptoms, describe an explicit conceptualisation of the problem, introduce the basic principles and

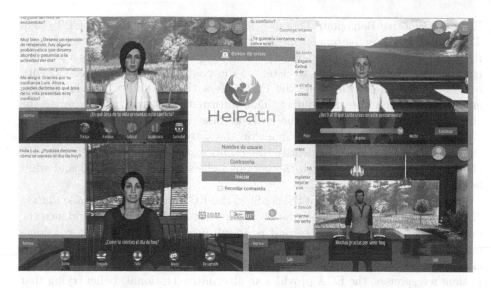

Fig. 3. The different ECAs of the HelPath mobile application.

goals of CBT, and how it can help them [36]. So, the first time that the patient enters into HelPath, a psychoeducative video is played where a combination of cartoonish images in movement with a narrator explaining the main components of the CBT including some cognitive, emotional and behavioural factors and how they are related with a dysfunctional condition. In subsequent sessions, the patient can access the video at any moment through the main menu of HelPath.

Monitoring of the Emotional State. A key element in CBT is to support the patient with the ability to be self-aware and reflective of his/her emotional states, thoughts and behaviours. A useful strategy -for both: the clinician and patient- is to maintain a constant monitoring of these elements to understand better how they are interrelated and influenced. In HelPath, the first activity after the ECA's welcome is to ask the patients about their feelings. The ECA questions about what emotion is the patient feeling today and the GUI offers five basic emotions (sad, angry, happy, disgust and fear) and the "none of these" option for the patient makes a selection. Once the emotion is selected, the ECA asks the user about the intensity of that emotion offering a slider for the patient to select a 1–10 value. When the patient does not select any of the five basic emotions, the ECA asks "How is your mood today?" and the patient responds by using a slider representing values from bad to good mood. The self-reported emotions/mood and their intensities are stored for the further assessment of the patient's condition and for the summary reports that are integrated into the patient's electronic psychological record.

Cognitive Modification. HelPath supports patients with cognitive modification by implementing some activities based on the *ABC-DEF* framework of the

Rational-Emotive Behaviour Therapy - REBT (a particular form of CBT) [34]. The first part, the *activating event (A)*, starts when the ECA asks the area (family, work, academic, social or partner) where the patient could identify a possible conflict. A second question is to detect if the conflict is with him/herself, with others or with life. After that, the ECA offers the possibility for the patient enters text to describe the conflict. This information is used to categorise the (irrational) *belief (B)* allowing the ECA to offer a set of 5–7 irrational beliefs (IB), according to the selected area, for the patient to choose the one more related with the conflict. To identify the -emotional- *consequences (C)* of the IB, the ECA asks about how much the patient beliefs in the selected IB and what is the emotion elicited by it.

Once identified the *ABC* of the conflict, the ECA implements the *disputation (D)* of the IB by asking three questions. The first one is about the evidence the patient has on that IB. The second is about how much the patient considers useful the IB, and with the third one, the ECA guides the patient towards thoughts' flexibility by requesting some other explanation to the IB. After the patient's responses, the ECA provides an alternative (rational) belief trying that the patient replaces the IB by an *effective (E) new belief.* Finally, to promote the co-construction of more *functional (F) emotions and responses*, the ECA suggests the execution of an activity related to the offered rational belief to practice and reinforce it. Moreover, the ECA asks about what the patient has learned, how much believability the patient now has on the original IB and whether there was some change in the original reported emotion or mood. All this information is used for the assessment of a possible cognitive change in the patient.

Behavioural Activation. A complementary strategy to the cognitive change is the promotion of activities that help patients to develop protective factors against suicidality risks. The behavioural activation focuses on activity scheduling to encourage patients to approach relevant and satisfactory activities [40]. Thus, the ECA offers a set of activities to schedule a maximum of five during the current week aiming to get a commitment from the patient. The activities are divided into two categories: those directed to develop personal and social abilities (such as interpersonal relationships, self-discovery or conflict resolution); and those for activation such as sports, movies, art, nature, or religion among some others. Once the week's activities are set, HelPath sends reminders highlighting the importance to execute them and offers the option to re-schedule those activities not reported as performed on the planned day. When the deadline of each activity arrives, the ECA questions the patient whether he/she performed the activity, what were the obstacles faced during its (no) execution, and for the cases of the executed activities, what was the obtained satisfaction level.

Relaxation Techniques. The relaxation is one of the procedures that have benefits to a variety of mental health problems. The main goal of relaxation is to reduce the physiological activation produced by stressful events, facilitating the recovery of a well-being state. HelPath offers the patient with four relaxation exercises.

Two of these exercises are based on Jacobson's progressive muscle relaxation exercises (PMR) involving muscle tension and relaxation [1]. The other two exercises are based on controlled and deep-breathing relaxation techniques. The ECA explains the content and objective of each exercise, and when the patient selects one, a video with a pre-recorded voice guides the patient through the exercises while some images are displayed on the screen. After the exercise is finished, the ECA asks the patient about his/her current emotional state. If the patient reports a negative emotion with a higher intensity than the reported at the beginning of the session, the ECA offers another relaxation exercise, a cognitive modification exercise to identify the possible conflict, or suggests the calling to a contact person.

Suicide Risk Detection. The prediction of suicide in a person is difficult due that individual risk factors account for a small proportion of the variance in risk and lack sufficient specificity, which results in high rates of false positives [24]. Individual assessments need to be done to identify if suicide risk is present by recognising personal protective and risk factors. Then if suicide risk is present, further assessment should address the imminence of suicidal behaviour [13]. Using the information collected during the screening and the filling of the electronic psychological record stages, and some of the self-reported information through HelPath, some risk factors associated with suicidal behaviour are identified taking as reference the SAD PERSONS scale [26]. If risk factors are detected, the Roberts' Suicide Ideation Scale [30] is applied to assess the imminence of suicidal behaviour and to minimise the occurrence of false positives. Depending on the results, alert messages are sent to pre-defined contacts promoting direct face-to-face support.

The SAD PERSONS Scale. This scale consists of 10 items (each one corresponding to each scale's name letter) assessing a risk factor for suicide: *S*ex, *A*ge, *D*epression, *P*revious attempt, *E*thanol abuse, *R*ational thinking loss, *S*ocial supports lacking, *O*rganised plan, *N*o spouse, and *S*ickness. Each factor is scored as 1 if present or 0 if absent, resulting in a cumulative score that is interpreted as conveying a specified level of risk. In HelPath The assessment of the patient through SAD PERSONS is triggered when any of the following conditions occurs:

1. **Drastic or sudden changes in the emotional state.** These changes are identified when the patient reports a high positive emotion/mood during three or more consecutive sessions, and then he/she reports a high negative emotion/mood. Also, if during the same session the initial emotion reported is highly positive but after the execution of some suggested activity the patient reports a high negative emotion, the scale is applied.
2. **Suicidal thoughts.** When the patient selects any of the irrational beliefs categorised as hopelessness, negative views about self, verbalisation about dead, or possibilities to commit suicide.

3. **Cognitive rigidity.** Identified when the patient reports a high level of believability on any IB, even when the ECA has offered an alternative rational
   belief.
4. **Recurrent negative thoughts.** When the patient selects three or more
   consecutive times the same IB, but not classified in any of the categories of
   the above point 2.
5. **Difficulties in the execution of planned activities.** When the patient
   reports three or more consecutive times that he/she found obstacles to execute the planned week activities, independently whether the activities were
   reported as completed or not completed.
6. **Vulnerability to stress or adverse events.** When the patient reports a
   high negative emotion/mood, he/she performs a relaxation exercise, and the
   reported emotion/mood after the exercise is still highly negative.

When any of the six above conditions is fulfilled, HelPath internally assesses
whether the patient can be considered within a high-risk population through
the SAD PERSONS scale considering a score equal to or greater than 7. Nine of
the ten items of the scale are obtained from the electronic psychological record
and the results of the screening questionnaires. The only item obtained from the
patient interaction with HelPath is the *rational thinking loss*, by assessing the
irrational beliefs selected by the patient using the same condition explained in
the above point 2. If the patient is assessed within the high-risk population, then
the Roberts' Suicide Ideation Scale is applied to assess the imminence of suicide
and to minimise the false positives. The only condition to apply the Roberts'
scale without considering the results of SAD PERSONS is when the patient
selects any of the IB related with verbalisation about dead.

The Roberts' Suicide Ideation Scale. This scale, validated in Mexican population
[32], consists of four items regarding thoughts about death and taking one's own
life over the previous seven days. The items include *"thoughts about death"*;
"family and friends better off if I were dead"; *"thought about killing myself"*;
and *"would kill myself if I knew a way"*. A four-point scale is used with the
options: $0 = 0$; 1–2 days = 1; 3–4 days = 2; and 5–7 days = 3. The overall score
ranges between 0 and 12 points. In HelPath, when the Roberts' scale is applied
the assessment of a high-risk situation results from a score equal to or greater
than five points. In these cases, the HelPath app sends an SMS to the patient's
contacts (defined by the patient in the settings of the app), recommending to
make a call to the patient. Moreover, if the patient authorises and the GPS
is activated, the SMS includes the location of the patient to facilitate direct
contact. In the app, the ECA also suggests to the patient to make a call and put
the mobile phone in a call mode showing his/her contact numbers including the
crisis line number, and then finishes the current session.

For those cases when the score of the Roberts' scale is lesser than five, the
ECA suggests the patient make a call looking for social support. In these cases,
no alert messages are sent and the session can continue and finalise normally. It is
important to mention that as a complement to the mechanism for the automatic

detection of suicidality risk, HelPath also implements a *crisis button* which is accessible from the app's menu or the login screen (see Fig. 3). When the patient pushes this button, HelPath shows the list of the pre-defined contacts for the patient to select the person to make a call. When the patient selects the specific contact, the mobile phone is put on call mode, and at the same time, the alert messages are sent to the whole list of contacts. In this way, we try to minimise the risk that the patient's selected contact is not available to answer the call and warn about the situation to the other pre-defined contacts.

4   Conclusions and Future Work

Suicide is a complex phenomenon that requires the collaboration of different disciplines and sectors to guide the implementation of effective preventable strategies. One of the disciplines that have the potential to contribute to the design and deployment of effective prevention strategies is the ICT. Different computer-based applications have been developed in recent years as technological tools to support diverse suicide prevention activities, from the screening of individuals in risk to the provision of self-help interventions. In this paper, we have presented the development of a computational platform composed of two main modules: a Clinical Decision Support System to help health-care professionals, and the HelPath mobile application to monitor and support individuals in risk.

The design and development of the two components were developed in close collaboration with health care specialists to facilitate their use and adoption by the clinicians at both, the primary care and specialised health care centres. The deployment of this platform to perform an initial evaluation is ongoing, and it includes the participation of four primary care centres and two centres with specialised mental health services. All these public health care centres are coordinated by the local Government of Nayarit's region in Mexico that can facilitate the addition of new centres in the near future. The initial set of testings include the assessment of the CDSS's usability and functionality to detect corrective and improvement actions according to the feedback obtained from the users with the different roles in the system, such as general practitioners at primary care, specialists (psychologists and psychiatrists), clinicians at the emergency department and epidemiologists.

Additionally, we are currently finalising a first pilot study to evaluate the usability and acceptability of HelPath. We recruited a total of 18 participants with antecedents of suicidal ideation, planning or attempt but excluding in this first pilot, for safety reasons, those individuals with recent (during the last six months) suicidal behaviour. The participants, under the supervision of a specialist, were asked to use HelPath for two months suggesting them to carry out a daily interaction. The objective of this initial study is to get qualitative and quantitative data about the use, acceptability, usability and adherence level from the user towards the app as a whole, towards the appearance and behaviour of the ECA, and towards the CBT-based contents provided by HelPath. At this moment, we are starting to collect and analyse the data provided by the participants. The details of the HelPath's pilot design, the evaluation protocol and the obtained results will be further reported.

In the mid and long term, when the platform has been deployed in the different healthcare centres, the expected outcome from both components is to support the clinicians with a better understanding of the different (e.g. socio-demographic, contextual, environmental, etc.) factors associated with suicidality. The nurturing of the central data repository with the information from the people detected and treated, would allow the further implementation of data mining techniques for the recognition and assessment of different patterns associated with these factors. Moreover, the platform will contribute to getting a better picture not only of the suicide cases (which is the focus of current surveillance systems) but also of the different suicidal behaviours (ideation, planning and attempt) that occur in a more significant number.

Acknowledgements. This work has been funded by the "Fondo Sectorial de Investigación en Salud y Seguridad Social – FOSISS/CONACyT" under the research project 2016-1-273163 *"Desarrollo de nuevas tecnologías y su integración al sector salud como ayuda a una estrategia integral de prevención del suicidio"*. The first author also acknowledges the "Cátedras CONACyT" program funded by the Mexican National Research Council (CONACyT).

References

1. Bernstein, D.A., Borkovec, T.D., Hazlett-Stevens, H.: New Directions in Progressive Relaxation Training: A Guidebook for Helping Professionals. Greenwood Publishing Group, Westport (2000)
2. de Beurs, D., Kirtley, O., Kerkhof, A., Portzky, G., O'Connor, R.: The role of mobile phone technology in understanding and preventing suicidal behavior. Crisis **36**(2), 79–82 (2015)
3. Bickmore, T., Trinh, H., Asadi, R., Olafsson, S.: Safety first: conversational agents for health care. In: Moore, R.J., Szymanski, M.H., Arar, R., Ren, G.-J. (eds.) Studies in Conversational UX Design. HIS, pp. 33–57. Springer, Cham (2018). https://doi.org/10.1007/978-3-319-95579-7_3
4. Calderón-Narváez, G.: Cuestionario clínico para el diagnóstico de los cuadros depresivos (Clinical questionnaire for the diagnosis of depressive profiles). Revista Médica del Instituto Mexicano del Seguro Social **30**(5), 377–380 (1992)
5. Department of Health: Connecting for life: Ireland's national strategy to reduce suicide 2015–2020. Technical report, National Office for Suicide Prevention (2015). https://www.healthpromotion.ie/hp-files/docs/HME00945.pdf. Accessed 13 Nov 2018
6. Etter, D.J., et al.: Suicide screening in primary care: use of an electronic screener to assess suicidality and improve provider follow-up for adolescents. J. Adolesc. Health **62**, 191–197 (2018)
7. Franklin, J.C., et al.: A brief mobile app reduces nonsuicidal and suicidal self-injury: evidence from three randomized controlled trials. J. Consult. Clin. Psychol. **84**(6), 544–557 (2016)

8. Gardner, W., et al.: Screening, triage, and referral of patients who report suicidal thought during a primary care visit. Pediatrics **125**(5), 945–952 (2010)
9. Gould, M.S., Marrocco, F.A., Hoagwood, K., Kleinman, M., Amakawa, L., Altschuler, E.: Service use by at-risk youths after school-based suicide screening. Child Adolesc. Psychiatry **48**(12), 1193–1201 (2009)
10. Guille, C., Zhao, Z., Krystal, J., Nichols, B., Brady, K., Sen, S.: Web-based cognitive behavioral therapy intervention for the prevention of suicidal ideation in medical interns: a randomized clinical trial. JAMA Psychiatry **72**(12), 1192–1198 (2015)
11. Hamilton, M.: The assessment of anxiety states by rating. Br. J. Med. Psychol. **32**(1), 50–55 (1959)
12. Hawton, K., et al.: Self-harm in England: a tale of three cities. Soc. Psychiatry Psychiatr. Epidemiol. **42**(7), 513–521 (2007)
13. Hawton, K., van Heeringen, K.: Suicide. Lancet **373**, 1372–1381 (2009)
14. Hill, R.M., Pettit, J.W.: Pilot randomized controlled trial of LEAP: a selective preventive intervention to reduce adolescents' perceived burdensomeness. J. Clin. Child Adolesc. Psychol. **48**(Sup1) (2019). https://doi.org/10.1080/15374416.2016.1188705
15. Horrocks, M., Michail, M., Aubeeluck, A., Wright, N., Morriss, R.: An electronic clinical decision support system for the assessment and management of suicidality in primary care. JMIR Res. Protoc. (2018, in press). http://eprints.nottingham.ac.uk/52831/. Accessed 03 Nov 2018
16. Kisser, R., Walters, A., Rogmans, W., Turner, S., Lyons, R.A.: Injuries in the European Union 2013–2015. Technical report, European Association for Injury Prevention and Safety Promotion (EuroSafe) (2017). http://www.eurosafe.eu.com/uploads/inline-files/IDB%202013-2015_suppl%20to%206th%20edition%20Injuries%20in%20the%20EU.pdf. Accessed 04 Nov 2018
17. Lobo, A., Chamorro, L., Luque, A., Dal-Ré, R., Badia, X., Baró, E.: Validación de las versiones en español de la montgomery-asberg depression rating scale y la hamilton anxiety rating scale para la evaluación de la depresión y de la ansiedad. Medicina Clínica **118**, 493–499 (2002)
18. Luxton, D.D., June, J.D., Chalker, S.A.: Mobile health technologies for suicide prevention: feature review and recommendations for use in clinical care. Curr. Treat. Options Psychiatry **2**(4), 349–362 (2015)
19. Martínez-Miranda, J.: Embodied conversational agents for the detection and prevention of suicidal behaviour: current applications and open challenges. J. Med. Syst. **41**, 135 (2017)
20. Mewton, L., Andrews, G.: Cognitive behavioral therapy for suicidal behaviors: improving patient outcomes. Psychol. Res. Behav. Manage. **9**, 21–29 (2016)
21. Mishara, B., Kerkhof, A.: Suicide Prevention and New Technologies: Evidence Based Practice. Palgrave Macmillan, New York (2013)
22. Morales-Ramírez, M., Ocampo-Andréyeva, V., de la Mora, L., Alvarado-Calvillo, R.: Validez y confiabilidad del cuestionario clínico del síndrome depresivo (Validity and reliability of the depressive syndrome clinical questionnaire). Archivos de Neurociencias **1**(1), 11–15 (1996)
23. Muñoz-Sánchez, J.L., Delgado, C., Sánchez-Prada, A., Pérez-López, M., Franco-Martín, M.: Use of new technologies in the prevention of suicide in europe: an exploratory study. JMIR Ment. Health **4**(2), e23 (2017)
24. Oquendo, M.A., Currier, D., Mann, J.J.: Prospective studies of suicidal behavior in major depressive and bipolar disorders: what is the evidence for predictive risk factors? Acta Psychiatr. Scand. **114**(3), 151–158 (2006)

25. Oyama, H., et al.: A community-based survey and screening for depression in the elderly: the short-term effect on suicide risk in Japan. Crisis J. Crisis Interv. Suicide Prev. **31**(2), 100–108 (2010)
26. Patterson, W.M., Dohn, H.H., Bird, J., Patterson, G.A.: Evaluation of suicidal patients: the SAD PERSONS scale. Psychosomatics **24**(4), 343–349 (1983)
27. Peña, J.B., Caine, E.D.: Screening as an approach for adolescent suicide prevention. Suicide Life Threat. Behav. **36**(6), 614–637 (2006)
28. Perry, I.J., Corcoran, P., Fitzgerald, A.P., Keeley, H.S., Reulbach, U., Arensman, E.: The incidence and repetition of hospital-treated deliberate self harm: findings from the world's first national registry. PLoS ONE **7**(2), e31663 (2012)
29. Plutchick, R., van Praga, H.M., Conte, H.R., Picard, S.: Correlates of suicide and violence risk: the suicide risk measure. Compr. Psychiatry **30**(4), 296–302 (1989)
30. Roberts, R.E., Chen, Y.W.: Depressive symptoms and suicidal ideation among mexican-origin and anglo adolescents. J. Am. Acad. Child Adolesc. Psychiatry **34**(1), 81–90 (1995)
31. Robinson, J., et al.: Can an internet-based intervention reduce suicidal ideation, depression and hopelessness among secondary school students: results from a pilot study. Early Interv. Psychiatry **10**(1), 28–35 (2016)
32. Rosales-Pérez, J.C., Córdova-Osnaya, M., Cortés-Granados, R.: Reliability and validity of Roberts' suicidal scale. J. Behav. Health Soc. Issues **7**(2), 31–41 (2016)
33. Rubio, G., et al.: Validación de la escala de riesgo suicida de plutchik en población española (Validation of the plutchik suicide risk scale in Spanish population). Archivos de Neurobiología **61**(2), 143–152 (1998)
34. Sarracino, D., Dimaggio, G., Ibrahim, R., Popolo, R., Sassaroli, S., Ruggiero, G.M.: When REBT goes difficult: applying ABC-DEF to personality disorders. J. Rational-Emot. Cognitive-Behav. Ther. **35**(3), 278–295 (2017)
35. Schwartz-Lifshitz, M., Zalsman, G., Giner, L., Oquendo, M.: Can we really prevent suicide? Curr. Psychiatry Rep. **14**(6), 624–633 (2012)
36. Stanley, B., et al.: Cognitive-behavioral therapy for suicide prevention (CBT-SP): treatment model, feasibility, and acceptability. J. Am. Acad. Child Adolesc. Psychiatry **48**(10), 1005–1013 (2009)
37. Tarrier, N., Taylor, K., Gooding, P.: Cognitive-behavioral interventions to reduce suicide behavior: a systematic review and meta-analysis. Behav. Modif. **32**(1), 77–108 (2008)
38. Tighe, J., Shand, F., Ridani, R., Mackinnon, A., Mata, N.D.L., Christensen, H.: Ibobbly mobile health intervention for suicide prevention in australian indigenous youth: a pilot randomised controlled trial. BMJ Open **7**(1), e013518 (2017)
39. Vancayseele, N., Jaegere, E.D., Portzky, G., van Heeringen, C.: De epidemiologie van suïcidepogingen in Groot Gent (The epidemiology of suicide attempts in bigger Gent). Technical report, Universiteit Gent (2012). https://www.eenheidzelfmoordonderzoek.be/pdf/14082014-083537-Jaarverslag%20Groot%20Gent%202012.pdf. Accessed 04 Nov 2018
40. Veale, D.: Behavioural activation for depression. Adv. Psychiatr. Treat. **14**, 29–36 (2008)
41. WHO: Preventing suicide: a resource for counsellours. Technical report, World Health Organisation (2006). http://apps.who.int/iris/bitstream/handle/10665/43487/9241594314_eng.pdf?sequence=1. Accessed 01 Nov 2018
42. WHO: Preventing suicide: a global imperative. Technical report, World Health Organisation (2014). http://apps.who.int/iris/bitstream/handle/10665/131056/9789241564779_eng.pdf?sequence=1. Accessed 01 Nov 2018

43. WHO: Practice manual for establishing and maintaining surveillance systems for suicide attempts and self-harm. Technical report, World Health Organisation (2016). http://www.who.int/mental_health/suicide-prevention/attempts_surveillance_systems/en/. Accessed 04 Nov 2018
44. WHO: World Health Statistics 2017 - Monitoring Health for the SDGs. Technical report, World Health Organisation (2017). http://apps.who.int/iris/bitstream/handle/10665/255336/9789241565486-eng.pdf?sequence=1. Accessed 01 Nov 2018
45. Witt, K., et al.: Effectiveness of online and mobile telephone applications ('apps') for the self-management of suicidal ideation and self-harm: a systematic review and meta-analysis. BMC Psychiatry 17(297), 1–18 (2017)
46. Zalsman, G., et al.: Suicide prevention strategies revisited: 10-year systematic review. Lancet Psychiatry 3(7), 646–659 (2016)

Anthropometry and Scan: A Computational Exploration on Measuring and Imaging

Michelle Toti[1(✉)], Cosimo Tuena[1], Michelle Semonella[1],
Elisa Pedroli[1], Giuseppe Riva[1,2], and Pietro Cipresso[1,2]

[1] Applied Technology for Neuro-Psychology Lab,
IRCCS Istituto Auxologico Italiano, 20145 Milan, Italy
michelletoti5@gmail.com, cosimotuena@gmail.com,
semonellamichelle@gmail.com,
{e.pedroli,p.cipresso}@auxologico.it
[2] Department of Psychology, Università Cattolica del Sacro Cuore,
20100 Milan, Italy
{pietro.cipresso,giuseppe.riva}@unicatt.it

Abstract. New developments in the field of technology have led to the use of scanners in order to obtain anthropometric measurements. As a matter of fact, anthropometry finds its roots in the seventeenth century, currently its usage has been strengthened by the employment of scanners. 3D whole-body scanners allow to collect reliable data and to visualise the exact human body shape. Thus, this paper aims at exploring the combination of these topics, anthropometry and scan, through an innovative tool, the scientometrics analysis. This technique provides a clear overview of the existing literature in the field investigated. In our study we examined 1'652 papers from the Web of Science Core Collection database. Network analyses have shown an interesting scenario, emphasising the research evolution over time. Specifically, endocrinology and metabolism emerged as the most active publication domains. Accordingly, the two most high-impact journals and the most cited paper regard nutrition issues and metabolic risk factors respectively. However, the predominance of the USA for number of publications has not been confirmed by the institution's analysis, which has shown the University of Copenhagen as the most influential one. On the other hand, Yumei Zhang currently appears as the main authority in the field and Leslie G. Farkas as the most influential author over the entire time span analysed. The relevant implications of the findings are discussed in terms of future research lines.

Keywords: Anthropometry · Scan · 3D scan · Anthropometric measurements · Scientometrics analysis · Network analysis

1 Introduction

Nowadays human body shape has increasingly become useful to assess in several research fields. Digital anthropometry exploits mathematical analyses to investigate and define the shape of the body. These evaluations are performed using optic measuring methods with 3D imaging modalities. These techniques ensure that reliable data are

© ICST Institute for Computer Sciences, Social Informatics and Telecommunications Engineering 2019
Published by Springer Nature Switzerland AG 2019. All Rights Reserved
P. Cipresso et al. (Eds.): MindCare 2019, LNICST 288, pp. 102–116, 2019.
https://doi.org/10.1007/978-3-030-25872-6_8

obtained, and that these can be used in studies aim at improving human quality of life. Body parts and proportions have been of great interest, especially for aesthetic and figurative purposes, however from the 17th century the study of body shapes shifted to the scientific and medical field. By definition, anthropometry is considered a branch of morphometry and is the study of size and form of the body and its variations [1]. Traditional anthropometry aims at providing information about linear measurements and ratios, these consist of lengths, widths and depths whereas geometric (modern) anthropometry gives geometric information of the structure and it is a coordinates-based method [1, 2]. In particular the use of anthropometry in medicine has been applied in the context of nutritional status, within this field different anthropometric variables are used to assess morphological status and body composition [3]: height, weight, Body Mass Index (BMI), Waist to Height Ratio (WHtR), waist, hip, mid-upper arm and mid-arm muscle circumference, Waist-Hip Ratio (WHR), Sagittal Abdominal Diameter (SAD) and skinfold measurements are the most common variables applied for the study of clinical nutrition. Recent proceeding in the field of anthropometry has yielded to remarkable change due to the introduction of new tools for the study of the body, such as 3D whole body scanners, that are now powerful competitors of simple anthropometric tools/measurements and calipers [1, 4]. These 3D scanners use infrared light to create high-quality images of the body with non-invasive optical method. So far, 3D scanner has been applied in different context, initially in the clothing industry, then in psychology (e.g. body image) and medicine (e.g. anthropometry and musculoskeletal condition) [5]. For instance, different study used 3D scanner to provide 3D avatars in combination with virtual reality (VR) to study body image distortion in patients with anorexia nervosa [6, 7]. In the medical field, 3D scanners can be used to study obesity, risk factors associated with metabolic syndrome and body composition [8, 9]. Moreover, recent development in radiology allowed the study of internal structures by means of imaging techniques such as Computed Tomography (CT), Dual-energy X-ray Absorptiometry (DXA) and Magnetic Resonance (MR) [1, 10]. 3D scanner images can be used in combination with these data. For instance, 3D scan can be used in combination with DXA and traditional measurements to cluster participants by age, height, weight, BMI, percentage of fat mass, free fat mass, lean mass and bone mass [11].

According to Heymsfield and colleagues [4] whole body scanner can be used to extract anthropometric measures (e.g. height, hip, waist) and body shapes and to predict body composition, health risk and DXA, CT and MR images; additionally, digital anthropometry is considered a faster, cheaper and safer technique compared to classic imaging methods and can provide additional variables useful for the study of body parts and shapes [4, 5].

Fields of applications and methods used in the context of 3D scanners are multiple and in order to clarify past and current literature and future directions. The present scientometrics analysis has the objective to summarize and outline an overview of this technology in the field of anthropometry. This analysis is a computational bibliometric exploration that allows to visualize the existing literature within the scientific domain selected and to identify trends and patterns within the field. Citespace is a freely available computer program written in Java useful in this purpose, it takes bibliographic information, especially from the Web of Science and generates interactive visualizations of nodes and links (i.e. networks).

2 Methods

2.1 Selection Criteria and Data Collection

The input data, for the analysis, were collected from Web of science Core Collection scientific database. The topics selected to carry out the computer-based research were "anthropometr*" and "scan*". The search regarded papers published over the period from 1970 to 2018. Web of Science Core Collection is composed of: Citation Indexes, Science Citation Index Expanded (SCI-EXPANDED) – 1970-present, Social Sciences Citation Index (SSCI) – 1970-present, Arts & Humanities Citation Index (A&HCI) – 1975-present, Conference Proceedings Citation Index- Science (CPCI-S) – 1990-present, Conference Proceedings Citation Index- Social Science & Humanities (CPCI-SSH) – 1990-present, Book Citation Index– Science (BKCI-S) – 2009-present, Book Citation Index– Social Sciences & Humanities (BKCI-SSH) – 2009-present, Emerging Sources Citation Index (ESCI) – 2015-present, Chemical Indexes, Current Chemical Reactions (CCR-EXPANDED) – 2009-present (Includes Institut National de la Propriete Industrielle structure data back to 1840), Index Chemicus (IC) – 2009- present, the last two citation indexes were excluded from the articles sampling. The final input dataset was composed of 1'652 records, the bibliographic records contained various fields, such as author, title, abstract, keywords and all the references (needed for the citation analysis). The research tool to visualize the networks was Cite space v.5.3. R7 SE (32 bit) [12] under Java Runtime v.8 update 91 (build 1.8.0_91-b15). Some figures were done with Microsoft Excel and MapChart (https://mapchart.net).

3 Results

The literature collected includes 1'652 articles, according to the document types analysis of WoS, specifically, 84.56% are articles, 15.17% proceeding papers, 1.63% reviews, 1.27% book chapters, 0.72% meeting abstracts, 0.18% letters and 0.06 of both data paper and editorial material. Figure 1 provides preliminary information about the beginning of scientific research in this area. From the 90's the anthropometric research has been enriched by the use of the scan. In fact, more than 100 articles have been published in the last years, with a peak in 2017.

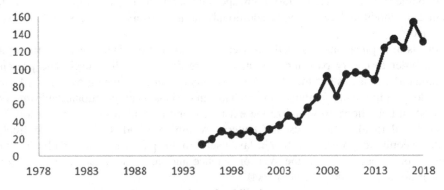

Fig. 1. Number of publications per year.

3.1   Categories

According to WoS categories analysis, the most ranked field of publications concerning anthropometry and scan is endocrinology and metabolism with a total record of 224 papers, following surgery with a total of 161 records, nutrition dietetics and sport science with at least more than 100 records.

On the other hand, categories based on research areas carried out with Citespace shows engineering as the most influent field, which constitutes the 16.74% of the total literature regarding the selected topics. Figure 2 illustrates the top ranked categories by citations count.

While, Fig. 3 represents the categories network assuming a threshold ≥ 10 citations per each category. Network analysis was conducted to calculate and to represent the centrality [13, 14].

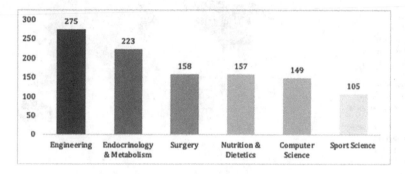

Fig. 2. Top ranked categories according to citations count.

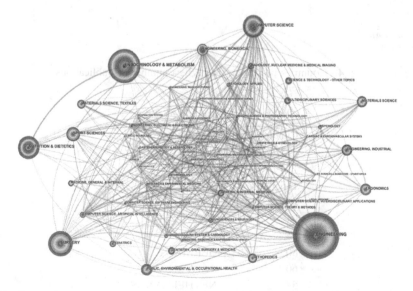

Fig. 3. Categories network. The dimensions of the nodes represent centrality, the dimensions of the characters represent the rank of the category.

3.2 Countries

Figure 4 displays the top ranked countries according to WoS records count. Table 1 shows the situation of the most influential countries in terms of publications calculated by citation count. Figure 5 illustrates a network of countries based on cited reference count and assuming a threshold of at least 35 citations for country. While, Table 2 provides indications about citation burst of each country. Bursts indicate the period in which a country has been most active in terms of scientific production. Bursts analysis represent a detection of a burst event, which can last for multiple years as well as a single year. A burst provides, for example, evidence that a particular publication is associated with a surge of citations. The burst detection is based on Kleinberg's algorithm [15].

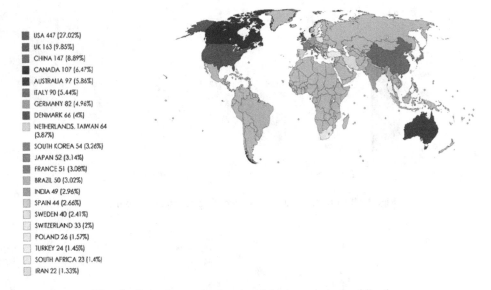

USA 447 (27.02%)
UK 163 (9.85%)
CHINA 147 (8.89%)
CANADA 107 (6.47%)
AUSTRALIA 97 (5.86%)
ITALY 90 (5.44%)
GERMANY 82 (4.96%)
DENMARK 66 (4%)
NETHERLANDS, TAIWAN 64 (3.87%)
SOUTH KOREA 54 (3.26%)
JAPAN 52 (3.14%)
FRANCE 51 (3.08%)
BRAZIL 50 (3.02%)
INDIA 49 (2.96%)
SPAIN 44 (2.66%)
SWEDEN 40 (2.41%)
SWITZERLAND 33 (2%)
POLAND 26 (1.57%)
TURKEY 24 (1.45%)
SOUTH AFRICA 23 (1.4%)
IRAN 22 (1.33%)

Fig. 4. Countries producing the highest number of publications

Table 1. Citations for countries.

Citations count	Country
423	USA
154	UK
146	CHINA
101	CANADA
94	AUSTRALIA
84	ITALY
80	GERMANY
60	TAIWAN
57	NETHERLANDS
55	DENMARK

Table 2. Top 10 countries with the strongest citation bursts.

Countries	Year	Strength	Begin	End	1990 - 2018
USA	1990	7.2673	1991	1998	
AUSTRALIA	1990	4.635	1997	2001	
SWEDEN	1990	4.9666	1999	2001	
JAPAN	1990	6.7446	2000	2011	
FINLAND	1990	5.1957	2001	2003	
CANADA	1990	3.7555	2005	2007	
TAIWAN	1990	4.333	2010	2011	
IRAN	1990	3.9249	2013	2018	
PORTUGAL	1990	4.0719	2014	2018	
BRAZIL	1990	4.486	2015	2018	

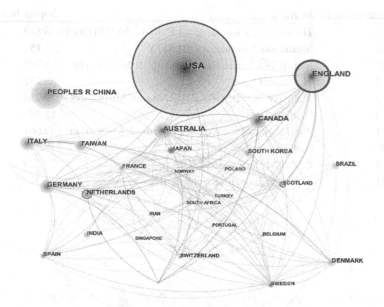

Fig. 5. Network of countries. The dimensions of the nodes represent centrality, the dimensions of the characters represent the rank of the country.

What emerges from countries analysis is that USA is the most authoritative country both in terms of scientific production and citation frequency. The network represented by Fig. 5 emphasizes the central position of USA. It displays a higher degree of connections with other countries and it's represented by the biggest node in the network.

Another interesting observation is that Brazil and Portugal got interested and to published in this field in the last four years, Brazil has produced over 50 publications in this period indeed.

3.3   Journals

Influential journals in the specific fields of anthropometry and scan are listed in Table 3, specifically, Fig. 6 represents the journals' co-citation analysis and the top five are represented by the biggest nodes on the right-hand side of the network. Co-citation is defined as the frequency with which two documents are cited together by other documents. In this case, if two journals are cited together by at least another journal, the two journals are defined as co-cited. If at least one other document cites two documents in common these documents are said to be co-cited. The more co-citations two documents receive, the higher their co-citation strength, and the more likely they are semantically related.

Table 3. Citations count and impact factors of journals.

Citation counts	Journals	Impact factor
445	The American journal of CLINICAL NUTRITION	6.549
358	International journal of OBESITY	5.151
330	Journal of Clinical Endocrinology & Metabolism	5.789
317	The Lancet	53.252
272	The NEW ENGLAND JOURNAL of MEDICINE	79.258
210	Diabetes Care	13.397
201	The Journal of the American Medical Association	47.661
187	Diabetes	7.273
187	British Medical Journal BJM	23.295
181	American Journal of Epidemiology	4.322

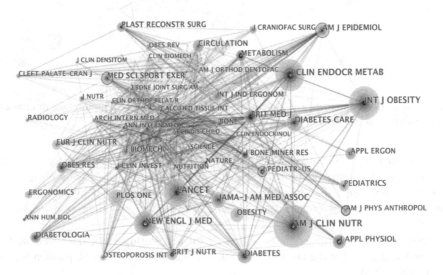

Fig. 6. Co-citation network of journals. The dimensions of the nodes represent centrality. The dimensions of the nodes represent centrality, the dimensions of the characters represent the rank of the journal.

3.4   References

The co-citation analysis allows to individualize the most cited references in the field investigated. We focused on the highly-cited documents in this area that are most influential papers in the area of anthropometry and scan domain [16–18]. We set a threshold of at least 7 citations per publication in the graphic representation in Fig. 7. While Table 4 reports the most influential publications in the domain from 1990 to 2018.

Table 4. Top ranked articles by citations count.

Citations count	Papers
20	Fox CS, 2007, CIRCULATION, 116, 39
16	Ball R, 2010, APPL ERGON, 41, 832
14	Daanen HAM, 2013, DISPLAYS, 34, 270
13	Wong JY, 2008, CLEFT PALATE-CRAN J, 45, 232
13	Han H, 2010, INT J IND ERGONOM, 40, 530
13	Robinette KM, 2006, APPL ERGON, 37, 259
13	Kouchi M, 2011, APPL ERGON, 42, 518
13	Witana CP, 2006, INT J IND ERGONOM, 36, 789
12	Lu JM, 2008, EXPERT SYST APPL, 35, 407
12	Aldridge K, 2005, AM J MED GENET A, 138A, 247

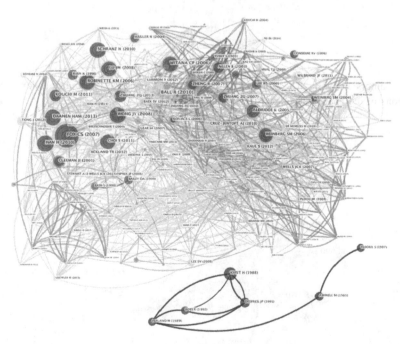

Fig. 7. Network of document co-citations. The dimensions of the nodes represent centrality, the dimensions of the characters represent the rank of the article rank.

3.5   Authors

In regards to the most active researchers in the topic of scan and anthropometry, clearly there are few authors that distinguish from others. ZHANG Y. with 9 citations, SFORZA C. with 7 citations, ZHANG X. with 7 citations and LI ZZ. with 6 citations. Figure 8 shows all authors in this field. While authors co-citation analysis (Fig. 9) highlights the authors in term of their impact on the literature over the entire time span of the field indeed [16, 19, 20].

The purpose of this analysis is to focus on the relations within the society of authors who contribute to this topic research. As for journals co-cited analysis in this case provides information about how two authors are semantically related in terms of topics addressed since they are mentioned together.

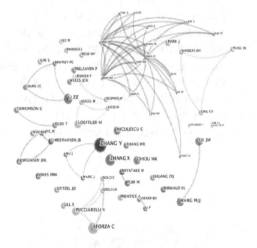

Fig. 8. Authors network. The dimensions of the nodes represent centrality index, and the dimensions of the characters represent the author's rank.

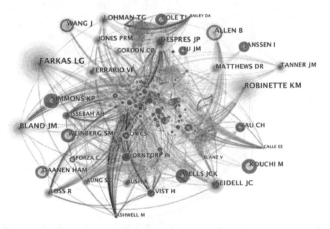

Fig. 9. Authors co-citation network. The dimensions of the nodes represent centrality index, and the dimensions of the characters represent the author's rank.

3.6   Institutions

In the same view as the countries analysis, according to Table 5 United States shows a clear predominance regarding the most influential universities in terms of citation count although University of Copenhagen holds the record for number of citations as it's graphically reported in Fig. 10.

Table 5. Citation counts for institution. The colors used in the histogram recall those used for nations in Fig. 2.

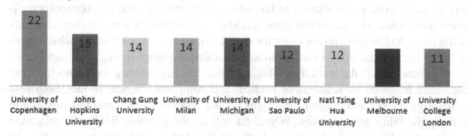

University of Copenhagen	Johns Hopkins University	Chang Gung University	University of Milan	University of Michigan	University of Sao Paulo	Natl Tsing Hua University	University of Melbourne	University College London
22	15	14	14	14	12	12		11

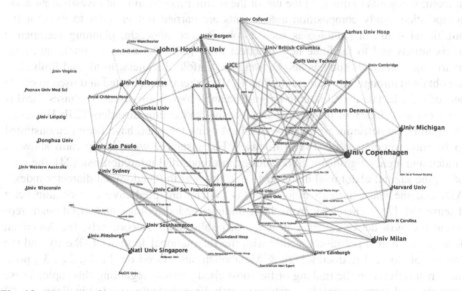

Fig. 10. Network of institutions. The dimensions of the nodes represent centrality index, and the dimensions of the characters represent the institution's rank.

4   Discussion

The study aims to analyse all the existing literature and citations about two topics, anthropometry and scan, that have been investigated together as a single field. The objective of this scientometrics analysis is to report all the information related to the current and future trends in this area.

Results highlight how the field of study investigated has expanded and evolved. Anthropometry research has developed since the 17th century [1, 21]; while, its association with scanner dates back to the nineties as displayed from the publication's years report. From nineties to nowadays, although the birth of anthropometry is much more dated, the use of the scans has allowed to obtain geometric measurements of the body, and in more recent times the use of 3D scanners has led to the achievement of three-dimensional body visualizations. Regarding the engineering field, continuous developments reflect the latest technological advances. Engineering represents the most cited area followed by subareas of medical and computer science. In fact, both new technological tools and clinical measurements are necessary to expand this research in both applicability and usability. While, among all the possible fields of application stands out medicine more than psychology and the clothing industry, meaning that the usefulness of these technologies has been widely exploited.

Specifically, endocrinology and metabolism constitute the most active publication domain, in regards to this field the use of the scanner mostly aims at investigating body composition. Body composition assessments are carried out in order to monitor the nutritional status in pathologies such as obesity and anorexia, planning therapeutic interventions and to facilitate new practical tools [22]. The most common anthropometric measurements such as height, weight, skinfold thickness, trunk and limb sizes are obtained through the scan employment. All of them are collected and used to create sets of reliable data useful in both prognostic and progression diseases' phases. BMI is the most used index in the domains of obesity and eating disorders [23]. However, other anthropometric measurements, obtained using the scan, have been demonstrated to be more predictive of several diseases. For instance, waist-to-hip ratio shows a graded and highly significant association with myocardial infarction risk [24], the ratio of supine sagittal abdominal diameter to mid-thigh girth ("abdominal diameter index"; AD) and the waist-to-thigh ratio of girths (WTR) are predictive of ischemic heart disease risk [25]. Therefore, from these findings endocrinology and metabolism represent the most active category in terms of publications. Accordingly, the American Journal of Clinical nutrition together with the International Journal of Obesity and the Journal of Clinical Endocrinology & Metabolism are placed on the 1_{st}, 2_{nd}, 3_{rd} positions respectively in the ranking of the most cited journals regarding this topic. These journals deal with arguments such as metabolic risk factors individualization, 3D whole-body scan applications and ergonomics fields.

Looking at the countries' investigation, USA currently holds the record for both citations and scientific production. In fact, this country owns two of the best scanners on the market. The first 3dMD body system is used in healthcare, mainly in digital dentistry, oral, maxillofacial and reconstructive plastic surgery; in research, for instance, in anthropology, biometrics, computer vision, ergonomic, product engineering, psychology, as well as others. The second is Canfiled Vectra XT, this scanner is mainly used in plastic surgery to help assess the risks and simulate the outcomes of plastic surgery interventions; it is able to capture in three dimensions the face, breast and the body images in ultra-high resolution within 3.5 ms capture time [26–28].

The bursts analysis has shown USA predominance in the literature panorama up to 2000, while, in more recent years other non-European and European countries catch the scene. While, considering the network institution, although USA is the most influential country in terms of citations and articles, so far, the University of Copenhagen is the most cited institution worldwide. This institution implies technologies such as DEXA scan in order to assess body composition [29, 30]. With respect to citations count, Yumei Zhang is the main authority within the field, affiliated to department of Nutrition of the School of Public Health of Beijing (China), his research predominantly focuses on nutritional problems and associated risk factors for metabolic and cardiovascular diseases among the Chinese population [31, 32]. On the other hand, the number two on this rank is an Italian researcher, Chiarella Sforza, affiliated to the Department of Biomedical Health Sciences, her studies are mainly related to human anatomy evaluation, such as three-dimensional analysis of human facial morphology [33, 34]. Authors with higher numbers of citations tend to be the scholars who drive the fundamental research in the field. While, from the authors co-cited network, which highlights authors in term of their impact on the literature over the entire time span considered and provides insights on most cited authors.

Farkas emerges as the most relevant one, he is considered the pioneer of craniofacial anthropometry. His lifelong devotion to research represents a major contribution to our understanding of the craniofacial complex. This author has collected more than 100 citations from other active authors in the field of scanner applications to anthropometry measures indeed.

The second most cited is Robinette, a researcher who focused on anthropometric differences comparing faces' morphology and analysing age-related changes [35–37]. Both authors have drawn the principles of anthropometric measurements, thus, their works are considered milestones in this area.

Turning to the citations' network the most cited papers investigate body composition, in order to define metabolism risk factors [38]; head shape anthropometric analysis through 3D scanner [39] and 3D whole body scanner usability and applicability [40, 41].

Therefore, it is reasonable to suppose that human body shape analysis deriving from 3D sensors has a real possibility to improve public health in a society where obesity and related metabolic and cardiovascular risks are pandemic.

Overall, the use of scanners for anthropometric analysis, specifically 3D whole body scanner, leads to quickly obtain body-shape reliable information providing high quality images with non-invasive optical methods. Since clinical applications and technologies developments are constantly evolving, many aspects should be further investigated within the area of research. In regards to all keys factors analysed, this paper provides information about the current state of art in this field, additionally, it may elucidate on perspectives and challenges expected in the future.

Acknowledgments. The present work was supported by the European funded project "Body-Pass"-API-ecosystem for cross-sectional exchange of 3D personal data (H2020-779780).

References

1. Utkualp, N., Ercan, I.: Anthropometric measurements usage in medical sciences. Biomed. Res. Int. **2015**, 7 (2015)
2. Breno, M., Leirs, H., Van Dongen, S.: Traditional and geometric morphometrics for studying skull morphology during growth in Mastomys natalensis (Rodentia: Muridae). J. Mammal. **92**(6), 1395–1406 (2011)
3. Madden, A.M., Smith, S.: Body composition and morphological assessment of nutritional status in adults: a review of anthropometric variables. J. Hum. Nutr. Dietietics **29**, 1–19 (2014)
4. Heymsfield, S.B., et al.: Digital anthropometry: a critical review. Eur. J. Clin. Nutr. **72**, 680–687 (2018)
5. Pedroli, E., et al.: The use of 3D body scanner in medicine and psychology: a narrative review. In: Cipresso, P., Serino, S., Ostrovsky, Y., Baker, Justin T. (eds.) MindCare 2018. LNICST, vol. 253, pp. 74–83. Springer, Cham (2018). https://doi.org/10.1007/978-3-030-01093-5_10
6. Mölbert, S.C., et al.: Assessing body image in anorexia nervosa using biometric self-avatars in virtual reality: attitudinal components rather than visual body size estimation are distorted. Psycholol. Med. **73**, 38–46 (2018)
7. Cornelissen, K.K., et al.: Body size estimation in women with anorexia nervosa and healthy controls using 3D avatars. Sci. Rep. **17**, 15773 (2017)
8. Wells, J.C.K., Ruto, A., Treleaven, P.: Whole-body three-dimensional photonic scanning: a new technique for obesity research and clinical practice. Int. J. Obes. **32**, 232–238 (2008)
9. Ng, B.K., et al.: Clinical anthropometrics and body composition from 3D whole-body surface scans. Eur. J. Clin. Nutr. **70**, 1265 (2016)
10. Haleem, A., Javaid, M.: 3D scanning applications in medical field: a literature-based review. Clin. Epidemiol. Glob. Health **7**, 199–210 (2018)
11. Pleuss, J.D., et al.: A machine learning approach relating 3D body scans to body composition in humans. Eur. J. Clin. Nutr. (2018)
12. Chen, C.: CiteSpace II: detecting and visualizing emerging trends and transient patterns in scientific literature. J. Am. Soc. Inf. Sci. Technol. **57**(3), 359–377 (2006)
13. Brandes, U.: A faster algorithm for betweenness centrality. J. Math. Sociol. **25**(2), 163–177 (2001)
14. Freeman, L.C.: A set of measures of centrality based on betweenness. Sociometry **40**(1), 35 (1977)
15. Kleinberg, J.: Bursty and hierarchical structure in streams. Data Min. Knowl. Discov. **7**(4), 373–397 (2003)
16. González-Teruel, A., González-Alcaide, G., Barrios, M., Abad-García, M.F.: Mapping recent information behavior research: an analysis of co-authorship and co-citation networks. Scientometrics **103**(2), 687–705 (2015)
17. Orosz, K., Farkas, L.J., Pollner, P.: Quantifying the changing role of past publications. Scientometrics **108**(2), 829–853 (2016)
18. Small, H.: Co-citation in the scientific literature: a new measure of the relationship between two documents. J. Am. Soc. Inf. Sci. **24**(4), 265–269 (1973)

19. Bu, Y., Liu, T.Y., Huang, W.B.: MACA: a modified author co-citation analysis method combined with general descriptive metadata of citations. Scientometrics **108**(1), 143–166 (2016)

20. White, H.D., Griffith, B.C.: Author cocitation: a literature measure of intellectual structure. J. Am. Soc. Inf. Sci. **32**(3), 163–171 (1981)

21. Ulijaszek, T.J. Lourie, J.A.: Intra- and inter-observer error in anthropometric measurement. Anthropometry, pp. 30–55

22. Madden, A.M., Smith, S.: Body composition and morphological assessment of nutritional status in adults: a review of anthropometric variables. J. Hum. Nutr. Diet. **29**(1), 7–25 (2016)

23. Cole, T.J., Bellizzi, M.C., Flegal, K.M., Dietz, W.H.: Establishing a standard definition for child overweight and obesity worldwide: international survey. BMJ **320**(7244), 1240–1243 (2000)

24. Yusuf, S., et al.: Obesity and the risk of myocardial infarction in 27 000 participants from 52 countries: a case-control study. Lancet **366**(9497), 1640–1649 (2005)

25. Kahn, H.S., Austin, H., Williamson, D.F., Arensberg, D.: Simple anthropometric indices associated with ischemic heart disease. J. Clin. Epidemiol. **49**(9), 1017–1024 (1996)

26. Treleaven, P., Wells, J.: 3D Body scanning and healthcare applications. Computer **40**(7), 28–34 (2007)

27. Tzou, C.-H.J., et al.: Comparison of three-dimensional surface-imaging systems. J. Plast. Reconstr. Aesthet. Surg. **67**(4), 489–497 (2014)

28. Weinberg, S.M., Naidoo, S., Govier, D.P., Martin, R.A., Kane, A.A., Marazita, M.L.: Anthropometric precision and accuracy of digital three-dimensional photogrammetry: comparing the Genex and 3dMD imaging systems with one another and with direct anthropometry. J. Craniofac. Surg. **17**(3), 477–483 (2006)

29. Haarbo, J., Gotfredsen, A., Hassager, C., Christiansen, C.: Validation of body composition by dual energy X-ray absorptiometry (DEXA). Clin. Physiol. **11**(4), 331–341 (1991)

30. Jensen, S.M., Mølgaard, C., Ejlerskov, K.T., Christensen, L.B., Michaelsen, K.F., Briend, A.: Validity of anthropometric measurements to assess body composition, including muscle mass, in 3-year-old children from the SKOT cohort. Matern. Child Nutr. **11**(3), 398–408 (2015)

31. Yu, K., Xue, Y., He, T., Guan, L., Zhao, A., Zhang, Y.: Association of spicy food consumption frequency with serum lipid profiles in older people in China. J. Nutr. Health Aging **22**(3), 311–320 (2018)

32. Zhao, A., et al.: Knowledge, attitude, and practice (KAP) of dairy products in Chinese urban population and the effects on dairy intake quality. Nutrients **9**(7), 668 (2017)

33. Ferrario, V.F., Sforza, C., Zanotti, G., Tartaglia, G.M.: Maximal bite forces in healthy young adults as predicted by surface electromyography. J. Dent. **32**(6), 451–457 (2004)

34. Sforza, C., de Menezes, M., Ferrario, V.: Soft- and hard-tissue facial anthropometry in three dimensions: what's new. J. Anthropol. Sci. **91**, 159–184 (2013)

35. Farkas, L.G., Eiben, O.G., Sivkov, S., Tompson, B., Katic, M.J., Forrest, C.R.: Anthropometric measurements of the facial framework in adulthood: age-related changes in eight age categories in 600 healthy white North Americans of European ancestry from 16 to 90 years of age. J. Craniofac. Surg. **15**(2), 288–298 (2004)

36. Farkas, L.G., Katic, M.J., Forrest, C.R.: International anthropometric study of facial morphology in various ethnic groups/races. J. Craniofacial. Surg. **16**(4), 615–646 (2005)

37. Robinette, K.M., Daanen, H., Paquet, E.: The CAESAR project: a 3-D surface anthropometry survey. In: Second International Conference on 3-D Digital Imaging and Modeling (Cat. No. PR00062), pp. 380–386. IEEE (1999)

38. Fox, C.S., et al.: Abdominal visceral and subcutaneous adipose tissue compartments: association with metabolic risk factors in the Framingham Heart Study. Circulation **116**(1), 39–48 (2007)
39. Ball, R., Shu, C., Xi, P., Rioux, M., Luximon, Y., Molenbroek, J.: A comparison between Chinese and Caucasian head shapes. Appl. Ergon. **41**(6), 832–839 (2010)
40. Daanen, H.A.M., Ter Haar, F.B.: 3D whole body scanners revisited. Displays **34**(4), 270–275 (2013)
41. Daanen, H.M., van de Water, G.J.: Whole body scanners. Displays **19**(3), 111–120 (1998)

Immersive Episodic Memory Assessment with 360° Videos: The Protocol and a Case Study

Claudia Repetto[1(✉)], Silvia Serino[2], Mauro Maldonato[3],
Teresa Longobardi[4], Raffaele Sperandeo[4], Daniela Iennaco[4],
and Giuseppe Riva[1,5]

[1] Department of Psychology, Università Cattolica del Sacro Cuore,
20100 Milan, Italy
{claudia.repetto,giuseppe.riva}@unicatt.it
[2] MySpace Lab, Department of Clinical Neurosciences,
University Hospital Lausanne (CHUV), 1011 Lausanne, Switzerland
silvia.serino@gmail.com
[3] Dipartimento di Neuroscienze, Scienze Riproduttive e Odontostomatologiche,
Università di Napoli Federico II, 80138 Naples, Italy
nelsonmauro.maldonato@unina.it
[4] School of Integrated Gestalt Psychotherapy, 80058 Torre Annunziata, Italy
{teresalongobardi,raffaelesperandeo,
danielaiennaco}@sipgi.it
[5] Applied Technology for Neuro-Psychology Laboratory,
Istituto Auxologico Italiano, 20149 Milan, Italy

Abstract. Episodic memory has been conceptualized as the memory for personal events with specific spatiotemporal components. The assessment of episodic memory is usually conducted by means of verbal recall tasks, in which the individual is required to repeat what (s)he remembers from a previously presented verbal material (either single words or a brief story). However, the need of a more ecological approach to memory assessment led researchers to investigate the potential use of 360° videos as a suitable tool to present real life scenes to be remembered. The present study presents the protocol of the assessment of episodic memory employing five 360° video that represent interpersonal, emotional experiences known to be altered in psychopathological conditions. Furthermore, a case study in which the assessment protocol is applied to a patient with Borderline Personality Disorder is described. The results of the case study seem to indicate that our 360° videos are able to detect anomalies in remembering the behaviors displayed, the connected emotion together with details regarding the "where" and "when" components of the episodic recall.

Keywords: 360° videos · Episodic memory · Assessment ·
Borderline Personality Disorder

© ICST Institute for Computer Sciences, Social Informatics and Telecommunications Engineering 2019
Published by Springer Nature Switzerland AG 2019. All Rights Reserved
P. Cipresso et al. (Eds.): MindCare 2019, LNICST 288, pp. 117–128, 2019.
https://doi.org/10.1007/978-3-030-25872-6_9

1 Introduction

A more ecological evaluation of episodic memory has challenged both researchers and clinicians in the last 20 years. From the pivotal definition of Tulving [1, 2], episodic memory has been traditionally conceptualized as the memory for personally first-person perspective events, with a specific spatiotemporal context. Typically, verbal paradigms are used to evaluate episodic memory function: participants are invited to remember a list of words, and then they are tested on that specific list. However, the need for a more naturalist approach to memory recently emerges, along with the use of self-relevant and everyday material, able to predict behaviors also in real-life contexts [3, 4]. A first trend is the use of Virtual Reality (VR) technology for developing an innovative assessment of episodic memory simulating everyday activities, but maintain also a strict control over the stimuli delivery [5–7]. Thanks to the use of VR, participants are completely immersed in highly ecological environments (i.e., a city, a park,) where it is possible to easily insert everyday events experienced in first-person perspective with their perceptual and affective details (i.e., a lady with a crying baby, a group of children playing soccer, etc.). Interesting examples were offered in Piolino's works [8–11]. In particular, Plancher et al. [11] exploited the potentiality of VR-based tools to better understand the cognitive profile of patients suffering from mild cognitive impairments and Alzheimer's Disease (AD). Participants were immersed in a virtual city (either in passive or active navigation) to remember a series of events; consistently with literature, they found that a deficit in remembering personally experienced events for patients with AD, but they also noted that active navigation was able to improve performance for all groups.

A more recent trend for the ecological evaluation of episodic memory function is the possibility to immerse participants in real environments and explore them from a first-person perspective thanks to the use of 360° technology [12, 13]. This technology records a circular fisheye view of the environment, and then participants can easily view the realistic 360° scenarios with a tablet (i.e., non immersive experience) or through a head mounted display (i.e., immersive experience). 360° technology allows the assessment of mnestic processes in a controlled and safe setting within real-life scenarios [13]. Moreover, it is a quite affordable technology, without any specific technical skills to be mastered. In the current work, we exploited the potentiality of 360° technology for episodic memory assessment focusing on individuals with borderline personality disorder (BPD). We studied BPD since previous studies have found specific memory biases in autobiographical recall for these patients [14, 15]. In particular, Winter et al. [16] highlighted the presence of a negative evaluation bias for positive, self-referential information in BPD. This bias did not influence the ability to store personal information, but their quality: it is related to self-attributions of negative events in daily life situations.

2 Methods

2.1 Materials

Five 360° videos were recorded for the purpose of the study. 360° videos are special videos recorded by omnidirectional cameras that capture images from all the space around. These videos can be played by wearing a head-mounted display (HMD) or they can be visualized by means of a smartphone provided with gyroscope and combined with a cardboard. Anyway, the user can explore the environment represented within the video by turning the head up-down-left and right, but (s)he cannot select the direction of the navigation (the navigation path is determined at the moment of the recording). Each video had been recorded in a different environment and included four actors, one of whom was always silent. The other three interacted among each other and the conversation focused on a specific topic, which constituted the core material to be remembered. Indeed, the content of four out of five video was a description of an interpersonal, emotional experience that is known to be altered in psychopathological conditions. In these videos functional and suitable behaviors are depicted in contexts of social and interpersonal relations challenging the coping abilities of psychopathological patients. The fifth video represented a control condition, in which a situation without emotional load and describing a very neutral personal exchange among characters is described. Table 1 illustrates the specific content of each video. Videos duration ranged from 40 s to 1 min and 10 s.

Table 1. Videos' content and dialogues.

	Context	Interpersonal/emotional function	Topic	Actors
Video name	ORAL EXAM	School class	Stable and coherent self consciousness within the boundaries suitable for the role assumed	To manage stunt attempts	1 professor (F); 3 students (2 F, 1 M)
Dialogue (synthesis)	Prof.: "Please tell me about the Second Global War"			
	Student 1: "Prof. I'm sorry but I did not understand that the topic had to be studied... Last week I was absent, you know... I told you that my grandmother had been admitted to the Hospital"			
	Prof: "Yes, I perfectly remember. However, I explained the Second Global War al least one month ago"			
	Student 1: "I know, but please, I am in troubles in this period, I feel confused... can you try with another question?			
	Prof. "Sorry, but this is the third time I test your knowledge, and you are always unprepared. Now I will give you an insufficient grade. You, instead, can you say something about the Second Global War?			
	Student 2: "The second Global War started in 1939... (*going further to give the complete and correct response*)			
Video name	COURTYARD	Yard with benches	Intimate reflection about past personal experiences, attributing meaning to them	To manage a conflict	4 friends (F)

(*continued*)

Table 1. (*continued*)

	Context	Interpersonal/emotional function	Topic	Actors
Dialogue (synthesis)	1: "I'm very disappointed… I did not expect this message from you… How could you blame me?"			
	2: "Actually I wrote that message because I was very angry with you. But now I'm thinking….			
	1: "Look, after this message I am very unwilling to listen to you!"			
	2: "Wait… It already happened to me to lose a fried for my fault. I friend of mine trusted me and I stupidly reported her secret to someone else. I did not apologize immediately and so I lose a very important friend. Therefore, Even though I am still angry with you, I apologize because I acknowledge my words sounded bad"			
	3: "It is important to be clear to each other, in order to save the friendship"			
	1: "You are right, our relation is very important to me too. I apologize as well…"			
Video name	HOUSE	Kitchen, around a table	Ability to acknowledge and respect others' points of views, even if not agreed	To disagree with others while being respectful	2 couples (wife and husband)
Dialogue (synthesis)	Wife 1: "Yesterday I discussed with my daughter …she wants to come home at midnight on Saturday, because Lucia is going to have a party for her birthday"			
	Wife2: "Also Chiara wants to go to the Lucia's party… Finally, we agreed, she can come home at 1 a.m."			
	Wife 1: "Really? I absolutely disagree…. I think we should set some limits at this age…."			
	Wife 2: "I understand your point of view and I respect it. But, in my opinion, it is also important trust adolescents and to see how they manage this freedom			
	Husband 1: "For me, it was important to grow up with limits. I learned a lot while negotiating with my parents"			
	Wife 1: "I understand you point… but I agree with my husband. Adolescents must earn the freedom they want			
Video name	OFFICE	office, desks and computers	Ability to collaborate for the common good	To give up your own benefits for the common good	1 man, 3 colleagues (F)
Dialogue (synthesis)	Man: "Great! I'm done. Now I can leave the office and enjoy the weekend…. I will go to the lake with my girlfriend			
	Colleague 1: "Lucky you! we are in the weeds…We have to accomplish the project by Monday… probably we will work all the weekend….			
	Man: "oh… I did not know about this deadline…. Well, then I will stay with you and working together we will finish sooner			
	Colleague 2: "It would be great if you could help us… but, unfortunately, I don't know whether we could put your name on the project….			
	Colleague 1: "thank you very much… I would not ask you to stay if this wouldn't be so important for the future of the whole company"			

(*continued*)

Table 1. (*continued*)

		Context	Interpersonal/emotional function	Topic	Actors
Video name	UNIVERSITY	Open space	Neutral	To provide/ask for information	2 boys 2 girls
Dialogue (synthesis)	Boy 1: "Did you read that the economy classroom has changed?"				
	Boy 2: "yes, the economy lesson will take place in room A3. I don't know where it is, let's ask someone…				
	Boy 1: "Excuse me, do you know where the room A3 is located?"				
	Girl 1: "sorry, I'm a freshman and I did not learn yet all the classes location"				
	Boy 2: "Don't worry, we will ask you the custodians who probably have a map."				

2.2 Protocol

The study is composed by two independent sessions that take place in different days to avoid interference effects of the materials. The order of the sessions is interchangeable and is counterbalanced across participants.

Neuropsychological Assessment. All the participants undergo a brief neuropsychological assessment to evaluate basic cognitive abilities. The battery includes an evaluation of short and long-term verbal memory [story recall "Anna Pesenti", [17]], sustained attention [Attention Matrices, [17]], attention shifting [Trail Making Test [18]] and verbal fluency with both semantic and phonetic cues [17].

Immersive Episodic Memory Assessment. At the beginning of this session the participant is introduced to the use of the cardboard/HMD and the 360° videos. Specifically, the experimenter illustrates the exploration capabilities of the device, underscoring the fact that the movement of the head allows the visualization of the correspondent portion of the environment. When the participant demonstrates to be familiar with the equipment the video administration can start. The experimenter provides the participants the following instructions: "*now you will be presented with 5 videos, each one set in a different location and involving 4 actors. Your job is to pay attention to the content of the conversation, to who is speaking and what (s)he is saying, and to whatever detail of the video. Upon video visualization, I will ask you to tell me what you remember*". All the videos are presented without breaks in the between, but before playing each video the experimenter clearly claims the video's title. The order of presentation is counterbalanced across participants, so that each video is seen in each of the five available positions. At the end of the last video, the Free Recall test starts. The participant is invited to described what (s)he remembers of each of the video presented, following the same presentation order. The recall is audiotaped. Afterwards, the Cued Recall is administered. This test includes 5 questions for each video, exploring the following topics: 1. the general content of the dialogue; 2. some details of the dialogue; 3. the spatial disposition of the actors; 4. the attitude of

one of the characters; 5. the timing of a given episode. The next step is the administration of a 3-questions survey investigating the following: 1. the extent to which while
remembering the video the participant had the subjective impression to re-live the
experience; 2. the evaluation of the valence of the emotion mostly represented within
the video; 3. the name of the emotion mostly represented within the video. After a
delay of 30 min, the Free Recall is repeated (Delayed Free Recall). During the pause,
the participants undergo an activity not involving memory abilities. Figure 1 depicts
the experimental protocol.

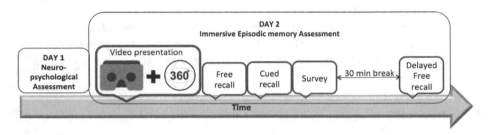

Fig. 1. The protocol of the study. Of note, the session order can be reversed.

Tests Scoring. The Free Recall grid score (see Table 2) includes 4 categories:

a. Main event represented: for each video 4 main elements, essential to understand and
   describe the content of the conversation, had been identified (see the list on
   Table 2). The score ranges from 0 to 4 according to the number of elements
   remembered.
b. Actors: the identity and number of actors represented in the video should be
   reported (score: 0–4)
c. Details: whatever detail remembered is worth 1 point (i.e.: specific people named
   during the conversation; details of the environment in which the scene is played,
   details about the actors, such as clothing, physical features; position of the actors); if
   the egocentric position of the actors is reported 1 additional point is attributed.
d. Errors: false memories are also recorded

The Cued Recall questionnaire is scored assigning 1 point to each correct response
(range: 0–20).

The post-video survey has 2 five- points Likert questions [n.1], "have you got the
impression to remember the details as if your were re-living the scene in your mind?"
ranging from 1 (not al all) to 5 (very much); n.2 "how do you rate the emotion
emerging from the interaction among actors?" ranging from 1 (very negative) to 5 (very
positive). The last question is open and the participant has to write down the name of
the prevalent emotion recognized in the video.

Table 2. The Free Recall scoring grid. In black the items C. remembered in the Free Recall, in red those remembered in the Delayed Free Recall.

		Category		
	Main event	**Actors**	**Details**	**Errors**
ORAL EXAM	Student's interrogation ☑☑	prof (F) ☑☑	5	1
	Adducing excuses	student (F) ☑☑	6	2
	Teacher's reply ☑☑	student (F) ☑		
	Second student's interrogation ☑☑	student (M) ☑☑		
COURTYARD	Accusation ☑☑	friend (F) ☑☑	5	0
	Reflection about past experience ☑☑	friend (F) ☑☑	6	1
	Apologizing ☑☑	friend (F) ☑☑		
	Reciprocating excuses	friend (F) ☑☑		
HOUSE	Discussion about time to come back home	wife ☑☑	1	2
	Two couples with different perspectives	husband ☑☑	2	1
	Birthday party ☑☑	wife ☑☑		
	Limits and their value	husband		
OFFICE	Person that wants to leave the office for the weekend ☑☑	colleague (M) ☑☑	5	0
	Claiming the workload ☑☑	colleague (F) ☑☑	7	1
	Man's change of mind ☑☑	colleague (F) ☑☑		
	Thanksgiving ☑☑	colleague (F) ☑☑		
UNIVERSITY	Classroom change	boy ☑☑	4	3
	Request to the girls ☑☑	boy ☑☑	1	4
	Stating to ignore the information ☑☑	girl ☑☑		
	Alternative strategy ☑	girl ☑		
	TOT (max 20): 14 13	TOT (max 20): 19 17	TOT: 20 26	TOT: 6 9

3 Case Study

Claudia (a pseudonym) is a 19-years-old university student. Her family is composed by mother, father and a 33-years-old brother who had problems with drug addiction up to 3 years ago. She reports that he has begun to experience frequent and apparently unexplained headaches, sudden hand and jaw tremors, and heartbeat acceleration;

for these reasons she carried out various investigations (MRI and blood tests) which, however, have not highlighted any problem. Although the symptoms are obvious, C. feels misunderstood. C. has been engaged for two years with A. He reports that he has a good relationship with the boy, even if he does not really understand her current state of suffering and distress. Presently, the girl has no friends, except for two schoolmates with whom she rarely talks. She tells of having gone through a difficult childhood and adolescence: indeed, during the years of elementary and middle schools her commitment was devalued and her difficulties, caused by strabismus, were confused with a lack of commitment and will. She is currently treated by a psychiatrist with paroxetine and diazepam; at the same time she is undergoing a psychotherapy with a male therapist she trusts a lot.

3.1 Psychological Examination

C. arrives at the evaluation on request of the psychiatrist. She is collaborative. The facial expression is marked by anxiety and restlessness. The state of consciousness is alert and sufficiently oriented in time and space. The course of thought is accelerated (tachipsychism) with frequent logical jumps, while the thought form is characterized by derailment (ideas deviate in a direction not apparently connected with the concept of departure) and tangentiality (response whose content is marginally, remotely or nothing at all related to the question). The language is characterized by logorrhea and incongruous syntax with respect to age and education (verbs declined incorrectly, need to repeat several times the questions, due to incongruent answers). She reports some disperceptive phenomena (auditory hallucinations: misperception of children voices in the street; perceptive hallucinations: moving objects; belief of being able to move objects with thought). The mood is labile (rapid alternation of opposite emotions - sudden transition from crying to smile) and dysphoric, characterized by variations due to low-relevance stimuli (access of uncontrolled rage). Furthermore, a marked anxious symptomatology is detected, characterized by agitation, restlessness, tension, fatigue and difficulty in concentration; in addition, a panic disorder with agoraphobia emerges. Current suicidal risk is high, and some suicide attempts are reported (strangulation with a headscarf).

The psychodiagnostic examination includes the Dissociative Experiences Scale (DES-II; [19]), the Symptom Checklist-90-R (SCL-90, [20]) and the Structured Clinical Interview for the *DSM* (SCID-II, [21]). The DES-II score is 57.14, indicative of numerous dissociative experiences. In the SCL-90 the patient obtained the highest scores in the following symptomatological dimensions: somatization (score = 41), obsession-compulsivity (score = 31), depression (score = 38), anxiety (score = 27), and psychoticism (score = 22). The *Global Severity Index (GSI)*, indicating the intensity of the psychological distress level complained of by the patient, is 2.61; the *Positive Symptom Total* (PST), that describes the number of symptoms reported by the subject, is 9; the *Positive Symptom Distress Index* (PSDI), indicating the response style index, is 2.9. The SCID-II questionnaire underscores the presence of a Borderline Personality Disorder. At least, five criteria are needed for the diagnosis of the Borderline Personality Disorder (BDP).

As a result of the clinical and psychodiagnostic examination the patient appears to meet 7 criteria of the Borderline Personality Disorder (BDP). The patient is characterized by:

- A pattern of unstable and intense interpersonal relationships, characterized by the alternation between extremes of hyperidealization and devaluation.
- Alteration of identity: self-image or self-perceptions markedly and persistently unstable.
- Recurrent behaviour or suicidal threats, and self-mutilating behaviour (self-harm, cuts on arms and legs, cigarette burns).
- Affective instability due to marked mood reactivity (e.g. episodic intense dysphoria, irritability or anxiety, which usually lasts a few hours, and only rarely more than a few days).
- Chronic feelings of emptiness.
- Inappropriate, intense anger, or difficulty controlling anger (e.g. frequent anger or constant anger, recurring physical fights).
- Transitional paranoid ideation, associated with stress, or severe dissociative symptoms.

3.2   Immersive Episodic Memory Assessment: Results and Discussion

Table 2 displays the summary of the Free Recall and Delayed Free Recall. Figure 2 represents the patient's performance in the Cued Recall task.

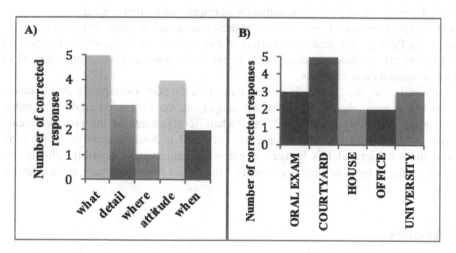

Fig. 2. The Cued Recall performance. In (A) The scores are calculated separately for the type of information requested: what, detail, where, attitude and when, aggregating the 5 vides. In (B) the performance in the different videos aggregating the type of information is displayed.

For what concerns the post-video survey, only the third question (the open one, investigating the prevalent emotion detected in each video) will be considered here.

C. identified the following emotions: fear (UNIVERSITY), anger (HOUSE), anger and compassion (COURTYARD), sadness (ORAL EXAM), and happiness (OFFICE).

As for the Free Recall, the patient remembered less than the 75% of the items pertaining the Main Event, at both the time points; the performance was better for the recall of the actors involved in the scenes (the characters not reported were usually those silent). Furthermore, more details as well as more errors were reported in the Delayed compared to the immediate recall. Looking at the differences among videos, it seems clear that in particular that titled "House" was less accurately recalled. Indeed, when describing the content of this video, C. missed all but one of the important elements of the conversation. This could indicate a specific difficulty in integrating coherently in personal memory behaviors demonstrating functional coping abilities in managing potential conflicting situations (of note, this specific video described a situation in which different points of view are presented and discussed respectfully, without anger). In the Cued Recall C. seemed to have more difficulties in remembering the "where" and "when" components of the episodic event, and the worst performance was obtained in the HOUSE (coherently with the Free Recall) and OFFICE videos. The post-video survey confirmed that C. is barely able to recognize the emotions and to catch the correct emotional content of the events represented. This is particularly true for the HOUSE video, in which C. states to have identified anger, but the actors discussed in a very respectful and calm way. Indeed, a recent study by Niedtfeld and colleagues [22] explained difficulties in emotional recognition in PBD with a general deficits in integrating social signals (i.e. speech content, variation in prosody, and facial expression) in a coherent way. Participants were invited to identify emotions in different short video clips (adapted from [23]) showing a person telling a self-related story. These video clips were specifically manipulated to represent different combinations of the three social signals: facial expression, speech content, and prosody. They found that PBD patients made more errors in emotion recognition compared to healthy controls whenever stimuli contained only facial expressions, and for combination of all three communication channels.

In conclusion, this case study demonstrates that the 360° videos were able to detect anomalies in remembering the behaviors displayed, the connected emotion together with details regarding the "where" and "when" components of the episodic recall. Further studies, with psychiatric samples compared to healthy controls will inform about the reliability of this immersive episodic memory test, possibly allowing to classify different types of diagnoses based on the different performances at the different videos.

References

1. Tulving, E.: Episodic memory: from mind to brain. Annu. Rev. Psychol. 53, 1–25 (2002). https://doi.org/10.1146/annurev.psych.53.100901.135114
2. Tulving, E.: Episodic memory and common sense: how far apart? Philos. Trans. R. Soc. Lond. Ser. B Biol. Sci. 356, 1505–1515 (2001). https://doi.org/10.1098/rstb.2001.0937

3. Parsons, T.D.: Virtual reality for enhanced ecological validity and experimental control in the clinical, affective and social neurosciences. Front. Hum. Neurosci. **9**, 660 (2015). https://doi.org/10.3389/fnhum.2015.00660

4. Parsons, T.D., Carlew, A.R., Magtoto, J., Stonecipher, K.: The potential of function-led virtual environments for ecologically valid measures of executive function in experimental and clinical neuropsychology. Neuropsychol. Rehabil. **27**, 777–807 (2017). https://doi.org/10.1080/09602011.2015.1109524

5. Bohil, C.J., Alicea, B., Biocca, F.A.: Virtual reality in neuroscience research and therapy. Nat. Rev. Neurosci. **12**, 752–762 (2011). https://doi.org/10.1038/nrn3122nrn3122

6. Parsons, T.D., Gaggioli, A., Riva, G.: Virtual reality for research in social neuroscience. Brain Sci. 7 (2017). https://doi.org/10.3390/brainsci7040042

7. Rizzo, A.A., Schultheis, M., Kerns, K.A., Mateer, C.: Analysis of assets for virtual reality applications in neuropsychology. Neuropsychol. Rehabil. **14**, 207–239 (2004). https://doi.org/10.1080/09602010343000183

8. Compère, L., et al.: Gender identity better than sex explains individual differences in episodic and semantic components of autobiographical memory and future thinking. Conscious. Cogn. **57**, 1–19 (2018). https://doi.org/10.1016/J.CONCOG.2017.11.001

9. Plancher, G., Gyselinck, V., Nicolas, S., Piolino, P.: Age effect on components of episodic memory and feature binding: a virtual reality study. Neuropsychology **24**, 379–390 (2010). https://doi.org/10.1037/a0018680

10. Plancher, G., Gyselinck, V., Piolino, P.: The integration of realistic episodic memories relies on different working memory processes: evidence from virtual navigation. Front. Psychol. **9**, 47 (2018). https://doi.org/10.3389/fpsyg.2018.00047

11. Plancher, G., Tirard, A., Gyselinck, V., Nicolas, S., Piolino, P.: Using virtual reality to characterize episodic memory profiles in amnestic mild cognitive impairment and Alzheimer's disease: influence of active and passive encoding. Neuropsychologia **50**, 592–602 (2012). https://doi.org/10.1016/j.neuropsychologia.2011.12.013

12. Negro Cousa, E., Brivio, E., Serino, S., Heboyan, V., Riva, G., de Leo, G.: New frontiers for cognitive assessment: an exploratory study of the potentiality of 360° technologies for memory evaluation. Cyberpsychol. Behav. Soc. Netw. Cyber. **2017**, 0720 (2018). https://doi.org/10.1089/cyber.2017.0720

13. Serino, S., Repetto, C.: New trends in episodic memory assessment: immersive 360° ecological videos. Front. Psychol. **9**, 1878 (2018). https://doi.org/10.3389/fpsyg.2018.01878

14. Minzenberg, M.J., Fisher-Irving, M., Poole, J.H., Vinogradov, S.: Reduced self-referential source memory performance is associated with interpersonal dysfunction in borderline personality disorder. J. Pers. Disord. **20**, 42–54 (2006). https://doi.org/10.1521/pedi.2006.20.1.42

15. Schnell, K., Dietrich, T., Schnitker, R., Daumann, J., Herpertz, S.C.: Processing of autobiographical memory retrieval cues in borderline personality disorder. J. Affect. Disord. **97**, 253–259 (2007). https://doi.org/10.1016/J.JAD.2006.05.035

16. Winter, D., Herbert, C., Koplin, K., Schmahl, C., Bohus, M., Lis, S.: Negative evaluation bias for positive self-referential information in borderline personality disorder. PLoS ONE **10**, e0117083 (2015). https://doi.org/10.1371/journal.pone.0117083

17. Spinnler, H., Tognoni, G.: Italian group on the neuropsychological study of ageing: Italian standardization and classification of neuropsychological tests. Ital. J. Neurol. Sci. **8**, 1–120 (1987)

18. Giovagnoli, A.R., Del Pesce, M., Mascheroni, S., Simoncelli, M., Laiacona, M., Capitani, E.: Trail making test: normative values from 287 normal adult controls. Ital. J. Neurol. Sci. **17**, 305–309 (1996). https://doi.org/10.1007/BF01997792

19. Schimmenti, A.: Dissociative experiences and dissociative minds: exploring a nomological network of dissociative functioning. J. Trauma Dissociation. **17**, 338–361 (2016). https://doi.org/10.1080/15299732.2015.1108948

20. Derogatis, L.R.: Symptom Checklist-90-R: Administration, Scoring, and Procedures Manual, 3rd edn. National Computer Systems, Minneapolis (1994)

21. First, M.B.: Structured clinical interview for the DSM (SCID). In: The Encyclopedia of Clinical Psychology, pp. 1–6. John Wiley & Sons, Inc., Hoboken (2015)

22. Niedtfeld, I., et al.: Facing the problem: impaired emotion recognition during multimodal social information processing in borderline personality disorder. J. Pers. Disord. **31**, 273–288 (2017). https://doi.org/10.1521/pedi_2016_30_248

23. Regenbogen, C., et al.: The differential contribution of facial expressions, prosody, and speech content to empathy. Cogn. Emot. **26**, 995–1014 (2012). https://doi.org/10.1080/02699931.2011.631296

An Internet-Based Intervention for Depressive Symptoms: Preliminary Data on the Contribution of Behavioral Activation and Positive Psychotherapy Strategies

Sonia Romero[1]([✉]), Adriana Mira[1,2], Juana Bretón-Lopez[1,3],
Amanda Díaz-García[1], Laura Díaz-Sanahuja[1],
Azucena García-Palacios[1,3], and Cristina Botella[1,3]

[1] Department of Basic Psychology, Clinic and Psychobiology,
Universitat Jaume I, Castellón, Spain
soniarom90@gmail.com, lauradiazsanahuja@gmail.com,
{miraa,breton}@psb.uji.es,
{amdiaz,azucena,botella}@uji.es
[2] Department of Psychology and Sociology,
Universidad de Zaragoza, Teruel, Spain
[3] CIBER Fisiopatología Obesidad y Nutrición (CIBERobn),
Instituto Salud Carlos III, Santiago de Compostela, Spain

Abstract. Depression is one of the most prevalent mental disorders worldwide. Cognitive Behavioral Therapy is a well-known evidence-based therapy. However, interventions are multi-component, and we do not know the specific mechanisms responsible for the change produced by depression therapies. Therapeutic components of most interventions have focused on reducing negative symptoms rather than on improving positive affect, well-being, and character strengths. Positive Psychotherapeutic strategies (PPs) are designed to fill this gap. These PPs have shown efficacy in improving depressive symptoms. Nonetheless, we do not know the specific contribution of a PPs component. Internet-based interventions are effective in treating depression. Using a dismantling design, we are currently carrying out a randomized controlled trial with the objective of evaluating the efficacy of an Internet-based protocol for depressive symptoms (including Behavioral Activation and PPs), the protocol without the PPs component, and the protocol without the BA component. In the present paper, we present preliminary results of nine participants randomized to one of the three conditions, exploring the pre-treatment to post-treatment changes and presenting the qualitative data on the participants' opinions of the BA and PPs. Participants in the intervention groups with the BA component presented greater improvements in their negative affect and depression; and participants in the PPs improved their positive affect and resilience. Regarding usefulness, the BA group pointed to the improvement in their relationships and to knowing that the activity is related to their mood, and the PPs learned about their psychological strength and saw the positive side of things more.

Keywords: Depression · Dismantling studies · Internet-based intervention · Behavioral Activation · Positive Psychotherapy strategies

© ICST Institute for Computer Sciences, Social Informatics and Telecommunications Engineering 2019
Published by Springer Nature Switzerland AG 2019. All Rights Reserved
P. Cipresso et al. (Eds.): MindCare 2019, LNICST 288, pp. 129–146, 2019.
https://doi.org/10.1007/978-3-030-25872-6_10

1   Introduction

Major Depressive Disorder (MDD) is one of the most prevalent and disabling mental disorders in the general population [1, 2]. The total estimated number of people living with depression increased by 18.4% between 2005 and 2015, and in the case of Spain, prevalence data show that 5.2% of the population suffers from depression [3]. Among the many interventions for depression treatment, the evidence supporting Cognitive Behavioral Therapy (CBT) [4–6] is well known. Numerous randomized controlled studies have shown that CBT is superior to wait-list, non-specific controls, or treatment as usual [7]. CBT for MDD is based on promoting change in certain patterns of maladjusted thinking, focusing not only on the use of cognitive techniques, but also on the use of behavioral procedures, which are fundamental in this change [8].

Among the components of CBT, the literature shows that the Behavioral Activation (BA) component is essential in the treatment of depression, indicating that its efficacy is equivalent to that of the complete treatment [9, 10]. Many "behavioral activation" interventions, as formulated by Jacobson [11], are considered well-established treatments for major depression [6, 12].

As mentioned above, the BA component has been found to be important in depression treatment. However, interventions for MDD are multi-component, and we do not know much about the specific mechanisms responsible for the change produced by depression therapies [13, 14].

Furthermore, therapeutic components of most depression interventions have focused on reducing negative symptoms (depressive and anxiety symptoms, negative affect, anxiety, etc.), rather than on improving positive affect, well-being, and character strengths [15]. Depressive symptoms often involve lack of engagement and a lack of purpose in life, as well as low levels of positive emotions. Consequently, low levels of positive affect are more strongly linked to depression than to other emotional disorders [16]. For this reason, Positive Psychotherapeutic strategies (PPs) are designed to fill this gap. These interventions, particularly in depression, have shown efficacy in improving depressive symptoms and enhancing well-being [17, 18]. Therefore, many authors defend the need for positive interventions that promote gratitude, resilience, positive affect, and positive functioning [15], as important elements of depression treatments [19, 20].

Nonetheless, as in the case of the BA component, we do not know the specific contribution of a PPs component to the change experienced by patients in depression therapies [13, 14]. Carrying out component studies (dismantling or additive) may provide a more direct way to identify the active ingredients in psychotherapy [21], and find out whether a specific active ingredient in psychotherapy contributes to differential outcomes [22].

In addition, one of the most important challenges in CBTs for depression is to design new ways to apply treatments in order to maximize their efficiency and dissemination [23, 24]. The results obtained for Internet-based interventions show that these interventions are effective in treating depression [25–27]. Nevertheless, most Internet-based intervention programs for depression are also multi-component, and it is important to make progress in investigating the contribution of each isolated component to the intervention.

In order to find out the contribution of PPs in effective interventions for depression and improve their dissemination through Internet-based programs, our research group developed an Internet-based CBT program that also includes PPs for depressive symptoms. Its efficacy has been shown in different RCTs [28–30]. However, we do not know the specific contribution of each of its therapeutic components. A dismantling strategy could help us to identify the contribution of the main therapeutic components of the intervention to the therapeutic change. There are few studies with a dismantling design in interventions for depression [31]. A recent comprehensive systematic review and meta-analysis of dismantling studies of psychotherapies for adult depression included only 16 studies [32]. None of them used an Internet-based intervention or an intervention with a PPs component [32].

Using a dismantling design, we are currently carrying out a randomized controlled trial to evaluate the efficacy of this Internet-based Global protocol for depressive symptoms developed by our research group (including motivation, psychoeducation, cognitive restructuring, BA, PPs, Relapse prevention) [28–30]; the protocol for depressive symptoms without the PPs component; and the protocol for depressive symptoms without the BA component. All of them are administered through the Internet.

The purpose of the present article is to show the preliminary results we obtained in nine participants randomized to one of the three conditions. The objectives are to explore the pre-treatment to post-treatment changes in some different positive and negative functioning measures in the three intervention conditions and observe the differences between them. Furthermore, we also present the qualitative data on the opinions of the patients in the BA and PPs components.

2 Method

2.1 Design

The study presents preliminary data from a three-armed, simple-blinded, randomized controlled clinical trial with a dismantling design. Nine participants were randomly allocated to one of the three experimental conditions: Internet-based Global protocol condition (IGc), Internet-based BA protocol condition (IBAc), Internet-based PPs protocol condition (IPPc). This study is ongoing, and we are continuing to recruit participants. The participants' randomization was stratified according to levels of severity of depression symptomatology. Therefore, the randomization to each condition was carried out within each stratum in order to ensure that all the levels of depression were equally represented in the three intervention conditions. This study is being conducted following the CONSORT statement (Consolidated Standards of Reporting Trials, http://www.consort-statement.org) [33, 34], CONSORT-EHEALTH guidelines [35] and the SPIRIT guidelines (Standard Protocol Items: Recommendations for Interventional Trials) [36, 37]. The study has been approved by the Ethics Committee of University Jaume I (Castellon, Spain, approval number: 4/2017). The trial is registered at clinicalstrials.gov as NCT03159715.

2.2   Participants

The nine participants who have taken part in the study and carried out the treatment programs consist of five women and four men who contacted the Emotional Disorder Clinic at Universitat Jaume I. The average age of the nine participants was 45 years (SD = 13.30); 44.44% of the participants were single, and 55.56% were married. Regarding the level of studies, 77.78% of the participants had university studies, and 22.22% had secondary studies. The mean on the BDI-II at pre-treatment before starting the treatment program was 19 (SD = 6.67). Table 1 shows the main participant sociodemographic characteristics in each condition.

Table 1. Participants' sociodemographic characteristics by intervention conditions.

	IGc (n = 4)	IBAc (n = 3)	IPPc (n = 2)
Average	48.25	36.33	51.5
Sex	2 male, 2 female	2 male, 1 female	2 female
Marital status	2 single, 2 married	2 single, 1 married	2 married
Education	3 university studies, 1 secondary studies	2 university studies, 1 secondary studies	2 university studies

The following specific inclusion and exclusion criteria were required for enrollment. Inclusion criteria are: (a) age between 18 and 65 years old; (b) ability to understand and read Spanish; (c) access to the Internet at home and an email address; (d) Internet use: user level; and (e) experiencing depressive symptoms (no more than 28 on the Beck Depression Inventory-II [BDI-II]).

Exclusion criteria are: (a) receiving a psychological treatment during the study; (b) suffering from a severe Axis I mental disorder: alcohol and/or substance dependence disorder, psychotic disorder, or dementia; (c) the presence of ideation or a significant suicide plan (assessed by the MINI and item 9 on the BDI-II).

2.3   Interventions

The three intervention protocols we developed for this study present some distinctive features. Nonetheless, they share some aspects, such as a "Welcome" initial module that provides the participant with general information about the protocol and its objectives, as well as recommendations for benefiting from it. After this "Welcome" module, initial online questionnaires are presented as the pre-treatment assessment.

The three intervention conditions we developed are briefly described below:

Internet-Based Global Protocol Condition (IGc). We carried out a treatment protocol for depressive symptoms called "Sonreír es Divertido" (Smiling is Fun). It is an Internet-based treatment protocol developed within the framework of the European online predictive tools for intervention in mental illness project [28]. Smiling is Fun includes traditional therapeutic components of evidence-based treatments for depression:

Motivation for change, Psychoeducation, Cognitive Therapy, BA, and Relapse Prevention. The program also includes a PP component, offering strategies to enhance positive mood and promote psychological strengths. The intervention protocol consists of eight interactive modules. Four of them are based on CBT, three on PPs, and one on Relapse prevention. For more information about the specific intervention content see [29, 38].

Internet-Based Behavioral Activation Protocol Condition (IBAc). This intervention protocol has the CBT components of the original protocol (IGc), mentioned above, but the PP component is not included in this protocol. The intervention protocol consists of eight interactive modules. Four of them are based on CBT, three on BA, and one on Relapse prevention. The modules related to the BA component in this intervention condition teach the same tools and strategies as the module dedicated to the BA component in IGc.

Internet-Based Positive Psychotherapy Protocol Condition (IPPc). This intervention protocol has the CBT components from the original protocol (IGc), mentioned above, but the BA component is not included in this protocol. The intervention protocol consists of eight interactive modules. Four of them are based on CBT, three on PPs, and one on Relapse prevention. The modules related to the PPs component in this intervention condition teach the same tools and strategies as the module dedicated to the PPs component in IGc.

All the modules are delivered through a web platform designed by our research group (https://www.psicologiaytecnologia.com/). The web platform has different transversal tools that accompany the person throughout the entire intervention process. These transversal tools are: "Home" (the starting point of the protocol); "Calendar" (allows the participant to know where he/she is in the program); "How am I?" (offers several graphs that make it possible to monitor the participant's progress); "Diary register" (collects the everyday data about different variables and shows them graphically on the "How am I?" tool; "Review" (used to review the treatment modules already completed).

Moreover, we provide human and ICT support to all participants. In the case of human support, one trained pre-doctoral student in our group makes several brief phone calls at four points in time: an initial telephone session (diagnostic interview); an initial telephone call in the Welcome module (encouraging participants); a brief phone call when the participants reach the mid-point of the intervention; and a final post-call after the post assessment (qualitative assessment). ICT support consists of several multiple-choice questions about the contents seen in each module in order to provide the participant with the correct feedback for their responses and a detailed explanation. Furthermore, the participants receive an automated email encouraging them to continue with the modules if they have not accessed the program for a week.

2.4 Measures

Diagnostic Interview

Mini International Neuropsychiatric Interview Version 5.0.0 (MINI): The MINI [39] is a short, structured clinical interview that enables researchers to make diagnoses of psychiatric disorders according to the DSM-IV or ICD-10. It was designed to be used by clinicians or even by nonclinical personnel after brief training. It has an administration time of approximately 15 min, The MINI has excellent interrater reliability (K = .88–1.00), and it has been translated and validated in Spanish [40].

Self-assessment Measures

Beck Depression Inventory (BDI-II): The BDI-II is a 21-item self-report multiple-choice inventory that is widely used to detect and assess depression severity. On each item, the person has to choose from four alternatives, ranging from less to more severity, the statement that best describes his/her state in the past two weeks, including the day the person completes the inventory. The items are scored on a scale ranging from 0 to 3, and they cover the different symptoms characterizing major depression disorder in the DSM-IV [41]. The scores on the scale range from 0 to 63 (0–13 minimal depression, 14–19 mild depression, 20–28 moderate depression, 29–63 severe depression). The internal consistency of the BDI-II is high (alpha = 0.76 to 0.95), and for the Spanish version of the instrument (alpha = 0.87), for both general and clinical populations (alpha = 0.89) [42].

Positive and Negative Affect Scale (PANAS). The PANAS [43] is a brief self-report questionnaire and one of the most widely used measures of affectivity. It consists of two 10-item mood scales, one that measures positive affect (PA) and the other that measures negative affect (NA). Each scale contains 20 items, and scores range from 10 to 50 (the maximum score). The PANAS has excellent psychometric properties, internal consistency (alpha between 0.84 and 0.90), and convergent and divergent validity. The Spanish version has also demonstrated high internal consistency (α = 0.89 and 0.91 for PA and NA in women, respectively, and α = 0.87 and 0.89 for PA and NA in men, respectively) in college students [43].

Connor-Davidson Resilience Scale (CD-RISC). The CD-RISC [44] is a brief scale that consists of 25 items. The person must indicate to what extent each statement has been true for him/her in the past month on a scale from 0–4, where 0 = "has not been true at all" and 4 = "true almost always". The total scores range from 0 to 100; higher scores indicate greater resilience. Previous studies have shown that the CD-RISC has good internal consistency (Cronbach alpha above 0.70) [45, 46].

Qualitative Interview. A qualitative semi-structured interview with open-ended questions was developed ad hoc for the present study to ask participants their opinions about the therapeutic components of the program (Motivation for change, Psychoeducation, Cognitive Therapy, BA, PPs component, and Relapse Prevention). In the interview, the opinion about the main components of each intervention is assessed through three questions: aspects of the specific component that have been *useful*; *satisfaction* with the component; and *recommending* the component to other people.

In the IBAc and IPPc conditions, where one of the components is not included, first the participants are informed about the main characteristics and strategies of the component that is not in their intervention. After that, the participants are asked whether it would have been useful for them to have this component, satisfactory, and whether they would recommend it. This qualitative semi-structured interview was developed based on the principles specified in the Consensual Qualitative Research (CQR) guidelines [47]. One of the main objectives of the CQR is to gather diverse information within certain thematic areas. As in other qualitative semi-structured interviews, we ask questions that allow us to delve into the participant's opinion [48].

2.5 Procedure

First, the adult volunteer participants contacted the Clinic of Emotional Disorders at Universitat Jaume I by phone or by sending an email to a specific address created for the study. Then, the participants completed a short evaluation on the Internet (https://www.surveymonkey.com) to find out if they met the exclusion and inclusion criteria. After that, the Mini International Neuropsychiatric Interview Version 5.0.0 (MINI) was administered by telephone by experienced clinical psychologists (with at least a master's degree or PhD) trained in CBT and with extensive experience in treatments using Internet-based interventions. After being assured that they were potential participants for the study, they signed an informed consent and were randomized to one of the three experimental conditions using a computer-generated random number sequence to ensure that we obtained a homogeneous distribution across the conditions. This randomization was performed by an independent researcher who was unaware of the characteristics of the study and communicated the allocation schedule to the study researchers by phone. Participants do not know to which intervention condition they have been assigned, and they are informed that they can withdraw from the treatment or the study without giving any explanation.

Regarding the data presented in the present study (9 participants), four participants were assigned to the IGc, three to the IBAc and two to the IPPc. After randomization, they were registered in the online treatment program, and they performed the pre-evaluation before starting the program. After the pre-treatment assessment, participants started the intervention modules. The treatment program lasts approximately 4 months (16 weeks), and the participants were advised to advance through the program by completing a module every two weeks. When they finished the program, they performed the post-treatment assessment within the web platform, and they were called to complete the qualitative interview. As mentioned above, the study is ongoing, and the total sample size needed, considering an additional 30% to anticipate potential dropouts, is 191 participants (63 per intervention group). Sample size calculations were carried out with the statistical program G*Power 3.1.9.2 [49].

2.6 Data Analysis

To estimate the clinical importance of the changes shown in the post-treatment, the clinically significant change (CSC) was calculated using the Jacobson and Truax index for all measures. This method involves, firstly, establishing a cut-off score that the patient must achieve in order to move from a dysfunctional to a functional distribution. Secondly, the method implies estimating whether the change indicated by the scores of the instruments is not due to its measurement error but reflects a reliable real change in the patient's symptomatology. Regarding that, these authors proposed the reliable change index (RCI) [50]. Moreover, participants were classified in one of the groups proposed by Kupfer: "Recovered", "Improved", "Stable", and "Deteriorate" [51]. "Recovered" group includes participants who showed a CSC in the outcome measure and had a score in the post within the functional or normal population range. In the "Improved" group were the participants who have achieved a CSC but are within dysfunctional or clinical population range. If the participants did not achieve CSC, or this CSC was in the direction of greater dysfunctionality, they were classified in "Stable" and "Deteriorate" group, respectively.

3 Results

3.1 Differences from Pre-treatment to Post-treatment in the Assessment Measures in the Different Conditions

Table 2 shows the results obtained at pre-treatment and post-treatment in each condition on the different assessment measures (negative functioning measures and positive functioning measures). The scores correspond to the means, standard deviations, and differences in the mean pre to post treatment. The results show improvements on all the assessed measures.

Table 2. Pre-post scores in each condition in the assessment measures.

	Measure	IGc n = 4			IBAc n = 3			IPPc n = 2		
		M	SD	Difference pre-post (M)	M	SD	Difference pre-post (M)	M	SD	Difference pre-post (M)
Negative functioning measures	BDI									
	Pre	22.0	5.6	14.25	20.3	5.50	13	11.0	5.7	5.5
	Post	7.8	6.1		7.3	6.80		5.50	.71	
	NA									
	Pre	31.5	2.9	9.25	23.7	1.52	8.67	19.5	.70	4.5
	Post	22.3	5.7		15.0	6.08		15.0	7.1	
Positive functioning measures	PA									
	Pre	19.5	4.7	−2.75	26.7	11.5	−5.66	28.0	2.8	−9
	Post	22.3	2.6		32.3	10.8		37.0	9.9	
	CD-RISC									
	Pre	32.3	15.6	−9.75	49.0	17.4	−5.67	53.5	3.5	−19.5
	Post	42.0	12.8		54.7	11.1		73.0	4.2	

Note. *BDI-II: Beck Depression Inventory, PA: positive affect, NA: negative affect, CD-RISC: Connor-Davidson Resilience Scale, M: Mean, SD: Standard Deviation, IGc: Internet Global protocol condition, IBAc: Internet-based Behavioral Activation protocol condition, IPPc: Internet-based Positive Psychotherapy protocol condition*

Regarding the negative functioning measures (BDI-II and negative affect in PANAS scale), the participants in the IGc and IBAc showed similar improvements in depressive symptoms (pre-post score differences respectively 14.25 and 13). In the case of the IPPc, the results showed less improvement in depressive symptoms (pre-post score differences 5.5). Furthermore, the improvements in negative affect were similar in the IGc and IBAc conditions: 9.25 in the IGc, and 8.67 in the IBAc. In this case, participants in the IPPc showed less improvement in negative affect (pre-post score differences 4.5).

Regarding the positive functioning measures (positive affect on the PANAS scale and CD-RISC), on positive affect, the participants who received the protocol based on the PPs component (IPPc) showed a greater increase (pre-post score differences 9), compared to the other two conditions (IGc 2.75 and IBAc 5.66). In the case of resilience, both participants in the conditions with the PP component (IGc and IPPc) improved more than the participants in the IBAc (9.75 and 19.5, respectively, compared to 5.67 in the IBAc). It is important to mention that the improvement in resilience was greater in the participants in the IPPc (pre-post score differences 19.5).

The RCI analyses are shown graphically in Fig. 1. The results showed that no participants of the three conditions were in the "Deteriorate" group in any clinical variable.

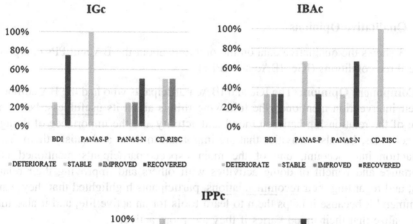

Fig. 1. Pre-treatment to post-treatment clinically significant change (CSC) in the assessed measures. (Note. *BDI-II: Beck Depression Inventory; PANAS −: Negative affect of the Positive and Negative affect Scale; PANAS +: Positive affect of the Positive and Negative affect Scale, CD-RISC: Connor-Davidson Resilience Scale, IGc: Internet Global protocol condition, IBAc: Internet-based Behavioral Activation protocol condition; IPPc: Internet-based Positive Psychotherapy protocol condition.*)

Regarding negative functioning measures, participants in the IGc and IBAc showed a clinically significant decrease in depressive symptoms. Specifically, 75% of participants in the IGc, and 33% in the IBAc were in the "Recovered" group. Furthermore 33% of the participants in the IBAc were in the "Improved" group. In the IPPc, participants did not achieve this CSC, being in the "Stable" group.

Regarding the negative affect, participants of the three conditions showed a clinically significant decrease in this measure. In the IGc and IPPc, 50% were in the "Recovered" group, and 63% of the participants in IBAc were also in this "Recovered" group". Furthermore, 25% of the participants in the IGc were in the "Improved" group.

Regarding positive functioning measures, the results showed that only the participants of the IBAc and IPPc had a CSC in positive affect: 33% of the participants in the IBAc and 50% in the IPPc were in the "Recovered" group. In the IGc the 100% of the participants were in the "Stable" group.

In resilience measure, the results showed a CSC in the IPPc: the 100% of the participants were in the "Recovered" group. Furthermore, 50% of the participants in the IGc achieved a CSC, coming into the "Improved" group. In the IBAc all the participants were in the "Stable" group.

3.2 Qualitative Opinions

Table 3 shows the qualitative data on the opinions about the BA and PPs components in the three conditions (IGc, IBAc and IPPc).

BA Component Opinion: The IGc and IBAc participants who had the BA component in their intervention mentioned the following things about its usefulness: being more aware of the relationship between mood and activity and the importance of doing not only activities, but also activities that are important to them and satisfy them. Taking satisfaction into account, one of the main aspects participants mentioned is the importance and benefit of doing activities with others and improving their relationships; and regarding their recommendations, participants highlighted that they want to recommend it because it helps them to learn tools for an active life, and it also makes them realize that their mood varies if they are more active.

In the IPPc condition where the BA component is not included, participants mentioned similar ideas to those of the other two conditions: Regarding usefulness, they said it would help them to improve their emotions. In the case of satisfaction, they pointed out that it would have been useful for talking to and knowing other people. We observe that in the IPPc, the participants emphasized that they would recommend it because it would help them to have more practice interacting with others.

PPs Component Opinion: The main things the IGc and IPPc participants who had the PPs component in their intervention mentioned with regard to its usefulness were: learning to recognize not only their weaknesses, but also their strengths, and thinking about the good parts of each person. In the case of satisfaction, participants pointed out the importance of knowing their own strengths. They wanted to recommend it because they learned that everybody has strengths, which can help more in bad times, and they have learned to see the positive side of things more. In the IBAc in which the PPs component is not included, participants said it would have been useful for learning to

Table 3. Qualitative information regarding the BA and PP components in each condition.

Component		IGc	IBAc	IPPc
BA	• Utility	• *"More aware of my mood in relation to what I had done during the week"* • *"The importance of the action to feel better and carry out activities that satisfy you"*	• *"Sometimes you think that your mood is not going to improve. whatever you do. but if you do nice things, it improves"* • *"It has been useful not only to do activities. but also to do activities that I like especially"*	• *"It would have benefited me more by having more activity"* • *"It would have helped me to be better emotionally"*
	• Satisfaction	• *"Identify the tasks and activities I like, and I can do to improve my self-esteem and thinking". "I can do something to improve"* • *"Realize what carrying out these activities generates and how important people's support is"*	• *"It has encouraged me to do a little more activity"* • *"Improving my relationships with people who I did not have a relationship with before"*	• *"I would have had more security"* • *"More practice talking and knowing others"*
	• Recommendation	• *"Yes. It gives simple tools to improve your mood"* • *"Yes. Because knowing the activities that are satisfactory to you strengthen you for the future"*	• *"Yes. Realize that the mood varies if you get more activity and do things that are nice to you"* • *"Yes. An active life helps you in your relationships and to feel better about yourself"*	• *"Yes. Because by doing that you can have more practice, and that helps you to have more emotional strength"* • *"Yes. To have more practice interacting with others"*
PP	• Utility	• *"The concept of flow". It helped me understand that state"* • *"It helped me see that I saw weaknesses in strengths, and identifying your strengths is beneficial"*	• *"It would have been good for me. because I am negative. and to learn to be more positive"* • *"I would have taken advantage of it. because it's important to know each self"*	• *"To move forward if a problem arises, to do things that satisfy"* • *"To think about the good in each person"*
	• Satisfaction	• *"To be able to give a word to that emotion"* • *"To know you more. The satisfaction of being aware that you have your strengths too and not all of this are weaknesses"*	• *"Maybe more self-confidence"* • *"The positivity that depends on knowing one's own emotions and knowing how to regulate them"*	• *"Get up, move, to feel better despite having a problem"* • *"Finding myself better doing things that I like with people who happen the same that happen to me"*
	• Recommendation	• *"Yes. Because it is very useful to identify your strengths and not just your weaknesses. It helps you more in the moments when you are emotionally worse"* • *"Yes. So that each person can see what he/she can contribute to society through his/her strengths"*	• *"I guess so. To have more security and think more positively"* • *"Yes. To know your own strengths and look more at them and work on them, not the weaknesses so much"*	• *"Yes. To be better"* • *"Yes. To look more at the positive side and not at the negative side of things"*

be more positive. Regarding <u>satisfaction</u>, participants pointed out the importance of knowing their own emotions and strengths and learning to have more self-confidence. Finally, they wanted to recommend it because it could help them to have more security, to think more positively, and to know their own strengths.

4 Discussion

The present work shows the preliminary results for 9 participants with depressive symptoms who were randomly assigned to one of three conditions in a dismantling randomized controlled trial (IGc, IBAc or IPPc). First, we examine the pre- to post-treatment changes in the different variables assessed in the three intervention conditions and the CSC. Furthermore, qualitative data on the opinions about the BA and PP components are reported.

Regarding the first objective, in the case of the negative functioning measures, the results showed that they improved in the three intervention conditions. Specifically, on depressive symptoms, there was less improvement in the participants in the IPPc condition than in the other two conditions, as these participants didn't show a CSC in this symptomatology. However, it is important to mention that, in this condition, the participants had lower levels of depressive symptoms at pre-treatment, which means there was less room for improvement. In addition, there are only 2 participants in this condition. The ongoing RCT will allow us to have the same level of severity in the three conditions at pre-treatment because the randomization is stratified by levels of depression severity.

The same pattern occurred in the case of negative affect. Participants of the three conditions showed a clinically significant decrease in this measure, but the least improvement occurred in the IPPc. Nevertheless, the participants in this condition also had lower levels of negative affect at pre-treatment. However, it is important that participants in all three conditions improved their depressive symptomatology and negative affect, essential aspects of depression treatment. With a larger sample, differences in these measures among the three groups can be further explored. The results are consistent with the line of research on the efficacy of Internet-based interventions in improving clinical symptomology [25, 52].

Regarding positive functioning measures, the biggest improvement is in the IPPc. Positive affect improves substantially more in the IPPc than in the other two conditions. Regarding resilience, it is important to consider that the biggest changes occurred in the two conditions that include the PP component (IGc and IPPc). The RCI analysis showed that there is a clinically significant change in these conditions where the PPs component is worked. However, there is a much greater improvement in the IPPc, as in this condition all participants were in the "Recovered" group. In this condition there are four specific modules in which the PP component is worked on in greater depth.

Because it is well known that depression often involves low levels of positive affect [15, 53], and that these low levels increase the severity of the problem [54], it is important to have treatment that works on these aspects (as the IGc and IPPc). It is essential to continue to work in this direction because current psychological treatments for depression focus largely on reducing excessive affect, rather than on specifically improving deficits in positive affect and well-being [17, 53]. The interventions need to have strategies that directly and primarily build positive emotions, positive affect, character strengths, and meaning [55, 56], considering well-being and positive functioning to be core elements of the treatment for depression.

Regarding resilience, it is worth noting that a great change occurs in the IPPc condition, where the PP strategies are learned in a deeper way. Resilience refers to an individual's ability to properly adapt to stress and adversity, overcome the negative effects of risk exposure, or cope successfully with traumatic experiences [57]. It is also essential for maintaining quality of life, emotional well-being, and functional independence. Thus, it is relevant to see the effects of the PP strategies on resilience in the preliminary results. The PP component could help patients to directly build up positive resources in order to counteract negative symptoms and buffer against their future reoccurrence. However, we should wait to obtain more conclusive results after analyzing these measures in a broader sample.

Regarding the qualitative data, we observe that, in general terms, the participants in the three conditions agree on the main ideas about the usefulness, satisfaction, and recommendations about the two main components, BA and PP.

Taking the BA component into account, we observed that the importance of carrying out meaningful activities with other people is an idea highlighted by the participants who carry out the intervention with the BA component, and this is something the participants in the IPPc (without BA component) would like to work on more. We know that carrying out significant activities is a key aspect of depression treatment and helps with symptom improvement [58]. It is important to know that the intervention programs with the BA component help patients to do these meaningful activities.

Focusing on the aspects worked on in the PP modules, the qualitative data showed that learning to be more positive and knowing how to identify one's own strengths, and not only the weaknesses, are main ideas when we ask participants. This aspect is also pointed out by the participants in the IBAc, where the PP component was not included.

We observe that working on positive aspects is something demanded by the participants, and this is consistent with developing interventions that improve positive affect, well-being, and character strengths [15], rather than components focused on reducing negative symptoms [17, 18]. We can observe that the qualitative data presented in this article only give us a general idea because they correspond to a sample of 9 participants. We have only analyzed the topics shared in the participants' opinions in a subjective way. Our objective in the future is to carry out more exhaustive qualitative analyses with a larger sample of participants, following the lines of the Consensual Qualitative Research (CQR) developed by Hill, Thompson and Nutt-Williams [59]. CQR is considered a viable qualitative method [47] whose structure includes two essential aspects. The first is to set up a team with at least three members, two judges who analyze the data from multiple perspectives and the auditor who supervises the work done by the judges. The second aspect is to follow specific steps to establish the domains, core ideas, and cross categories to classify and analyze the data. At the moment, the qualitative interviews are being recorded, after receiving informed consent from the participants, in order to later carry out their transcription and analyze the data following this methodology and draw more solid conclusions [60].

The dismantling design of the study we are carrying out will allow us to explore the contribution of each treatment component. More specifically, it will allow us to know how PPs and emotional regulation strategies centered on positive affect function, resulting in a significant shift towards optimizing treatments for depression. In addition, with the ongoing study, it will be possible to analyze the mediators of changes in depressive symptoms and the acceptability of each intervention. Moreover, this study is consistent with one of the most important challenges in the field of depression treatment, which is to design new ways to apply treatments to maximize their therapeutic efficiency. Undoubtedly, the use of technology and the Internet can help to achieve this goal and contribute to the dissemination and accessibility of evidence-based treatments.

The present study has some limitations. The sample size is small; for this reason it was not possible to perform statistical analyses, and so the results are only exploratory. Because of the small sample size in the present study, no analysis of differences among groups in baseline depressive symptomatology was conducted. However, as the recruitment is on-going, the sample size is going to increase, and we will be able to carry out these analyses. Another aspect is that, regarding the qualitative data, we do not ask about aspects of the main components of the treatment (BA and PP) that have not been useful and satisfactory, and if there is any reason they would not recommend them. Because this is also important, we are going to include these aspects in the qualitative interview. Furthermore, we do not have data on the participants at the 3-, 6-, and 12-month follow-ups. Moreover, because we only have two participants in the IPPc, the BDI-II severity in this condition was lower than the other two conditions. Our aim is to continue to increase the sample size of the study in order to draw firmer conclusions and include the data from the different follow-ups in order to observe whether the results obtained are maintained in the long term.

Acknowledgments. CIBERobn, an initiative of Institute of Health Carlos III (ISCIII); UJI-A2016-14 Program, Project 16I336.01/1 (Universitat Jaume I).

References

1. Gabilondo, A., Rojas-Farreras, S., Vilagut, G., Haro, J.M., Fernández, A., Pinto-Meza, A., et al.: Epidemiology of major depressive episode in a Southern European country: results from the ESEMeD-Spain project. J. Affect. Disord. **120**, 76–85 (2010)
2. Haro, J.M., Ayuso-Mateos, J.L., Bitter, I., Demotes-Mainard, J., Leboyer, M., Lewis, S.W., et al.: ROAMER: roadmap for mental health research in Europe. Int J Methods Psychiatr Res. **23**(S1), 1–14 (2014). http://www.ncbi.nlm.nih.gov/pubmed/24375532
3. World Health Organization: Depression and Other Common Mental Disorders. CC BY-NC-SA 30 IGO, no. 1, pp. 1–22 (2017)
4. Cuijpers, P., Andersson, G., Donker, T., van Straten, A.: Psychological treatment of depression: results of a series of meta-analyses. Nord. J. Psychiatry **65**(6), 354–364 (2011). http://www.tandfonline.com/doi/full/10.3109/08039488.2011.596570
5. Nakagawa, A., Sado, M., Mitsuda, D., Fujisawa, D., Kikuchi, T., Abe, T., et al.: Effectiveness of cognitive behavioural therapy augmentation in major depression treatment (ECAM study): study protocol for a randomised clinical trial. BMJ Open **4**(10) (2014). http://www.ncbi.nlm.nih.gov/pubmed/25335963

6. National Collaborating Centre for Mental Health (Great Britain): Royal College of Psychiatrists. Depression : The treatment and management of depression in adults. Royal College of Psychiatrists 705 p. (2010)
7. Cuijpers, P., Berking, M., Andersson, G., Quigley, L., Kleiboer, A., Dobson, K.S.: A meta-analysis of cognitive-behavioural therapy for adult depression, alone and in comparison with other treatments. Can. J. Psychiatry **58**(7), 376–385 (2013). http://journals.sagepub.com/doi/10.1177/070674371305800702
8. Beck, A.T., Rush, A., Shaw, B., Emery, G.: Cognitive Therapy of Depression, 425 p. Guilford Press, New York (1979)
9. Dimidjian, S., Hollon, S.D., Dobson, K.S., Schmaling, K.B., Kohlenberg, R.J., Addis, M.E., et al.: Randomized trial of behavioral activation, cognitive therapy, and antidepressant medication in the acute treatment of adults with major depression. J. Consult. Clin. Psychol. **74**(4), 658–670 (2006). http://doi.apa.org/getdoi.cfm?doi=10.1037/0022-006X.74.4.658
10. Spates, C.R., Pagoto, S.L., Kalata, A.: A qualitative and quantitative review of behavioral activation treatment of major depressive disorder. Behav. Anal. Today **7**(4), 508–521 (2006)
11. Jacobson, N.S.: Contextualism is dead: long live contextualism. Fam. Process **33**(1), 97–100 (1994)
12. Pérez Álvarez, M., Fernández Rodríguez, C., Amigo, I.: Guía de tratamientos psicológicos eficaces I, pp. 161–196 (2003)
13. Kazdin, A.E.: Mediators and mechanisms of change in psychotherapy research. Annu. Rev. Clin. Psychol. **3**(1), 1–27 (2007). http://www.annualreviews.org/doi/10.1146/annurev.clinpsy.3.022806.091432
14. Kazdin, A.E.: Understanding how and why psychotherapy leads to change. Psychother. Res. **19**(4–5), 418–428 (2009). https://www.tandfonline.com/doi/full/10.1080/1050330080244-8899
15. Ruini, C.: Positive Psychology in the Clinical Domains. Springer, Cham (2017). https://doi.org/10.1007/978-3-319-52112-1
16. Watson, D., Naragon-Gainey, K.: On the specificity of positive emotional dysfunction in psychopathology: evidence from the mood and anxiety disorders and schizophrenia/schizotypy. Clin. Psychol. Rev. **30**(7), 839–848 (2010). https://doi.org/10.1016/j.cpr.2009.11.002
17. Bolier, L., Haverman, M., Westerhof, G.J., Riper, H., Smit, F., Bohlmeijer, E.: Positive psychology interventions: a meta-analysis of randomized controlled studies. BMC Public Health **13**(1), 119 (2013)
18. Sin, N.L., Lyubomirsky, S.: Enhancing well-being and alleviating depressive symptoms with positive psychology interventions: a practice-friendly meta-analysis. J. Clin. Psychol. **65**(5), 467–487 (2009). http://www.ncbi.nlm.nih.gov/pubmed/19301241
19. Pressman, S.D., Jenkins, B.N., Moskowitz, J.T.: Positive affect and health: what do we know and where next should we go? Annu. Rev. Psychol. **70**(1), 627–650 (2019). https://www.annualreviews.org/doi/10.1146/annurev-psych-010418-102955
20. Werner-Seidler, A., Banks, R., Dunn, B.D., Moulds, M.L.: An investigation of the relationship between positive affect regulation and depression. Behav. Res. Ther. **51**(1), 46–56 (2013). https://linkinghub.elsevier.com/retrieve/pii/S0005796712001623
21. Borkovec, T.D., Castonguay, L.G.: What is the scientific meaning of empirically supported therapy? J. Consult. Clin. Psychol. **66**(1), 136–142 (1998)
22. Bell, E.C., Marcus, D.K., Goodlad, J.K.: Are the parts as good as the whole? A meta-analysis of component treatment studies. J. Consult. Clin. Psychol. **81**(4), 722–736 (2013)
23. Kazdin, A.E., Blase, S.L.: Rebooting psychotherapy research and practice to reduce the burden of mental illness. Perspect. Psychol. Sci. **6**(1), 21–37 (2011). http://journals.sagepub.com/doi/10.1177/1745691610393527

24. Kazdin, A.E.: Technology-based interventions and reducing the burdens of mental illness: perspectives and comments on the special series. Cogn. Behav. Pract. **22**(3), 359–366 (2015). https://linkinghub.elsevier.com/retrieve/pii/S1077722915000292
25. Johansson, R., Andersson, G.: Internet-based psychological treatments for depression. Expert Rev. Neurother. **12**(7), 861–870 (2012)
26. Karyotaki, E., Riper, H., Twisk, J., Hoogendoorn, A., Kleiboer, A., Mira, A., et al.: Efficacy of self-guided internet-based cognitive behavioral therapy in the treatment of depressive symptoms a meta-analysis of individual participant data. JAMA Psychiatry **74**(4), 351–359 (2017)
27. Karyotaki, E., Kemmeren, L., Riper, H., Twisk, J., Hoogendoorn, A., Kleiboer, A., et al.: Is self-guided internet-based cognitive behavioural therapy (iCBT) harmful? An individual participant data meta-analysis. Psychol Med. **48**(15), 2456–2466 (2018). https://www.cambridge.org/core/product/identifier/S0033291718000648/type/journal_article
28. Botella, C., Mira, A., Moragrega, I., García-Palacios, A., Bretón-López, J., Castilla, D., et al.: An internet-based program for depression using activity and physiological sensors: efficacy, expectations, satisfaction, and ease of use. Neuropsychiatr. Dis. Treat. **12**, 393 (2016). https://www.dovepress.com/an-internet-based-program-for-depression-using-activity-and-physiologi-peer-reviewed-article-NDT
29. Mira, A., Bretón-López, J., García-Palacios, A., Quero, S., Baños, R.M., Botella, C.: An internet-based program for depressive symptoms using human and automated support: a randomized controlled trial. Neuropsychiatr. Dis. Treat. **13**, 987 (2017)
30. Montero-Marín, J., Araya, R., Pérez-Yus, M.C., Mayoral, F., Gili, M., Botella, C., et al.: An internet-based intervention for depression in primary care in Spain: a randomized controlled trial. J. Med. Internet Res. **18**(8), e231 (2016). http://www.ncbi.nlm.nih.gov/pubmed/27565118. Accessed 20 Oct 2018
31. Vazquez, F.L., Torres, A., Di-az, O., Otero, P., Blanco, V., Hermida, E.: Protocol for a randomized controlled dismantling study of a brief telephonic psychological intervention applied to nonprofessional caregivers with symptoms of depression. BMC Psychiatry **15**(1), 1–9 (2015). https://doi.org/10.1186/s12888-015-0682-8
32. Cuijpers, P., Cristea, I.A., Karyotaki, E., Reijnders, M., Hollon, S.D.: Component studies of psychological treatments of adult depression: a systematic review and meta-analysis. Psychother. Res. **29**(1), 15–29 (2019). https://doi.org/10.1080/10503307.2017.1395922
33. Moher, D., Schulz, K.F., Altman, D.G.: The CONSORT statement: revised recommendations for improving the quality of reports of parallel group randomized trials. BMC Med. Res. Methodol. **1**(1), 2 (2001). http://bmcmedresmethodol.biomedcentral.com/articles/10.1186/1471-2288-1-2
34. Moher, D., Hopewell, S., Schulz, K.F., Montori, V., Gøtzsche, P.C., Devereaux, P.J., et al.: CONSORT 2010 explanation and elaboration: updated guidelines for reporting parallel group randomised trials. BMJ 340 (2010)
35. Eysenbach, G., CONSORT-EHEALTH Group: CONSORT-EHEALTH: improving and standardizing evaluation reports of web-based and mobile health interventions. J. Med. Internet Res. **13**(4) (2011)
36. Chan, A., Tetzlaff, J.M., Gøtzsche, P.C., Altman, D.G., Mann, H., Berlin, J.A., et al.: Research methods and reporting SPIRIT 2013 explanation and elaboration : guidance for protocols of clinical trials. BMJ Res. Methods Rep. 1–42 (2013)
37. Chan, A.-W., Tetzlaff, J.M., Altman, D.G., Laupacis, A., Gøtzsche, P.C., Krleža-Jerić, K., et al.: SPIRIT 2013 statement: defining standard protocol items for clinical trials. Ann. Intern. Med. **158**(3), 200 (2013). http://www.ncbi.nlm.nih.gov/pubmed/23295957

38. Mira, A., Bretón-López, J., Enrique, Á., Castilla, D., García-Palacios, A., Baños, R., et al.: Exploring the incorporation of a positive psychology component in a cognitive behavioral internet-based program for depressive symptoms results throughout the intervention process. Front Psychol. **9**, 2360 (2018). http://www.ncbi.nlm.nih.gov/pubmed/30555384

39. Sheehan, D.V., Lecrubier, Y., Sheehan, K.H., Amorim, P., Janavs, J., Weiller, E., et al.: The Mini-International Neuropsychiatric Interview (M.I.N.I.): the development and validation of a structured diagnostic psychiatric interview for DSM-IV and ICD-10. J. Clin. Psychiatry. **59** (Suppl 2:22–33), 34–57 (1998)

40. Ferrando, L., Bobes, J., Gibert, J.: MINI. Mini International Neuropsychiatric Interview. Versión en Español 5.0.0 DSM-IV. Instrumentos detección y orientación diagnóstica. 2–26 (2000). http://www.fundacionforo.com/pdfs/mini.pdf

41. Beck, A.T., Steer, R.A., Brown, G.K.: Manual for the Beck Depression Inventory-II. Psychological Corporation, San Antonio (1996)

42. Sanz Fernández, J., Navarro, M.E., Vázquez Valverde, C.: Adaptación española del inventario para la depresión de Beck-II: 1. Propiedades psicométricas en estudiantes universitarios. Análisis y Modif Conduct. **29**(124), 239–288 (2003)

43. Sandín, B., Chorot, P., Lostao, L., Joiner, T.E., Santed, M.E., Valiente, R.: Escalas PANAS de afecto positivo y negativo: validación factorial y convergencia transcultural. Psicothema **11**(1), 37–51 (1999)

44. Connor, K.M., Davidson, J.R.T.: Development of a new resilience scale: the Connor-Davidson Resilience Scale (CD-RISC). Depress Anxiety. **18**(2), 76–82 (2003). http://doi.wiley.com/10.1002/da.10113

45. Yu, X., Zhang, J.: Factor analysis and psychometric evaluation of the Connor-Davidson Resilience Scale (CD-RISC) With Chinese people. Soc. Behav. Personal. Int. J. **35**(1), 19–30 (2007). http://openurl.ingenta.com/content/xref?genre=article&issn=0301-2212&volume=35&issue=1&spage=19

46. Singh, K., Yu, X.: Psychometric evaluation of the Connor-Davidson Resilience Scale (CD-RISC) in a sample of Indian students. J. Psychol. **1**(1), 23–30 (2010). https://www.tandfonline.com/doi/full/10.1080/09764224.2010.11885442

47. Hill, C.E., Knox, S., Thompson, B.J., Williams, E.N., Hess, S.A.: Consensual qualitative research: an update. J. Couns. Psychol. **52**, 196 (2005)

48. Knox, S., Burkard, A.W.: Qualitative research interviews. Psychother. Res. **19**(4–5), 566–575 (2009)

49. Faul, F., Erdfelder, E., Lang, A.-G., Buchner, A.: G*Power 3: a flexible statistical power analysis program for the social, behavioral, and biomedical sciences. Behav. Res. Methods **39**(2), 175–191 (2007)

50. Jacobson, N.S., Truax, P.: Clinical significance: a statistical approach to defining meaningful change in psychotherapy research. J. Consult. Clin. Psychol. **59**(1), 12–19 (1991). http://www.ncbi.nlm.nih.gov/pubmed/2002127

51. Kupfer, D.J.: Long-term treatment of depression. J. Clin. Psychiatry **52**, 28–34 (1991). http://www.ncbi.nlm.nih.gov/pubmed/1903134

52. Andersson, G., Cuijpers, P.: Internet-based and other computerized psychological treatments for adult depression: a meta-analysis. Cogn. Behav. Ther. **38**(4), 196–205 (2009). http://www.tandfonline.com/doi/full/10.1080/16506070903318960

53. Fredrickson, B.L.: The role of positive emotions in positive psychology. The broaden-and-build theory of positive emotions. Am. Psychol. **56**(3), 218–226 (2001)

54. Lopez-Gomez, I., Chaves, C., Hervas, G., Vazquez, C.: Comparing the acceptability of a positive psychology intervention versus a cognitive behavioural therapy for clinical depression. Clin. Psychol. Psychother. **24**(5), 1029–1039 (2017). http://doi.wiley.com/10.1002/cpp.2129

55. Ryff, C.D.: Psychological well-being revisited: advances in the science and practice of eudaimonia. Psychother. Psychosom. **83**(1), 10–28 (2014). https://www.karger.com/Article/FullText/353263
56. Seligman, M.E.P., Rashid, T., Parks, A.C.: Positive psychotherapy. Am. Psychol. **61**(8), 774–788 (2006). http://doi.apa.org/getdoi.cfm?doi=10.1037/0003-066X.61.8.774
57. Southwick, S.M., Bonanno, G.A., Masten, A.S., Panter-Brick, C., Yehuda, R.: Resilience definitions, theory, and challenges: interdisciplinary perspectives. Eur. J. Psychotraumatol. **5** (1), 25338 (2014). http://www.eurojnlofpsychotraumatol.net
58. Furukawa, T.A., Imai, H., Horikoshi, M., Shimodera, S., Hiroe, T., Funayama, T., et al.: Behavioral activation: is it the expectation or achievement, of mastery or pleasure that contributes to improvement in depression? J. Affect. Disord. **238**, 336–341 (2018). https://www.sciencedirect.com/science/article/pii/S0165032718300338?via%3Dihub
59. Hill, C.E., Thompson, B.J., Williams, E.N.: A guide to conducting consensual qualitative research. Couns. Psychol. **25**(4), 517–572 (1997). http://journals.sagepub.com/doi/10.1177/0011000097254001
60. Fernández-Álvarez, J., Díaz-García, A., González-Robles, A., Baños, R., García-Palacios, A., Botella, C.: Dropping out of a transdiagnostic online intervention: a qualitative analysis of client's experiences. Internet Interv. **10**, 29–38 (2017)

Usability of a Transdiagnostic Internet-Delivered Protocol for Anxiety and Depression in Community Patients

Amanda Díaz-García[1(✉)], Alberto González-Robles[1],
Javier Fernández-Álvarez[2], Diana Castilla[3], Adriana Mira[3],
Juana María Bretón[1], Azucena García-Palacios[1,4],
and Cristina Botella[1,4]

[1] Universitat Jaume I, Castellón, Spain
{amdiaz, vrobles, breton, azucena, botella}@uji.es
[2] Università Cattolica del Sacro Cuore, Milán, Italy
javier.fernandezkirszman@unicatt.it
[3] Universidad de Zaragoza, Zaragoza, Spain
{castilla, miraa}@unizar.es
[4] CIBER Fisiopatología Obesidad y Nutrición (CIBERObn),
Instituto Salud Carlos III, Madrid, Spain

Abstract. Internet-based psychological treatments have shown to be a promising solution to increase the accessibility to evidence-based treatments. However, the implementation of these interventions is still a challenge in health care settings. The study of the acceptability of these interventions may be a key aspect to reach successful implementation. Specifically, the study of usability may help to ensure that the interventions are well-designed and therefore increase the interest and number of people who can benefit from a psychological treatment. The present work aims to assess the usability of a transdiagnostic Internet -based treatment for emotional disorders among 87 patients who participated in it. The online program was considered well-accepted in terms of usability. This study analyzes the usability of an Internet-based treatment for emotional disorders, based on the transdiagnostic perspective and including a specific therapeutic component to address positive affect. Further research is needed in order to promote adherence and achieve the dissemination of evidence-based Internet-delivered psychological treatments.

Keywords: Usability · Internet-based treatments · Emotional disorders

1 Introduction

Internet-based treatments (IBTs) have shown to be effective in the treatment of depression and anxiety disorders [1], being also considered as evidence-based treatments for numerous psychological disorders [2]. Moreover, some meta-analyses reveal that these treatments are as efficacious as face-to-face traditional treatments [3]. Several advantages have been indicated in Internet interventions regarding the recruitment of patients, assessment and diagnosis, accessibility to evidence-based treatments,

© ICST Institute for Computer Sciences, Social Informatics and Telecommunications Engineering 2019
Published by Springer Nature Switzerland AG 2019. All Rights Reserved
P. Cipresso et al. (Eds.): MindCare 2019, LNICST 288, pp. 147–156, 2019.
https://doi.org/10.1007/978-3-030-25872-6_11

disse-mination and comorbidity management [4]. In addition, the literature has pointed out that the use of IBTs can help to solve several mental health problems to overcome common treatments barriers such as safety, geographical reach, acceptability and convenience [5].

Although Internet-based treatments seem to be a very promising solution to treat psychological disorders, it is essential to acquire more knowledge about its implementation and the acceptability of such interventions. In this regard, investigating the acceptability of the interventions delivered online may help to reach successful implementation in the routine clinical practice.

Treatment acceptability refers to the degree to which users are satisfied or at ease with a service and willing to use it [6], and it has been identified as an important aspect for ethical, methodological and practical reasons in IBTs [7]. Furthermore, acceptability also refers to perceive the treatment as appropriate, fair, reasonable, and non-intrusive for a given problem [8].

Focusing on the acceptability, the literature suggests that the evaluation of the usability of these interventions is crucial in order to ensure that the system design is effective [9]. Usability testing has been described as a method for evaluating user performance and acceptance of a product during its development process [9]. Following the International Organization for Standardization guidelines, usability is measured by its effectiveness (i.e. the ability of the user to complete tasks using the system), efficiency (i.e. the resources expended in performing a task), and satisfaction (i.e. users' subjective reactions to using the system) [10]. Moreover, different usability characteristics have been accepted as part of any software project such as *learnability* (i.e. to learn and interact rapidly with the system), *efficiency* (i.e. to achieve a high level of productivity), *memorability* (i.e. to retain knowledge about the system after a period of non-use), *rate of errors* (i.e. to have few errors while using the system), and *satisfaction* (i.e. to make the system pleasant to use it) [11]. The use of a well designed platform to deliver psychological treatments can have a great impact on increasing the interest and number of people who can benefit from them. However, few studies have assessed usability in Internet- and Computer-based treatments [12–15]. In this regard, the usability of these interventions should be further explored.

The aim of this study is to evaluate the usability of a transdiagnostic Internet-based treatment for patients suffering from one or more emotional disorder (ED), including a specific therapeutic component to address positive affect.

2   Method

2.1   Participants

This study is a secondary analysis of data collected as part of a clinical trial of a transdiagnostic Internet-based treatment for ED with a specific component to address positive affect [16]. Those participants interested in the study contacted via personal visits or phone calls to the Emotional Disorders University Clinic, through emails, or leaving their data on the clinic website. All participants were recruited from a community sample of patients diagnosed with one or more diagnosis of ED: major depressive disorder (MDD), dysthymic disorder (DD), (unipolar) mood disorder not otherwise specified, obsessive-compulsive disorder (OCD), and five anxiety disorders: panic disorder (PD), agoraphobia (AG), generalized anxiety disorder (GAD), social anxiety disorder (SAD), anxiety disorder not otherwise specified (ADNOS) [17]. Individuals were eligible for the study if they were 18 years or older, met the DSM-IV diagnostic criteria for one or more of the aforementioned ED, had the ability to understand and read Spanish, had access to Internet at home and an email address, and provided online informed consent. Exclusion criteria were: (a) suffering from Schizophrenia, bipolar disorder, or alcohol and/or substance dependence disorder; (b) the presence of high risk of suicide; (c) medical disease/condition that prevents the participant from carrying out the psychological treatment; (d) receiving another psychological treatment during the study; or e) an increase and/or change in the pharmacological treatment during the study period (in the case of being in pharmacological treatment). All the participants included in this study participated in the transdiagnostic intervention protocol (described below). The treatment protocol from which these data were drawn was approved by the Ethics Committee of Universitat Jaume I (Castellón, Spain) and was registered at clinicaltrial.gov as NCT02578758.

The sample was composed of 87 participants. Participants' mean age was 36.75 years old (SD = 11.12, range 20–63), the majority were female (67%, 58/87), and most of them were single (54%, 47/87) and had higher studies (71%, 62/87). In addition, most participants suffered from GAD (31%, 27/87), followed by SAD (30%, 26/87) and MDD (12%, 10/87). Regarding the patterns of comorbidity in the sample, 42% of the participants had at least one comorbid diagnosis, with 11 individuals (13%) meeting criteria for two comorbid diagnoses, and 7 (8%) meeting criteria for three comorbid diagnoses.

2.2 Measures

Diagnostic Interview
Mini International Neuropsychiatric Interview Version 5.0.0 (MINI) [18]. The MINI is a short, structured, diagnostic psychiatric interview for DSM-IV and ICD-10 diagnoses. This interview can be used by clinicians after a brief training session and has excellent inter -rater reliability (k = .88–1.00) and adequate concurrent validity with the Composite International Diagnostic Interview [18].

Usability Questionnaire
System Usability Scale (SUS) [19, 20]. This scale assesses the usability of a service or product and the acceptance of technology by the people who use it. The SUS is a simple, ten -item scale that indicates the degree of agreement or disagreement with the statements on a 5-point scale (1 = strongly disagree; 5 = strongly agree). The final score is obtained by adding the scores on each item and multiplying the result by 2.5. Scores range from 0–100, where higher scores indicate better usability [21]. Following [21], the scores are replaced for adjectives and classified according to their acceptability, being not acceptable if the mean score is less than 50 and acceptable if the score is higher than 70. A score between 50 and 70 is classified as marginal acceptability (see Fig. 1). The Usability and Acceptability Questionnaire is currently being validated by

our research group, and a short- form consisting of 7 items was used in a previous study, showing a Cronbach's Alpha of .94 [14].

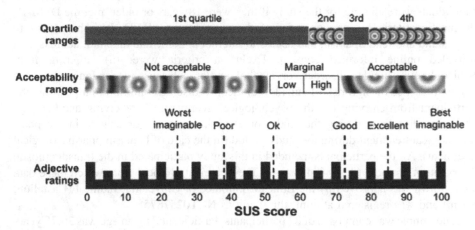

Fig. 1. SUS scores by quartile ranges, acceptability ranges, and adjective ratings [19].

2.3   Treatment Protocol

The treatment protocol is based on the classic transdiagnostic perspective derived from the Unified Protocol [22, 23] and some strategies from Marsha Linehan's protocol [24]. The program includes core components, mainly designed to down-regulate negative affect (present-focused emotional awareness and acceptance, cognitive flexibility, behavioral and emotional avoidance patterns, and interoceptive and situational exposure) and a positive affect regulation component to promote psychological strengths and enhance well-being [25]. The treatment protocol also includes therapeutic components of evidence-based treatment for ED: psychoeducation, motivation for change, and relapse prevention. All these treatment components were developed through two self-applied protocol modalities with 12 (Transdiagnostic Internet-based protocol, TIBP) and 16 modules (Transdiagnostic Internet-based protocol + Positive Affect component, TIBP + PA), respectively. The description of the modules for each protocol modality have been described elsewhere [16].

Regardless of treatment modality, all participants completed the intervention through a multimedia web platform using videos, vignettes, audios, images, etc., in order to make the therapeutic content more attractive to the patients (https://www. psicologiaytecnologia.com). The program was designed to be completely self-applied via the Internet through a PC or a tablet and with a linear navigation in order to optimize the treatment structure, allowing participants with less experience in handling technologies to know how to keep moving forward at any time (Fig. 2).

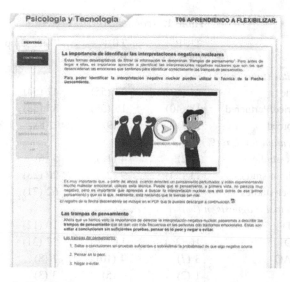

Fig. 2. "Screenshot" of one of the modules of the Internet-based treatment for emotional disorders

2.4 Statistical Analyses

Participant's descriptive statistics of all sociodemographic characteristics and Student's *t*-test for usability were examined. All statistical analyses were conducted using IBM SPSS Statistics for Windows, version 22.

3 Results

3.1 Socio-Demographic Data

Details about participants' sociodemographic characteristics are presented in Table 1.

Table 1. Sociodemographic characteristics of participants

	TIBP (N = 45)	TIBP + PA (N = 42)	Total sample
Age (years)			
Mean (SD)	38.99 (12.38)	34.36 (9.15)	36.75 (11.12)
Range	21–63	20–52	20–63
Gender, n (%)			
Male	13 (29)	16 (38)	29 (33)
Female	32 (71)	26 (62)	58 (67)

(continued)

Table 1. (*continued*)

	TIBP (N = 45)	TIBP + PA (N = 42)	Total sample
Marital status, n (%)			
Single	24 (53)	23 (55)	47 (54)
Married/Partnered	18 (40)	15 (36)	33 (38)
Divorced	3 (7)	4 (9)	7 (8)
Education level, n (%)			
Basic studies	1 (2)	4 (10)	5 (6)
Medium studies	11 (24)	9 (21)	20 (23)
Higher studies	33 (73)	29 (69)	62 (71)
Principal diagnosis, n (%)			
MDD	6 (13)	4 (10)	10 (12)
GAD	16 (36)	11 (26)	27 (31)
PD/AG	3 (7)	4 (10)	7 (8)
PD	1 (2)	2 (5)	3 (3)
AG	4 (9)	3 (7)	7 (8)
SAD	11 (24)	15 (35)	26 (30)
OCD	2 (4)	1 (2)	3 (3)
ADNOS	2 (4)	2 (5)	4 (5)
Number of comorbid diagnoses, n (%)			
None	22 (49)	10 (24)	32 (37)
1	16 (35)	21 (50)	37 (42)
2	4 (9)	7 (17)	11 (13)
3	3 (7)	4 (9)	7 (8)

Note: SD = Standard deviations.

3.2 Usability of the Program

Usability scores are shown in Table 2. According to [21], results showed that the program obtained high acceptability levels among participants in terms of usability. The overall score was 82.67/100 (SD = 12.53). The Student's *t*-test analysis did not reveal statistical differences between groups ($t = -.60$; $p = .55$), this result indicates that the levels of usability achieved in both experimental conditions are equal.

Table 2. System Usability Scale: Means and standard deviations

	TIBP (N = 45)	TIBP + PA (N = 42)	Total sample
1. I think that I would like to use this system frequently	3.16 (.90)	3.38 (.79)	3.26 (.86)
2. I found the system unnecessarily complex	3.49 (.82)	3.14 (1.34)	3.32 (1.10)

(*continued*)

Table 2. (*continued*)

	TIBP (N = 45)	TIBP + PA (N = 42)	Total sample
3. I thought the system was easy to use	3.27 (1.23)	3.33 (1.28)	3.30 (1.25)
4. I think that I would need the support of a technical person to be able to use the system	3.18 (1.21)	3.19 (1.25)	3.18 (1.23)
5. I found the various *functions in this system* were well integrated	3.13 (1.12)	3.71 (.67)	3.41 (.97)
6. I thought there was too much inconsistency in this system	3.18 (1.13)	3.17 (1.21)	3.17 (1.16)
7. I would imagine that most people would learn to use this system very quickly	3.38 (.96)	3.76 (.91)	3.56 (.95)
8. I found the system very cumbersome to use	3.13 (1.46)	2.67 (1.73)	2.91 (1.60)
9. I felt very confident using the system	3.47 (.84)	3.86 (.65)	3.66 (.78)
10. I needed to learn a lot of things before I could get going with this system	3.38 (1.19)	3.19 (1.31)	3.29 (1.25)
Overall score	81.89 (12.43)	83.51 (12.72)	82.67 (12.53)

Note: TIBP: Transdiagnostic Internet-based protocol; TIBP + PA: Transdiagnostic Internet-based protocol + Positive Affect component.

4 Discussion

The present study aimed to evaluate the usability of a transdiagnostic Internet-based treatment for patients suffering from one or more ED. The program was composed of a multimedia web platform including videos, images, vignettes, and audios, specifically designed to optimize the understanding of all the therapeutic content.

Results from the SUS scale revealed that the program obtained high scores, between the third and fourth quartile indicating that the program was considered very usable. According the literature, a worse performance at usability level could have an impact on the effectiveness of a treatment [26]. The user characteristics can influence performance, user experience and satisfaction [27]. Low usability results may indicate that users have experienced use difficulties during treatment (i.e. if they cannot use the system properly, how can we be sure about they will access the content of the treatment successfully?). Our results revealed no differences rating on the Usability adjective rating scale in both treatment conditions. That is an important result because indicate both conditions were equals at this level and platform usability have the same impact on both experimental conditions.

In this regard, participants expressed willingness to use the system frequently, reported that the system was easy to use, and that it had functions that were well integrated. In addition, participants reported that people could learn to use the system very quickly and that they felt confident using the system.

In summary, the results showed that the program was well-accepted, in terms of usability. The literature has suggested that the ease of use along with usefulness, service excellence, aesthetics, and playfulness is one the five key factors involved in the use of a system in the future [28]. Therefore, it is important to consider the study of the usability of Internet-based interventions as an important aspect in psychological treatments. Furthermore, other variables related to acceptability such as expectations, satisfaction, and treatment preference should also be considered.

The present study represents an initial attempt to evaluate the acceptability of an Internet-based treatment for ED. However, this study presents some limitations that should be mentioned. First, this study only provides data about the usability of the Internet-based treatment. Information about satisfaction or treatment preferences had significantly contributed to the program's acceptability. Second, participants in the study answered the usability scale with quantitative data but no qualitative feedback about the program was collected. Future studies should complement quantitative and qualitative analyses in order to obtain more information about participant's impressions of the program.

In sum, to the best of our knowledge, the aim of this study is to analyze the usability of a transdiagnostic Internet-based treatment for ED that includes a specific therapeutic component to address positive affect. This program is presented as a well-accepted online treatment in terms of usability. Further research is needed in this field in order to improve Internet-based programs and therefore increase the acceptance and dissemination of evidence-based Internet-delivered psychological treatments.

References

1. Andersson, G., Cuijpers, P.: Internet-based and other computerized psychological treatments for adult depression: a meta-analysis. Cogn. Behav. Ther. **38**(4), 196–205 (2009)
2. Andersson, G.: Internet-delivered psychological treatments. Annu. Rev. Clin. Psychol. **12**(1), 157–179 (2016)
3. Andrews, G., Cuijpers, P., Craske, M.G., McEvoy, P., Titov, N.: Computer therapy for the anxiety and depressive disorders is effective, acceptable and practical health care: a meta-analysis. PLoS ONE **5**(10), e13196 (2010)
4. Andersson, G., Titov, N.: Advantages and limitations of Internet-based interventions for common mental disorders. World Psychiatry **13**(1), 4–11 (2014)
5. Andrews, G., Newby, J.M., Williams, A.D.: Internet-delivered cognitive behavior therapy for anxiety disorders is here to stay. Curr. Psychiatry Rep. **17**(1), 1–5 (2014)
6. Peñate, W., Fumero, A.: A meta-review of Internet computer-based psychological treatments for anxiety disorders. J. Telemedicine Telecare **22**(1), 3–11 (2016)
7. Kaltenthaler, E., Sutcliffe, P., Parry, G., Beverley, C., Rees, A., Ferriter, M.: The acceptability to patients of computerized cognitive behaviour therapy for depression: a systematic review. Psychol. Med. **38**(11), 1521–1530 (2008)

8. Kazdin, A.E.: Acceptability of alternative treatments for deviant child behavior. J. Appl. Behav. Anal. **13**(2), 259–273 (1980)
9. Kushniruk, A.: Evaluation in the design of health information systems: application of approaches emerging from usability engineering. Comput. Biol. Med. **32**(3), 141–149 (2002)
10. ISO 9241-11:1998 - Ergonomic requirements for office work with visual display terminals (VDTs) – Part 11: Guidance on usability (1998)
11. Shneiderman, B.: Designing the User Interface : Strategies for Effective Human-Computer Interaction. Addison-Wesley, Boston (2010)
12. Anderson, P., Zimand, E., Schmertz, S.K., Ferrer, M.: Usability and utility of a computerized cognitive-behavioral self-help program for public speaking anxiety. Cogn. Behav. Pract. **14**(2), 198–207 (2007)
13. Botella, C., Mira, A., Moragrega, I., García-Palacios, A., Bretón-López, J., Castilla, D., et al.: An Internet-based program for depression using activity and physiological sensors: efficacy, expectations, satisfaction, and ease of use. Neuropsychiatric Dis. Treat. **12**, 393 (2016)
14. Castilla, D., Garcia-Palacios, A., Miralles, I., Breton-Lopez, J., Parra, E., Rodriguez-Berges, S., et al.: Effect of Web navigation style in elderly users. Comput. Hum. Behav. **55**, 909–920 (2016)
15. Currie, S.L., McGrath, P.J., Day, V.: Development and usability of an online CBT program for symptoms of moderate depression, anxiety, and stress in post-secondary students. Comput. Hum. Behav. **26**(6), 1419–1426 (2010)
16. Díaz-García, A., González-Robles, A., Fernández-Álvarez, J., García-Palacios, A., Baños, R. M., Botella, C.: Efficacy of a transdiagnostic internet-based treatment for emotional disorders with a specific component to address positive affect: study protocol for a randomized controlled trial. BMC Psychiatry **17**(1), 145 (2017)
17. American Psychological Association. Diagnostic and statistical manual of mental disorders (4th ed. Rev.). American Psychiatric Association, Washington, DC (2000)
18. Lecrubier, Y., Sheehan, D.V., Weiller, E., Amorim, P., Bonora, I., Sheehan, K.H., et al.: The Mini International Neuropsychiatric Interview (MINI). A short diagnostic structured interview: reliability and validity according to the CIDI. Eur. Psychiatry **12**(5), 224–231 (1997)
19. Bangor, A., Kortum, P.T., Miller, J.T.: An empirical evaluation of the system usability scale. Int. J. Hum. Comput. Interact. **24**(6), 574–594 (2008)
20. Brooke, J.: SUS - A quick and dirty usability scale. In: Usability Evaluation in Industry, vol. 189, no. 194, pp. 4–7 (1996)
21. Bangor, A., Kortum, P., Miller, J.: Determining what individual SUS scores mean: adding an adjective rating scale. J. Usability Stud. **4**(3), 114–123 (2009)
22. Ellard, K.K., Fairholme, C.P., Boisseau, C.L., Farchione, T.J., Barlow, D.H.: Unified protocol for the transdiagnostic treatment of emotional disorders: protocol development and initial outcome data. Cogn. Behav. Pract. **17**(1), 88–101 (2010)
23. Barlow, D., Allen, L.B., Choate, M.L.: Toward a unified treatment for emotional disorders. Behav. Ther. **35**, 205–230 (2004)
24. Linehan, M.: Cognitive-Behavioral Treatment of Borderline Personality Disorder. Guilford Press, New York City (1993)
25. Sin, N.L., Lyubomirsky, S.: Enhancing well-being and alleviating depressive symptoms with positive psychology interventions: a practice-friendly meta-analysis. J. Clin. Psychol. **65**(655), 467–487 (2009)

26. Zapata, B.C., Fernández-alemán, J.L., Idri, A., Toval, A.: Empirical studies on usability of mHealth apps: a systematic literature review. J. Med. Syst. **39**(1), 1–19 (2017). https://doi.org/10.1007/s10916-014-0182-2
27. Georgsson, M., Staggers, N.: Quantifying usability: an evaluation of a diabetes mHealth system on effectiveness, efficiency, and satisfaction metrics with associated user characteristics. J. Am. Med. Inform. Assoc. **23**(1), 5–11 (2016). https://doi.org/10.1093/jamia/ocv099
28. Huang, T.L., Liao, S.: A model of acceptance of augmented-reality interactive technology: the moderating role of cognitive innovativeness. Electron. Commer. Res. J. **15**(2), 269–295 (2015)

How Can We Implement Single-Case Experimental Designs in Group Therapy and Using Digital Technologies: A Study with Fibromyalgia Patients

Carlos Suso-Ribera[1]($\boxtimes$), Guadalupe Molinari[2],
and Azucena García-Palacios[1,2]

[1] Jaume I University, 12007 Castellón de la Plana, Castelló, Spain
{susor, azucena}@uji.es
[2] CIBER of Physiopathology of Obesity and Nutrition CIBERobn,
CB06/03 Instituto de Salud Carlos III (Spain), Madrid, Spain
molinari@uji.es

Abstract. Single case designs (SCDs) have been argued to reduce or eliminate some of the problems of large-scale, randomized controlled trials, including the focus on average scores, the need for control groups, the difficulties in modifying treatment protocols after study onset, and the use of a reduced number of assessment points. To date, however, SCDs have been rare due to methodological difficulties (i.e., need for repeated assessment), which is now feasible with technology. It is also rare to find SCDs in group therapy research, again due to methodological and conceptual barriers. Our aim was to set up a SCD within the context of a group delivery psychological intervention for fibromyalgia patients (FM). An app developed by our team, Pain Monitor, was used for ecological momentary assessment. The treatment protocol integrates CBT techniques with positive psychology, pain acceptance, and mindfulness exercises. In this study, we intend to discuss how SCDs can be construed in the context of group therapy. We will present benefits and shortcomings of this methodology in this context and finally we will expose a real case with FM patients from our on laboratory which is currently running. In this investigation, a multiple baseline design was selected, but examples using other designs, such as ABAB (A = baseline; B = treatment), changing criterion, or alternating treatments, will be discussed with the same sample to provide an overview of different possibilities to address group treatment research using SCDs.

Keywords: Singe case experimental design · Smartphone app · Fibromyalgia

1 Introduction

Clinical research in the past decades has been dominated by large-scale, randomized controlled trials that investigate the effectiveness of one or more interventions compared to a control condition (i.e., waiting list or a well-established treatment to be used for comparison). In such designs, a number of assessment points (i.e., pretreatment, posttreatment, and a varying number of follow-ups) is usually included to demonstrate

© ICST Institute for Computer Sciences, Social Informatics and Telecommunications Engineering 2019
Published by Springer Nature Switzerland AG 2019. All Rights Reserved
P. Cipresso et al. (Eds.): MindCare 2019, LNICST 288, pp. 157–167, 2019.
https://doi.org/10.1007/978-3-030-25872-6_12

treatment effectiveness. By doing this, because of the reduced number of evaluation points, treatment effectiveness is compared at the mean level at the group level [1].

While randomized controlled trials have certainly contributed to the advance of clinical research, important limitations of this methodology should not be ignored. For instance, the limited number of assessment points frequently included in large-scale studies affects the reliability of measurements at the individual level, especially when outcomes can easily fluctuate (i.e., mood). Additionally, the focus on the average level of change makes the validity of findings limited for the individual and the need for a control group results in ethical concerns. Finally, the use of this methodology is problematic when disorders or outcomes of interest are infrequent in daily practice or not prevalent in the population and when a new treatment for which there is no previous evidence is to be tested, as there is risk for low efficacy or even side effects that would affect large samples [2].

Single case designs (SCDs) are an alternative to large-scale, randomized controlled trials in clinical research. Different to large-scale interventions, SCDs require repeated assessment over time (at least five measurements in the baseline phase and five measurements in the treatment phase), evaluate the effectiveness of interventions in the individual as opposed to averaging group scores, eliminates the need for control conditions (each individual acts as his/her own control in the baseline phase), and is suitable when disorders or outcomes are infrequent or when a new treatment is being tested (it can be used with a single individual). Regarding the latter, while SCDs are usually seen as having limited external validity because they can be applied to a single individual, replications of the single effect in an increased number of subjects is perfectly possible (and recommended), thus increasing the generalizability of findings [3, 4].

Despite the use of SCDs in clinical research has important benefits, their use has been limited, arguably due to methodological difficulties. For instance, repeated assessment was initially made using paper diaries and more recently with telephone calls. Both procedures are problematic as resulted in frequent missing or unreliable information (i.e., paper diaries) or they were very time- and cost-consuming (i.e., phone calls). The explosion of smartphones and the increasing use of apps have renewed interest in SCDs as they facilitate ecological momentary assessment with reduced costs. The previous has resulted in a significant increase in the number of single case investigations in clinical research in a variety of conditions [5].

The application of SCDs in group therapy, however, is still rare, which we believe is due to the difficulties in designing a study that fits the assumptions and requirements of SCDs in a group delivery context. For instance, SCDs need three attempts to replicate treatment effect, so AB (A = baseline; B = treatment) and ABA designs are not considered adequate experimental studies. Only ABAB, multiple baselines with three baselines, changing criterions with three criteria, and alternating treatments with three treatment effect replications would be acceptable [6].

Our goal is to discuss how SCDs can be effectively implemented within a group therapy context. An example of an ongoing study from our group using multiple baselines with fibromyalgia patients will be presented, but the remaining designs will also be described for the same sample to provide the reader with different design options for group treatment. Fibromyalgia is a prevalent and disabling syndrome characterized by generalized pain, fatigue, and stiffness which presents with a high comorbidity of affective disorders [7]. Fibromyalgia patients were selected because psychological intervention, such as cognitive behavioral therapy, mindfulness-based treatments, or acceptance and commitment therapy, in a group format is very frequent in this population [8, 9] and because a new treatment including components of other well-established interventions was to be tested. The feasibility of using this methodology including apps for repeated assessment is also discussed in the paper according to our experience.

2   Method

2.1   Participants

Five patients were referred by a rheumatologist from the Rheumatology Unit of the General Hospital of Castellon, Spain. After the screening interviews, three patients were accepted into the study (two of them had difficulties in attending group sessions weekly) and further assessments were conducted. The three patients were women. P1 has 62 years old and a disease duration of 10 years. She is married, has basic levels of education, and is an active worker. P2 has 44 years old and a fibromyalgia (FM) duration of 2 years. She is married, has basic levels of education, and she currently does not work due to a sick leave. P3 has 36 years old and a disease duration of 2 years. She is single, has a university degree, and is an active worker.

2.2   Measures: Ecological Momentary Assessment with Pain Monitor

Assessment was made with a smartphone app developed and validated by our team [10]. In the app, the initial evaluation consists of a set of sociodemographic and pain- and health-related outcomes, including pain localization, average pain intensity and interference in the past two weeks, and overall perceived health status, among others. This group of questions is administered once after downloading and using the app for the first time.

EMA begins the day after the first evaluation and occurs twice a day (10 am and 7 pm with two-hour response flexibility) throughout the study duration. Morning and evening evaluations share a number of items, such as pain intensity and mood (i.e., sadness, anxiety, anger, and happiness), because these variables can vary within the same day. Other constructs are either evaluated in the morning (i.e., interference of pain on sleep) or in the evening only (i.e., interference of pain on daily activities, use of rescue medication during the day, and symptoms experienced during the day). Finally, psychological variables (i.e., pain acceptance, catastrophizing, and fear of pain) are either included in the morning or the evening administration to balance the duration of the evaluations.

At the end of study (i.e., after the 11 weekly sessions), a final assessment is made. Similar to the initial evaluation, this final assessment is administered once only. This includes some sociodemographic information to explore changes compared to the initial assessment (i.e., marital and job status), but also explores additional variables that are important for the evaluation of the treatment effectiveness (i.e., perceived change after treatment and stressful life events experienced during the study).

2.3 Treatment

The psychological treatment program integrates CBT techniques with positive psychology, acceptance, and mindfulness tools, which have shown evidence in the treatment of chronic pain [11]. The therapeutic components of the program are: Motivation for Change, Psychoeducation, Cognitive Flexibility, Behavioral Activation, Positive Psychology strategies, Mindfulness, Self-compassion, and Relapse Prevention.

The first session of the treatment is "Motivation for Change" and it was delivered individually in order to establish the multiple baselines. This session focused on each participant's motivation to participate in the psychological treatment. Participants set individual goals to be achieved during and at the end of treatment. The rest of the treatment consists of 11 weekly sessions of an approximate duration of 2 h applied in a group format. Every session is held at the University and is conducted by a psychologist. A more detailed description of this multicomponent treatment can be seen in Table 1.

2.4 Procedure

The rheumatologist of the local public hospital provided the participants' with general information about the study and referred FM patients interested in participating. Patients had to fulfill the American College of Rheumatology criteria for primary FM [12]. Also important for the present study, inclusion criteria included having access to a smartphone using Android operating system, having Internet connection, and not presenting a severe psychiatric condition.

At the start of the first week, participants attended an individual information and assessment session on different days to establish the multiple baselines. In this initial session they were informed about the characteristics of the study and were asked to download the app. All participants attended voluntarily and received no economic compensation to participate. All the sessions took place in a therapy room at the Jaume I University and all the appointments were set at the same day to fulfil the requirements of this type of design. Once the participants gave written informed consent to participate, a brief structured interview was conducted in order to assess pain history and previous treatments. After this initial assessment, the psychologist and lead author, GM, who has been trained and is experienced in this type of treatments and population, explained the use of the Pain Monitor App to the patients and helped them to download it from the Google Play Store. Once the Pain Monitor App was installed on the participants' smartphone, they completed the initial assessment with the support of the psychologist. No technical or usability problems were detected at this stage, so further assessments were made without the supervision of the lead researcher.

Previous to recruitment, all participants were randomly assigned to one of the three study conditions (i.e., 5 days, 7 days, or 9 days of baseline assessment). This meant that participants recorded their responses to the app daily in their natural environments for 5, 7, and 9 days prior to the treatment onset. The random assignment of the participants

Table 1. Description of each of the sessions of the psychological treatment

Session	Content	Objective
Session 1	**Motivation for change**	To analyze the advantages and disadvantages of change, emphasizing the importance of being motivated
Session 2	**Psychoeducation**	Provide information about fibromyalgia taking into account related medical, psychological and social aspects. Explanation of the rationale of treatment and group therapy rules
Session 3	**Acceptance**	Recognition of one's own physical limitations and changes in habits caused by fibromyalgia. Learn to be in contact with one's own experience, even when it is not pleasant, and accept it as it is. Acceptance of this "new self"
Session 4	**Activity Programming**	Increase the number and intensity of positive emotions through an appropriate level of activity to better cope with pain. Each participant has to select a list of meaningful activities to perform during the treatment
Session 5	**Mindfulness**	Practice of mindfulness meditations to lower the perception of pain, reduce tension, and improve functioning and well-being
Session 6	**Cognitive flexibility**	Learn to identify and modify maladaptive thoughts, and to generate other alternative interpretations to different situations
Session 7	**Communication strategies**	Learn to identify the main communication problems to move towards more effective communication. Improve interpersonal relationships, self-esteem and put into practice assertiveness
Session 8	**Self-compassion**	Learn the need to take care of ourselves, to be kind to ourselves, seeking well-being and the relief of suffering
Session 9	**Relapse prevention**	Review all the skills learned during treatment and see how to maintain and continue with the progress made so far. Assess the way to act in future risk situations

to the different experimental conditions was generated by an independent researcher according to a randomization list created by an online randomizing program [13].

After the baseline assessment period, participants attended to the first treatment session individually (i.e., "Motivation to Change" session) after 5, 7, or 9 days of study onset in order to establish the multiple baselines (see Fig. 1 for a summary of the design). Participants set individual goals to be achieved during treatment. The following week, participants started group treatment. Weekly sessions were also held at the University and had an approximate duration of 2 h. All sessions were conducted by a clinical psychologist.

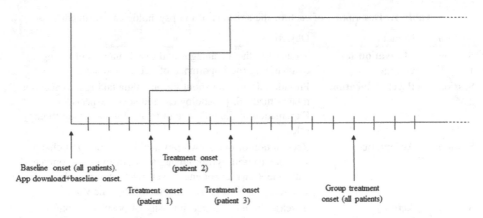

Fig. 1. Graphical representation of the multiple baseline study design. The first treatment session, which occurs at different moments to establish the multiple baselines, is individual and addresses content related to motivation to change. After the group treatment onset, the subsequent group sessions occur on a weekly basis and are not shown in the Figure to facilitate its interpretation. The x axis represents days and the y axis represents each participant.

3 Discussion

3.1 Advantages and Barriers to the Implementation of a Multiple Baseline SCD in a Group Format Supported by Technologies

The present study is currently ongoing (four therapy sessions have been delivered so far), but positive aspects and difficulties in the design and implementation of a SCD in a group format supported by an app have been already revealed. First, an advantage of using a SCD has been that the study could be implemented with a reduced number of women and that a control group was not required (the baseline phase is used as the control for each individual). We calculated that, with an anticipated effect size of 0.40, an alpha level of .005, a power of .80, two conditions (treatment vs control), and 10 measurement points only (5 for the A phase and 5 for the B phase), we would need more than 110 patients using a traditional randomized controlled trial [14]. Additionally, this would mean having a control group, which is ethically problematic. Another advantage of the SCD is that treatments can be modified if an issue emerges (i.e., the treatment is causing side effects or not being effective). In the present study, this has not been necessary, but the treatment could be adapted for the whole group if required. Finally, repeated assessment tends to be a challenge in SCDs, which was efficaciously minimized with the use of a smartphone application. In the past, paper diaries and telephone calls have been used but proven to be unreliable or inefficacious. Our experience in the present and past research is that the use of apps finally makes EMA feasible.

While acknowledging the benefits of this design for group psychological treatment in particular and clinical research in general, we also noted some difficulties in the present investigation. For instance, the multiple baseline design, which we believe best suited the study goals (see the next point for further discussion), implies that participants had to start the treatment phase on different days, which might be difficult in group treatment. We have proposed a solution for this problem, but other studies might need a different strategy to manage this requirement. Another limitation that we have observed when implementing a SCD in a group psychological treatment for FM is that technology is still a barrier for a number of individuals, especially older ones. The physicians who referred the patients to us indicated that some potential participants had very old phones with no Internet connection, so their inclusion was not possible. This is certainly a problem we will face in the next years when using technology for research, but the increasing availability of smartphones is likely to minimize this difficulty [15].

3.2   Alternatives to a Multiple Baseline Design for Group Delivery Using Technologies

In the present investigation, a multiple baseline SCD was selected because we believed this design had the best fit to the study purposes and characteristics. However, we will now present other SCDs and discuss how they could be implemented in the same study presented above (i.e., group psychological treatment of FM patients), together with their advantages and disadvantages.

ABAB Design. An ABAB design is a straightforward SCD that consists of a baseline phase (A), followed by treatment phase (B), a withdrawal phase (A), and a final treatment phase (B). Simpler forms of this design are AB or ABA designs, but these do not meet the requirements for adequate SCDs (i.e., three replications of the treatment effect). In the present investigation, an ABAB design for the psychological treatment of FM patients in a group format with the help of technology for EMA could have been easily implemented [16]. First, all patients should have started the baseline assessment with the app on the same day. Next, at least five days after the initial assessment (five assessments are the minimum to meet the requirements of excellent SCDs) [6] all patients would start the treatment in a group format (note that this is largely different from the multiple baseline design). After a number of treatment sessions (this might vary depending on the treatment), the treatment would be withdrawn and a return to baseline scores in the outcome measure (i.e., mood or pain intensity or interference) would be expected. A new treatment phase is then started to obtain the third evidence of treatment effect (improvement from A to B, worsening from B to A, and new improvement from A to B).

As described above, this is a straightforward design to be used in group (and individual) format is one is to implement a SCD, which is one of the strengths of this design. However, in the present study an ABAB design would have been problematic because the return to baseline levels after treatment withdrawal is rare in psychological treatments [17]. In fact, increasing the patient's ability to deal with difficult situations outside the therapy context and in a large number of settings (i.e., generalization) is one of the main goals of psychological interventions, so this design is not suitable when a return to baseline levels is not expected in the transition from B to A.

Changing Criterion Design. In the changing criterion design, participants are required to reach a specific goal (i.e., criterion) that changes at different stages of the study (i.e., when the goal is repeatedly met). Similar to the previous design, three replications of a treatment effect are required to meet the standards for SCDs, which means that at least three different criteria are needed [6]. In the present investigation, the three criteria could have been: a reduction of 10% in pain interference compared to baseline levels, a reduction of 20% in pain interference compared to baseline levels, and a reduction of 30% in pain interference compared to baseline levels. This means that a first study goal would be to achieve and maintain a reduction of 10% in pain interference during five or more days after the onset of treatment. Once this was achieved, a more difficult criterion of 20% reduction would be set and, again, this should be maintained for five days or more. Finally, the third replication of treatment effect should be achieved with a 30% reduction of pain interference.

While this design is perfectly feasible for the present investigation and has important benefits (i.e., only one participant or group of participants are needed), a barrier for using this method is that goals have to be successively achieved at the established criterion, but not further [18]. Therefore, if a patient or group of patients showed a large reduction in pain interference of 30% in the first step (when the criterion was 10%), we could not conclude that the reduction was due to the effect of treatment or due to an external event that occurred at the same time as treatment onset (i.e., obtained a sick leave or there was a change in the tasks assigned at work). Therefore, if the treatment was "too effective", this would become an AB design which prevents us from drawing causal conclusions. Because we anticipated that the change obtained with our treatment would be difficult to restrict to a specific criterion (i.e., it is difficult to indicate pain patients in the group that they should improve functioning despite the pain, but to a certain extent only), a changing criterion design was not felt like the most appropriate design for our purposes.

Alternating Treatments Design. In an alternating treatments design, two or more interventions are provided alternatively after a baseline phase. Next, the treatment that appears to provide the smaller effect (i.e., when graphically representing the evolution on the outcome of interest or after overlap calculations) is withdrawn and the most effective treatment is left alone to ensure that the efficacy revealed when both treatments were provided together is maintained when the arguably most effective one is presented alone [19].

In the present investigation, our goal was not to compare the effectiveness of two interventions, so this design was not suitable. However, we discuss how this could have been implemented if two treatments, such as cognitive behavioral-therapy (CBT) and acceptance and commitment therapy (ACT), were to be compared. After a baseline phase, CBT and ACT sessions would be randomly alternated (2 CBT sessions, 1 ACT session, 1 CBT session, 2 ACT sessions, 2 CBT sessions, 3 ACT sessions, etc.) until the full treatment is delivered. All group members would attend all sessions. Assessments would be made during the whole study duration and a graphical representation would evidence whether the outcome of interest (i.e., depressive symptoms) was more largely improved after the delivery of one of the treatments (e.g., CBT). Finally, to ensure that the effectiveness of CBT was not due to the interaction with ACT, CBT would be provided alone and the graphical analysis would indicate whether the effect on the outcome was maintained after removing ACT.

3.3 Analytic Strategies

An in-depth discussion of the analytic strategies for SCDs is out of the scope of the present investigation. However, we believe that a brief overview of this topic, including some recommended references will be important for the reader. Early studies using SCDs mostly relied on visual analysis (i.e., analysis of changes in trend and slope) between phases, with an emphasis on clinically meaningful changes in outcomes [6, 20]. While graphical visualization is clearly informative, more rigorous procedures have emerged in the past decades. Note, first, that the presence of autocorrelation in SCDs (time series data) means that traditional tests, both parametric and non-parametric, are not appropriate for the calculation of treatment effects, so a different analytic approach is required for SCDs. Some of the most frequently used analytic strategies in SCDs include calculations of overlap between baseline and treatment phases [21]. Several overlap methods exist, which mostly differ in the number of baseline measurement points included in the analyses (i.e., some take the median, while others use non-overlapping data only). However, the *non-overlap of all pairs*, a strategy that includes the comparison of every measurement in the baseline phase and every measurement in the treatment phase, is the procedure that has shown to be more robust to bias [22]. In addition to an analysis of overlap, randomization in SCDs (i.e., of both participants and duration of baseline phases), as performed in the present investigation, allows for more sophisticated calculations, such as the analysis of randomized tests, a nonparametric of treatment effect size [23, 24].

4   Conclusions

The present study aimed at presenting a SCD for group psychological treatment of patients. The use of SCDs is gaining ground in clinical research, arguably to the explosion of smartphones, which have made EMA a feasible alternative to episodic, onsite assessment. Despite this increasing interest in these designs, the literature in this field is still scarce, especially in relation to group treatment formats. We have presented the four most commonly used SCDs and we have provided an example of how group psychological treatment of FM could be implemented with each design. In doing so, we have discussed the advantages and barriers to implementing each design in a group format, as well as the methodological requirements for each method.

We believe the present work will provide new light into clinical research using group formats and SCDs and will encourage researchers to implement these designs in future research.

References

1. Perez-Gomez, A., Mejia-Trujillo, J., Mejia, A.: How useful are randomized controlled trials in a rapidly changing world? Glob. Ment. Heal. **3**, e6 (2016). https://doi.org/10.1017/gmh. 2015.29

2. Blampied, N.M.: The third way: single-case research, training, and practice in clinical psychology. Aust. Psychol. **36**, 157–163 (2001). https://doi.org/10.1080/00050060108259648
3. Ray, D.C., Schottelkorb, A.A.: Single-case design: a primer for play therapists. Int. J. Play Ther. **19**, 39–53 (2010). https://doi.org/10.1037/a0017725
4. Smith, J.D.: Single-case experimental designs: a systematic review of published research and current standards. Psychol. Methods **17**, 1–70 (2012). https://doi.org/10.1037/a0029312
5. Suso-Ribera, C., et al.: Improving pain treatment with a smartphone app: study protocol for a randomized controlled trial. Trials **19**, 145 (2018). https://doi.org/10.1186/s13063-018-2539-1
6. Kratochwill, T.R., et al.: Single-case intervention research design standards. Remedial Spec. Educ. **34**, 26–38 (2012). https://doi.org/10.1177/0741932512452794
7. Queiroz, L.P.: Worldwide epidemiology of fibromyalgia topical collection on fibromyalgia. Curr. Pain Headache Rep. **17** (2013). https://doi.org/10.1007/s11916-013-0356-5
8. Glombiewski, J.A., Sawyer, A.T., Gutermann, J., Koenig, K., Rief, W., Hofmann, S.G.: Psychological treatments for fibromyalgia: a meta-analysis. Pain. Int. Assoc. Study Pain **151**, 280–295 (2010). https://doi.org/10.1016/j.pain.2010.06.011
9. Häuser, W., Thieme, K., Turk, D.C.: Guidelines on the management of fibromyalgia syndrome – a systematic review. Eur. J. Pain **14**, 5–10 (2010). https://doi.org/10.1016/j.ejpain.2009.01.006. European Federation of International Association for the Study of Pain Chapters
10. Suso-Ribera, C., Castilla, D., Zaragozá, I., Ribera-Canudas, M.V., Botella, C., García-Palacios, A.: Validity, reliability, feasibility, and usefulness of pain monitor, a multidimensional smartphone app for daily monitoring of adults with heterogeneous chronic pain. Clin. J. Pain **34**, 1 (2018). https://doi.org/10.1097/AJP.0000000000000618
11. Jenny, M.Q., Isabel Casado, Mª.: Terapias psicológicas para el tratamiento del Dolor Crónico. Clín. Salud. **22**, 41–50 (2011). https://doi.org/10.5093/cl2011v22n1a3
12. Wolfe, F., et al.: The American College of Rheumatology 1990 criteria for the classification of fibromyalgia. Report of the Multicenter Criteria Committee. Arthritis Rheum. **33**, 160–172 (1990). https://doi.org/10.1016/j.pain.2008.02.009
13. Urbaniak, G.C., Plous, S.: Research Randomizer (Version 4.0) [Computer software] (2013)
14. Faul, F., Erdfelder, E., Lang, A.-G., Buchner, A.: G*Power 3: a flexible statistical power analysis program for the social, behavioral, and biomedical sciences. Behav. Res. Methods **39**, 175–191 (2007). https://doi.org/10.3758/BF03193146
15. Dallery, J., Cassidy, R.N., Raiff, B.R.: Single-case experimental designs to evaluate novel technology-based health interventions. J. Med. Internet Res. **15** (2013). https://doi.org/10.2196/jmir.2227
16. Horner, R.H., Swaminathan, H., Sugai, G., Smolkowski, K.: Considerations for the systematic analysis and use of single-case research. Educ. Treat. Child. **35**, 269–290 (2012). https://doi.org/10.1353/etc.2012.0011
17. Sexton-Radek, K.: Single case designs in psychology practice. Heal. Psychol. Res. **2** (2014). https://doi.org/10.4081/hpr.2014.1551
18. Belles, D., Bradlyn, A.S.: The use of the changing criterion design in achieving controlled smoking in a heavy smoker: a controlled case study. J. Behav. Ther. Exp. Psychiatry **18**, 77–82 (1987). http://www.ncbi.nlm.nih.gov/pubmed/3558855
19. Cannella-malone, H., Sigafoos, J., Reilly, M.O., De, Cruz B., Lancioni, G.E.: Comparing video prompting to video modeling for teaching daily living skills to six adults with developmental disabilities. Educ Train. **41**, 344–356 (2006)

20. Kratochwill, T.R., Levin, J.R.: Meta- and statistical analysis of single-case intervention research data: quantitative gifts and a wish list. J. Sch. Psychol. **52**, 231–235 (2014). https://doi.org/10.1016/j.jsp.2014.01.003. Society for the Study of School Psychology

21. Sanz, J., García-Vera, M.P.: Técnicas para el análisis de diseños de caso único en la práctica clínica: ejemplos de aplicación en el tratamiento de víctimas de atentados terroristas. Clin Salud **26**, 167–180 (2015). https://doi.org/10.1016/j.clysa.2015.09.004. Colegio Oficial de Psicólogos de Madrid

22. Parker, R.I., Vannest, K.: An improved effect size for single-case research: nonoverlap of all pairs. Behav Ther. **40**, 357–367 (2009). https://doi.org/10.1016/j.beth.2008.10.006. Elsevier B.V.

23. Bulté, I., Onghena, P.: An R package for single-case randomization tests. Behav. Res. Methods **40**, 467–478 (2008). https://doi.org/10.3758/BRM.40.2.467

24 Levin, J.R., Ferron, J.M., Kratochwill, T.R.: Nonparametric statistical tests for single-case systematic and randomized ABAB... AB and alternating treatment intervention designs: New developments, new directions. J. Sch. Psychol **50**, 599–624 (2012). https://doi.org/10.1016/j.jsp.2012.05.001. Society for the Study of School Psychology

An Attempt to Estimate Depressive Status from Voice

Yasuhiro Omiya[1,2(✉)], Takeshi Takano[1,3], Tomotaka Uraguchi[1],
Mitsuteru Nakamura[2], Masakazu Higuchi[2], Shuji Shinohara[3],
Shunji Mitsuyoshi[3], Mirai So[4], and Shinichi Tokuno[2]

[1] PST Inc., Industry & Trade Center Building 905, 2 Yamashita-cho, Naka-ku,
Yokohama, Kanagawa, Japan
{omiya, takano, uraguchi}@medical-pst.com
[2] Graduate School of Medicine, The University of Tokyo, Tokyo, Japan
{m-nakamura, higuchi, tokuno}@m.u-tokyo.ac.jp
[3] Graduate School of Engineering, The University of Tokyo, Tokyo, Japan
{shinohara, mitsuyoshi}@bioeng.t.u-tokyo.ac.jp
[4] Ginza Taimei Clinic, Tokyo, Japan
mirai.so@keio.jp

Abstract. In the whole world especially developed countries, increasing mental
health disorders is a serious problem. As a countermeasure, the main objective
of this paper is an attempt to estimate depressive status from voice. In this study,
we gathered patients with major depressive disorders in the hospital's consulting
room. Several questionnaires including "the Hamilton Depression Rating Scale"
(HAM-D) were administered to evaluate the patients' depressed state. Voices
corresponding to three long vowels were recorded from the subjects. Next, the
acoustic feature quantity was calculated based on the voice. We developed the
HAM-D score estimation algorithm from the voice using one of three types of
long vowel audio content. As a result, there was a correlation between the
"Actual HAM-D Score" and the "Estimated HAM-D Score". We found that the
algorithm is effective in estimating depression state and can be used for estimating the disease state based on voice.

Keywords: Vocal analysis · Depressive status estimation ·
The Hamilton Depression Rating Scale (HAM-D)

1 Introduction

In the whole world especially developed countries, increasing mental health dis-orders is
a serious problem, and thus various screening techniques and countermeasures have been
studied. For diagnostic support, medical interviews by specialists (e.g., using "the
Hamilton Rating Scale for Depression" [HAM-D] [1]), self-report type psychometric
tests (e.g., "the Patient Health Questionnaire" [PHQ-9] [2], and "the Beck Depression
Inventory" [BDI] [3, 4] are used to screening depressive status of patients with mental
health disorders. However, medical interviews by specialists are limited by the number of
patients that can be evaluated, and though self-report type psychometric tests are useful in

determining mental health status at their early stages and in complementing diagnoses, there are issues of reporting biases. Regarding evaluations with biomarkers such as saliva [5, 6] and blood [7, 8], they are invasive, and the tests reagent may be required or analysis may take time, and the tests are expensive. Therefore, those methods are not appropriate as easy or simple solutions. In contrast, voice-based evaluation methods have several advantages; for example, they provide diagnostic support to doctors, are almost non-invasive, no needs special equipment, and there can be used remotely and easily. It is thought that depression is triggered by psychological stress that causes the brain to lose its balance with the stress. We conducted studies to estimate stress condition in patients and support the diagnosis of disease using voice [9, 10]. Research on the relationship analyzed the pose from question to the answer and analyzed the relationship with mental health disorders, as well as the vocal fundamental frequency (F0) [11]. However, in the analysis of conversation, it is necessary to have a talk partner, the test cannot be performed alone, and it is time-consuming.

Because patients can provide false information in interviews and questionnaires, objective indicators are effective for diagnostic support. If the depression state of a patient can be estimated from the voice obtained during examination, the burden on the examiner can be reduced and possibly support the diagnosis. In this paper, our aim was to estimate the depression state of patients from their voicing of long vowels, which do not depend on the native language.

2 Materials and Methods

2.1 Experiment

We recorded the voice of patients with major depressive disorder (MDD) in a hospital's consulting room. In addition, HAM-D was conducted to screen for depressed mood. Further, patients were excluded if they had been diagnosed with serious physical disorders or organic brain disease diagnosed by a psychiatrist using The Mini-International Neuropsychiatric Interview [12]. Subjects vocalized three types of the long vowels, such as /Ah/, /Eh/, and /Uh/ approximately three seconds. The voices recorded as 24bit/96 kHz pcm audio files, using the Portable Recorder "R-26" (Roland, Japan), and a pin microphone "ME-52 W" (OLYMPUS, Japan). As for the utterance content, long vowels were selected because they do not depend on the native language. After the time of second visit, we collected the subjects voice and conducted HAM-D at each visit to observe the progress of the patient's recovery. Since the patients were undergoing treatment by a doctor, in many cases, the symptoms improved. As some patients did not revisit the hospital when their condition improved, their voice could not be recorded.

The data were collected from 28 subjects and the total number of data were 42 (Table 1).

This study was approved by the University of Tokyo, Clinical Research Review Board and informed consent was obtained from all the subjects.

Table 1. Collected subjects information.

Gender	Number of recordings			Age		Number of data	HAM-D score	
	Once	Twice	3 times	Mean ± S.D.	t-test		Mean ± S.D.	t-test
Male	5	5	1	32.5 ± 5.9	n.s.	20	23.3 ± 11.1	n.s.
Female	10	7	0	32.2 ± 8.6		22	25.0 ± 9.3	

2.2 Hamilton Depression Rating Scale (HAM-D)

"The Hamilton Rating Scale for Depression" (HRSD), also called "the Hamilton Depression Rating Scale" (HDRS), abbreviated as HAM-D, is a multi-item questionnaire used to indicate signs of depression, and as a tool to evaluate recovery. HAM-D is used to conduct clinical surveys, and its examination by health care workers usually takes about 15 to 20 min. HAM-D has various items such as "HAM-D-17", "HAM-D-21", "HAM-D-24", and so on.

2.3 Analysis of Data

We used the openSMILE software [13], 6,552 acoustic features were calculated from the collected subjects voice.

The acoustic features were calculated as follows:

(A) Physical feature was calculated on the basis of a frame unit or 56 similar feature types.
(B) Three processing contents (moving average and time change) in the time direction concerning (A)
(C) After the process (B) is performed on (A), statistical quantities of 39 types

Then the feature selection was done by implementing "CfsSubsetEval" and "BestFirst" settings in Weka software [14]. "The Sequential Minimal Optimization" (SMO) algorithm and "the Support Vector Machines" (SVM) for regression algorithm were implemented [15] in Weka software. We used 10-fold cross-validation (10FCV) in order to develop the HAM-D score estimation algorithm, generated from voice associated with pronunciation of each long vowel.

In the analysis, the correlation coefficient between the "Actual HAM-D Score" and the "Estimated HAM-D Score", according to the generated algorithm, was evaluated.

3 Results and Discussion

Figures 1, 2 and 3 are scatter plots for the "Estimated HAM-D Score" versus the "Actual HAM-D Score" based on the acoustic features of /Ah/, /Eh/, and /Uh/.

The performance of the algorithm with 10FCV relative to the "Estimated HAM-D Score" using the acoustic features of /Ah/, /Eh/, and /Uh/, and the correlation coefficients with the "Actual HAM-D Score" were found to be 0.68, 0.83, and 0.68, respectively.

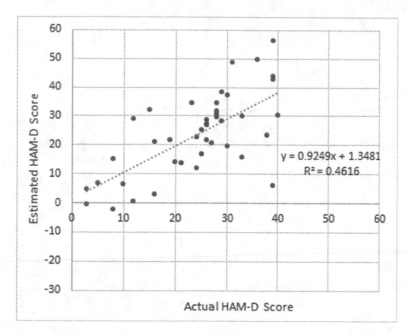

Fig. 1. Scatter plot for the "Estimated HAM-D Score" versus the "Actual HAM-D Score" based on the acoustic features of /Ah/.

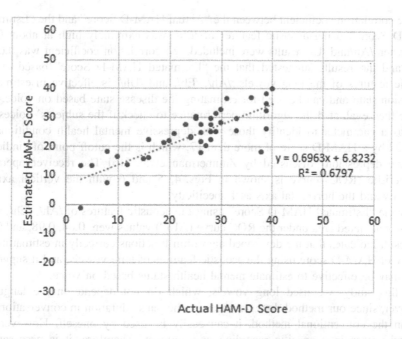

Fig. 2. Scatter plot for the "Estimated HAM-D Score" versus the "Actual HAM-D Score" based on the acoustic features of /Eh/.

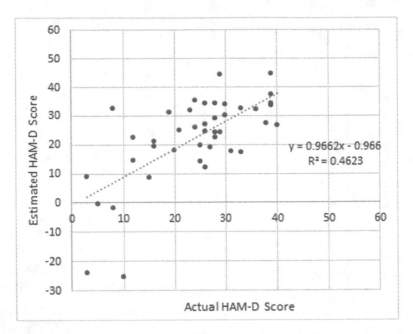

Fig. 3. Scatter plot the "Estimated HAM-D Score" versus the "Actual HAM-D Score" based on the acoustic features of /Uh/.

The correlation coefficient between the "Actual HAM-D Score" and the "Estimated HAM-D Score", using acoustic features of /Eh/, was extremely high at about 0.83. Even when /Ah/and /Uh/results were included, the correlation coefficient was 0.65 or more, and the results suggested that the "Estimated HAM-D Score" based on the acoustic features of the long vowels, /Ah/, /Eh/, and /Uh/, is effective in estimating depression state and can be used for estimating the disease state based on voice.

We then evaluated the algorithm performance to check if the subjects' voices can serve as a parameter to identify those with depressive mental health conditions, as indicated by a HAM-D score of more than 17, which is the cutoff point of "indicates moderate depression" discussed by Zimmerman et al. [16] The receiver operating characteristic (ROC) curve is shown in Figs. 4, 5 and 6 with the vertical axis as sensitivity and the horizontal axis as 1-specificity.

For the "Estimated HAM-D Score" using the acoustic features of /Ah/, /Eh/, and /Uh/, the calculated area under the ROC curve (AUC) values were 0.84, 0.98, and 0.87. This result indicates that the developed algorithm functions correctly in estimating the severity of HAM-D score using the acoustic features of long vowels, and it suggested that it may be effective to estimate mental health status based on voice.

In this study, we used long vowels, which do not depend on the language. Moreover, since our method does not measure the pause duration in conversations, as done in the conventional method, it can easily be used by oneself. However, we acquired voices in a specific recording environment. Therefore, it is necessary to evaluate our method in other recording environments.

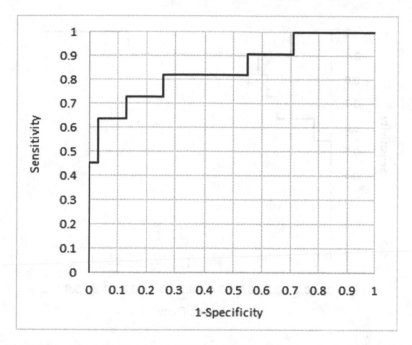

Fig. 4. ROC curve of the "Estimated HAM-D Score" using the acoustic features of /Ah/.

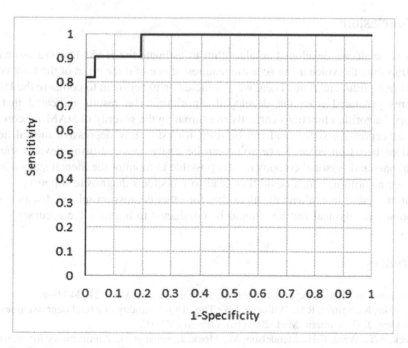

Fig. 5. ROC curve of the "Estimated HAM-D Score" using the acoustic features of /Eh/.

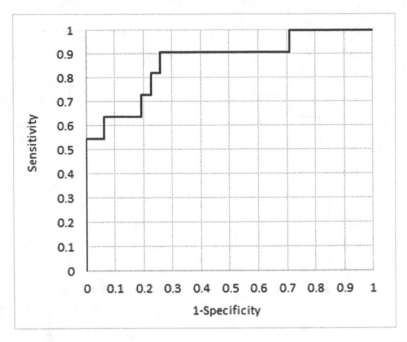

Fig. 6. ROC curve of the "Estimated HAM-D Score" using the acoustic features of /Uh/.

4 Conclusion

In this research, we developed an algorithm to estimate the HAM-D score estimation algorithm from the voice using acoustic features of one of three types of the long vowel such as /Ah/, /Eh/, and /Uh/. Then, we conducted an experiment to compare the HAM-D scores generated from the developed algorithm. The results indicated that the developed algorithm functions correctly in estimating the severity of HAM-D score that indicates depressive status, and can be used for estimating depressive mental health conditions based on voice. Since voice can be easily acquired using devices such as smartphones and personal computers, it is possible to monitor the mental state at home using our algorithm, which could then lead to a doctor's diagnostic support.

Future studies to evaluate the algorithm for other depression-related diseases, such as bipolar with atypical features should be conducted to improve the accuracy.

References

1. Hamilton, M.: Rating depressive patients. J. Clin. Psychiatry **41**, 21–24 (1980)
2. Kroenke, K., Spitzer, R.L., Williams, J.B.: The PHQ-9: validity of a brief depression severity measure. J. Gen. Intern. Med. **2001**(16), 606–613 (2001)
3. Beck, A.T., Ward, C.H., Mendelson, M., Mock, J., Erbaugh, J.: An inventory for measuring depression. Arch. Gen. Psychiatry **4**, 561–571 (1961)

4. Beck, A.T., Steer, R.A., Carbin, M.G.: Psychometric properties of the Beck Depression Inventory twenty-five years of evaluation. Clin. Psychol. Rev. **8**, 77–100 (1988)
5. Izawa, S., et al.: Salivary dehydroepiandrosterone secretion in response to acute psychosocial stress and its correlations with biological and psychological changes. Biol. Psychol. **79** (3), 294–298 (2008)
6. Ito, Y., et al.: Relationships between salivary melatonin levels, quality of sleep, and stress in young Japanese females. Int. J. Tryptophan Res. **6**(Suppl. 1), 75–85 (2013)
7. Sekiyama, A.: Interleukin-18 is involved in alteration of hipothalamic-pituitary-adrenal axis activity by stress. In: Society of Biological Psychiatry Annual Meeting, San Diego, USA (2007)
8. Kawamura, N., Shinoda, K., Ohashi, Y., Ishikawa, T., Sato, H.: Biomarker for depression, method for measuring a biomarker for depression, computer program, and recording medium. U. S. Patent, US2015126623 (2015)
9. Hagiwara, N., et al.: Validity of mind monitoring system as a mental health indicator using voice. Adv. Sci. Technol. Eng. Syst. J. **2**(3), 338–344 (2017)
10. Tokuno, S.: Pathophysiological voice analysis for diagnosis and monitoring of depression. In: Kim, Y.-K. (ed.) Understanding Depression, pp. 83–95. Springer, Singapore (2018). https://doi.org/10.1007/978-981-10-6577-4_6
11. Yang, Y., Fairbairn, C., Cohn, J.F.: Detecting depression severity from vocal prosody. IEEE Trans. Affect. Comput. **4**(2), 142–150 (2013)
12. Sheehan, D.V., et al.: The Mini-International Neuropsychiatric Interview (M.I.N.I): the development and validation of a structured diagnostic psychiatric interview for DSM-IV and ICD-10. J. Clin. Psychiatry **59**(Suppl. 20), 22–33 (1998)
13. Eyben, F., Wöllmer, M., Schuller, B.: Opensmile: the munich versatile and fast open-source audio feature extractor. In: Bimbo, A.D., Chang, S.F., Smeulders, A.W.M. (eds.) ACM Multimedia, pp. 1459–1462 (2010)
14. Hall, M., et al.: The WEKA data mining software: an update. ACM SIGKDD Explor. Newsl. **11**(1), 10–18 (2009)
15. Shevade, S.K., Keerthi, S.S., Bhattacharyya, C., Murthy, K.R.K.: Improvements to the SMO algorithm for SVM regression. IEEE Trans. Neural Netw. **11**, 1188–1193 (1999)
16. Zimmerman, M., Martinez, J.H., Young, D., Chelminski, I., Dalrymple, K.: Severity classification on the Hamilton depression rating scale. J. Affect. Disord. **150**(2), 384–388 (2013)

Usability, Acceptability, and Feasibility of Two Technology-Based Devices for Mental Health Screening in Perinatal Care: A Comparison of Web Versus App

Verónica Martínez-Borba[1]([⊠]), Carlos Suso-Ribera[1], and Jorge Osma[2,3]

[1] Universitat Jaume I, 12071 Castellón de la Plana, Spain
{al189588, susor}@uji.es
[2] Universidad de Zaragoza, 44003 Teruel, Spain
osma@unizar.es
[3] Instituto de Investigación Sanitaria de Aragón, 50009 Zaragoza, Spain

Abstract. The use of Information and Communication Technologies (web pages and apps) in mental health has boosted. However, it is unknown which of these two devices can be better in terms of feasibility and acceptability. Our aim is to compare the feasibility, usability, and user satisfaction of two devices (web vs mobile application) of an online program for perinatal depression screening called HappyMom. In total, 348 and 175 perinatal women registered into HappyMom web and app version, respectively. The assessment protocol included different biopsychosocial evaluations (twice during pregnancy and thrice in the postpartum) and a satisfaction questionnaire. Results showed that a higher percentage of women in the web sample (27.3–51.1%) responded to each assessment compared to the app sample (9.1–53.1%). A smaller proportion of women in web sample never responded to any assessments. By contrast, the percentage of women who responded to all assessments was higher in app sample (longitudinal retention sample was 4.6% of web users and 9.1% of app users). In general, high satisfaction was found in both web and app users. Our result showed that online assessment methods are feasible and acceptable by perinatal women. However, dropout rates are a real problem that urge a solution that will be discussed further in the paper. Web and App devices present different advantages and limitations. The choice of one of them must be made taking into account the study's objective, the sample characteristics, and the dissemination possibilities.

Keywords: Information and Communication Technologies ·
Dropouts · Satisfaction · Assessment · Perinatal women

1 Introduction

During the last decades, the use of Information and Communication Technologies (ICTs) in health (eHealth) have become widespread globally. The explosion of this technology is due to several factors. One of them is its low cost and high availability in

© ICST Institute for Computer Sciences, Social Informatics and Telecommunications Engineering 2019
Published by Springer Nature Switzerland AG 2019. All Rights Reserved
P. Cipresso et al. (Eds.): MindCare 2019, LNICST 288, pp. 176–189, 2019.
https://doi.org/10.1007/978-3-030-25872-6_14

the general population [1]. Other reasons include their advantages for the health service industry and research institutions. In the specific field of mental health, ICTs offer the possibility to overcome some barriers and limitations found in traditional face-to-face evaluations and interventions. Some of these advantages include accessibility and flexibility, reducing or eliminating the need to travel to the health center, anonymity, and the reduction of stigmatization associated with mental health consultation [2–5]. Not surprisingly, this has led to a great interest in the use of ICTs for mental and overall health-related issues in the past years [6–8].

Among the different ICTs that exist, the use of online platforms (i.e., web pages and mobile applications) has increased very quickly in health research and practice. As found in recent systematics reviews, apps and web pages have been used for delivering psychological treatment and routine monitoring in different populations with mental health problems, such as perinatal depression, chronic pain, social anxiety, eating disorders, borderline personality disorder, addictions, insomnia, stress, post-traumatic stress disorder, burnout, and suicidality, to name some examples [9–15].

In the specific field of perinatal depression, which is depressive symptoms that occur during pregnancy and up to 12 months postpartum [16], different web and app-based programs exist. Some of these screening, prevention, and treatment programs are web-based [17–21] while other are app-based [22–25]. Despite the wide use of these two online platforms, it is still unknown whether one of these two devices actually performs better in terms of feasibility (i.e., response rate), acceptability and usability (i.e., user satisfaction). Considering the widespread integration of smartphones into the daily life of individuals, mobile applications would be expected to present some advantages compared to web pages. For instance, mobile applications offer the possibility to conduct ecological momentary assessments (EMA), which involves repeated data collection (thoughts, behaviors and symptoms) in real time and in the natural environments of the individual [26, 27]. Additionally, smartphones allow collecting relevant antecedent information to the experience (i.e., localization or number of phone calls and SMS received). Consistent with this idea, a recent study showed that women who used a web-based treatment for perinatal depression would like the program to be available for its use on smartphones [3].

Although repeated assessment via ICTs might have important advantages, some possible limitations of this methodology should also be acknowledged. When assessments are made several times a day for a long period of time, dropout rates tend to occur [28], especially in self-administered online interventions [29]. Studies reporting attrition rates have found dropouts up to 50% in online treatment for depression and anxiety [30], showing that sample retention is one of the main concerns for studies using eHealth for monitoring and treatment [31]. In an effort to improve eHealth adherence, some authors have suggested that the psychological experience with the platform is important to determine usage and adherence to interventions [32], so acceptability and usability are key elements in this study.

In sum, the aim of this study was to compare the feasibility, usability, and user satisfaction of two devices (web vs mobile application) of an online program for perinatal depression screening called HappyMom (HM). We expect that feasibility, as measured by response rates and dropouts, as well as usability and acceptability will be better for mobile applications because this platform is more suited to be used in smartphones than the web version of Happymom.

2   Method

2.1   Participants

The sample was composed of 523 perinatal women who registered into HM. Of these, 348 women registered into the web version (HM-Web) and 175 participants used the app version (HM-App). Longitudinal assessments were carried out entirely with HM. Two evaluations were made during pregnancy (weeks 16–24 and 30–36 of gestation) and three in the postpartum (weeks 2, 4, and 12 after delivery). The assessment points were the same for both devices. The study was conducted between 2012 and 2015.

2.2   Procedure

The ethical committees of the Hospital Universitario La Plana de Villarreal and the Gobierno de Aragón approved the present study and its procedures.

HM is designed to evaluate mental well-being during perinatal period. The platform is composed by two devices: HM-Web and HM-App. A different procedure was followed depending on the device employed to better fit the characteristics of each device and to facilitate recruitment:

HM-Web. Participant recruitment was carried out at the health collaborating centers. Midwives offered the codes to pregnant women who met inclusion criteria. Adult women (>18 years) between week 16 and 36 of gestation were invited to participate if they had internet access (at home or on the phone). Exclusion criteria included not being able to read or answer to the questions in Spanish. Women who voluntarily agreed to participate registered into the HM-Web and responded to different biopsychosocial assessments during pregnancy and the postpartum. Women were contacted via e-mail to complete each assessment at the required gestational stage (i.e., two assessments during pregnancy and three after delivery). Women who finished the evaluations received feedback about their mental well-being and those with depressive symptoms received a recommendation to consult their public health care service.

HM-App. Dissemination campaigns for recruitment were carried out via press, posters, e-mail, radio, and television. The link to download the app was posted in these social media. The HM-App was available for free download at Play Store (Android system). No healthcare professional support is integrated into the app. No code access was needed, so women who were interested in participating only had to download the HM-App and start using it. Given the free download character of the application, the age variable could not be controlled as an exclusion criteria. Inclusion criteria were being between week 16 and 36 of gestation at the time of download and being able to read and answer to the questions in Spanish. Women who agreed to participate registered into the HM-App to complete the biopsychosocial assessments during pregnancy and the postpartum. Once the women had registered into the HM-App, the app sent reminders to complete each biopsychosocial assessment at the required gestational stage. At the end of the evaluations, women received feedback about the mental well-being. When depressive symptoms were present, they were recommended to consult their public health care service.

2.3 Measures

The distribution of questionnaires administered according to the perinatal period and the device employed (HM-Web/HM-App) is shown in Table 1.

Questionnaires could be grouped into blocks according to their biological (obstetric data), psychological (emotional disorders, personality, affect, self-esteem, emotion regulation, quality of life, and satisfaction with life), or social (social adjustment, perceived social support, marital adjustment, stressful events, and familism) characteristics. In the postpartum, when the last biopsychosocial assessment was completed, all HM users responded to satisfaction questions.

The biopsychosocial measures changed between HM-App and HM-Web because of the limitations inherent to the use of smaller devices such as smartphones, so the app assessment was shorter. For that reason, the questionnaires in the HM-Web were divided in three blocks so the users could stop answering the questionnaires at any time and continuing answering where possible. In addition, some questionnaires (EPQ-R, STAI-T, ERQ, CAE, QLI and SRSS)[1] were administered only during pregnancy.

Table 1. Measures according to the perinatal period and device employed.

Questionnaires	Perinatal period				
	Pregnancy		Postpartum		
	Weeks 16–24	Weeks 30–36	Week 2	Week 4	Week 12
Register	1 Web				
	1 App				
Sociodemographic	1 Web				
	1 App				
Obstetric	1 Web	1 Web	1 Web	1 Web	1 Web
	1 App	1 App	1 App	1 App	1 App
Depressive symptoms [33–37]	3 Web	3 Web	3 Web	3 Web	3 Web
	1 App	1 App	1 App	1 App	1 App
Psychological factors [38–56]	10 Web	10 Web	5 web	5 web	5 Web
	3 App	3 App	3 App	3 App	3 App
Social factors [57–65]	3 Web	3 Web	2 Web	2 Web	2 Web
	2 App	2 App	2 App	2 App	2 App
Satisfaction					1 Web
					1 App

---

[1] EPQ-R: Eysenck Personality Questionnaire Revised; STAI-T: State-Trait Anxiety Inventory (trait subscale); ERQ: Emotion Regulation Questionnaire; CAE: Cuestionario de Afrontamiento del Estrés; QLI: Quality of Life Index; SRSS: Social Readjustement Rating Scale.

2.4   Data Analysis

First, we conducted a descriptive analysis of the sample. Then, we analyzed dropout rates (proportion of women who completed each assessment in relation to women who were registered into the program). Finally, we explored women's usability reports and satisfaction with HM.

3   Results

3.1   Demographic Characteristics

The HM-App sample comprised 175 women between 16 and 44 years of age (mean = 28.96; SD = 6.34). The majority of them (78.9%) were Spanish, 64% had completed secondary education studies or higher, and 76% of them were in a relationship at the time of the first assessment. With regards to the HM-Web, 348 women registered to this platform, but only 151 of them provided demographic information. Their age ranged from 20 to 42 years (mean = 32.77; SD = 4.48). Almost all women (92.1%) were Spanish and the majority of them (78.8%) had completed secondary education studies or higher and were in a relationship (76.8%). Statistical differences between app and web users were found for age (t = 6.17; $p < .001$; 95% CI = 2.60, 5.02), nationality (χ^2 = 11.05; $p < .001$; 95% CI = 5.56, 20.62), and educational level (χ^2 = 8.57; p = .003; 95% CI = 4.94, 24.13). Women who used the web were older, they had a higher educational level, and were more likely to be Spanish. There were no statistical differences in marital status (χ^2 = 0.03; p = .866; 95% CI = −8.51,9.91).

3.2   Dropout Rates

HM-Web. Out of the 348 women who registered into HM-Web, 102 (29.3%) did not complete any evaluation. During pregnancy, the percentage of women who completed all the questionnaires was 32.2% in the first evaluation and 51.1% in second assessment. In the postpartum, the proportion of women who completed all the questionnaires during the first, the second, or the third postpartum assessments were 38.2%, 27.3%, and 28.7%, respectively. Only 16 women (4.6%) responded to all the assessments.

HM-App. Out the 175 women who downloaded HM-App and registered into the program, 82 (46.9%) did not complete any assessment. During pregnancy, the proportion of women who completed the first and the second evaluation was 53.1% and 21.7%, respectively. In the postpartum, the percentage of women who completed the first, the second, or the third assessments was 13.7%, 10.9%, and 9.1%, respectively. Again, only 16 women (9.1%) responded to all the evaluations.

As shown in Table 2, statistical differences in response rates between HM-App and HM-Web were found for all assessment points. Compared to HM-App users, more women registered into HM-Web and a larger percentage of women completed the assessments (i.e., second assessment during pregnancy and all of the postpartum evaluations) in the HM-Web. The proportion of women who completed all five assessments was higher in the HM-App, but the proportion of women who did not complete any evaluation was also higher in HM-App.

Table 2. Response rates according to the evaluation time and device used.

Assessment	Respondents n (%)		Chi-square test (p, 95% CI)
	HM-Web	HM-App	
Registration	348	175	
PRE 1	112 (32.2)	93 (53.1)	21.30 (p < .001; 11.94 to 29.53)
PRE 2	178 (51.1)	38 (21.7)	41.45 (p < .001; 20.91 to 36.95)
POST 1	114 (32.8)	24 (13.7)	21.82 (p < .001; 11.56 to 25.78)
POST 2	95 (27.3)	19 (10.9)	18.33 (p < .001; 9.36 to 22.61)
POST 3	100 (28.7)	16 (9.1)	25.90 (p < .001; 12.73 to 25.63)
All assessments	16 (4.6)	16 (9.1)	4.10 (p = .043; 0.11 to 9.97)
Any evaluation	102 (29.3)	82 (46.9)	15.78 (p < .001; 8.80 to 26.26)
Satisfaction	16 (4.6)	16 (9.1)	4.10 (p = .043; 0.11 to 9.97)

3.3 User's Satisfaction

We registered 99 HM-Web satisfaction responses and 16 responses from HM-App. However, since only 16 of the 99 women using HM-Web completed the five assessment points, the analyses will be made both when considering the women who none completed all longitudinal measures ($n = 16$ for HM-Web and $n = 16$ for HM-App) and the web non-completers ($n = 99$ for HM-Web and $n = 16$ for HM-App). There was no difference in satisfaction when considering non-completers and completers for web users.

As shown in Table 3, all women considered studying perinatal well-being important. General satisfaction with HM was high for both, HM-Web and HM-App. The majority of women were satisfied with the registration process and indicated that the questions and instructions were easy to understand. Only 12.2% of web users reported difficulties when using the device. Despite the longitudinal character of the study and the number of questionnaires included, most women did not consider the time they devoted to answering the questions to be excessive (86.9% in the HM-Web sample and 93.8% in the HM-App sample) and did not perceive their daily life had been altered (87.5% in the HM-Web sample and 100% in the HM-App sample). Half of the women (50% in HM-Web sample and 43.7% in HM-App sample) considered that the device was reliable for the assessment of mental well-being and about three fourths of women trusted the information received by HM.

The results regarding the perceived impact of HM in the mental well-being of participants and the future intention of use and willingness to recommend the platform to others revealed that one fourth of the sample perceived an improvement in their emotional well-being after using the platform. Additionally, between 50–75% of women (depending on the platform used) would use the application in a future pregnancy, while 62.5–75.8% of participants would recommend it to other women.

Significant statistical differences were found in the perceived usefulness of the reminders to complete the assessments during the five evaluation points. A greater percentage of women in the HM-Web sample valued the reminders to complete the assessments positively compared to women in the HM-App sample. No other significant statistical differences were found in terms of user's satisfaction when comparing app and web users.

Table 3. HappyMom satisfaction according to device used.

	Affirmative responses (%)		Chi-square test (p, 95%CI)
	HM-Web*	HM-App	
Ease of registration	100	93.7	1.01 (p= .316, -13.90 to 28.29)
	92		0.05 (p= .814, -20.74 to 10.44)
Enough information about HappyMom	62.5	56.2	0.13 (p= .721, -25.26 to 36.19)
	77.8		3.38 (p = .066, -0.99 to 45.72)
Ease of understand instructions	100	100	
	97		0.49 (p = .486, -16.48 to 8.48)
Reminders utility	100	68.7	5.75 (p = **.016**, 5.45 to 55.63)
	95		11.94 (p<**.001**,8.10 to 50.81)
Ease of web/app use	93.8	100	0.99 (p= .320, -13.84 to 28.25)
	91.9		1.38 (p= .240, -11.67 to 15.15)
Ease of understand questions	87.5	100	2.06 (p = .151, -8.87 to 36.01)
	84.9		2.75 (p=.097, -5.11 to 23.43)
Ease of respond questions	81.2	87.5	0.23 (p= .629, -20.19 to 32.18)
	81.8		0.31 (p=.579, -18.67 to 18.25)
Difficulties with web/app	0	0	
	12.2		2.16 (p= .142, -7.83 to 20.09)
Excessive time	0	6.2	0.94 (p=.331 -13.98 to 28.16)
	13.1		0.61 (p=.435, -15.79 to 16.42)
Importance of studying perinatal mental well-being	100	100	
	100		
Reliability of HappyMom	50	43.7	0.12 (p=.725, -25.58 to 36.47)
	67.7		3.43 (p=.064, -1.04 to 46.28)
Confidence in the feedback received	75	68.7	0.15 (p=.697, -23.58 to 34.80)
	82.8		1.75 (p= .186, -5.05 to 39.21)
Conflict in the routine due to the use of the device	12.5	0	2.02 (p =.155, -9.01 to 35.92)
	11.1		1.91 (p=.167, -9.01 to 18.70)
Positive influence of the device on well-being	18.8	25	0.17 (p=.676, -22.23 to 33.56)
	31.3		0.26 (p= .613, -19.56 to 24.01)
Future use of HappyMom	50	75	2.07 (p=.151, -7.93 to 51.52)
	74.7		0.01 (p= .980, -25.33 to 17.83)
HappyMom recommendation	62.5	62.5	
	75.8		1.25 (p= .263, -7.87 to 38.27)

*Note: shaded values corresponded to all web user's (n=99), web white values correspond to non-completers web user's (n=16).

4 Discussion

In recent year, an increasing number of eHealth programs, especially those based on web applications and smartphone applications, have emerged as an alternative to traditional face-to-face protocols as a result of the advantages of ICTs for health research and clinical purposes [9–15]. In relation to this literature on eHealth, some authors have highlighted the need to include participant engagement (i.e., acceptability and usability of the technology-based program) and retention rates as an key factors prior to the final implementation of ICT in routine practice [66]. In the field of perinatal depression, some studies have already reported encouraging acceptability and feasibility (i.e., dropout rates) results of eHealth, mostly after using web-based, online interventions [3, 18, 67, 68]. However, to the best of our knowledge no study had previously compared the usability, satisfaction, and feasibility of the two most popular forms of online applications, namely web-based and smartphone applications. Thus, the aim of this study was to compare the feasibility, acceptability, and user satisfaction of two devices (web vs mobile application) of a perinatal mental health screening program. We hypothesized that feasibility (response rates and dropouts) and acceptability and satisfaction would be higher for the mobile application because of the widespread use of smartphone applications.

Regarding feasibility, our hypothesis was mostly not confirmed by our findings. Contrary to our predictions, a higher proportion of women did not complete any evaluation in the HM-App and response rates during pregnancy and the postpartum were consistently higher across almost all assessment points in the HM-Web group. Additionally, the proportion of women who did not complete any assessment after registration was lower for the HM-Web (29.3%) compared to the HM-App (46.9%). Only retention occurred as expected, in the sense that a greater percentage of women using the HM-App completed all assessments.

Several reasons might explain these aforementioned findings regarding feasibility. For instance, it is possible that higher response rates in the HM-Web group are due to differences in the sample recruitment method. Recruitment in the HM-Web was conducted with the collaboration of health care professionals who delivered the web access codes to women, mainly midwives. By contract, the HM-App was available for free download, with no health care professional collaboration for its dissemination. It is possible that women were more motivated to use HM at least once when they perceived that health care professionals were involved in the program. As suggested in a recent study [69], it is possible that some women do not trust information from health-related websites and apps, so it is necessary to involve health care professionals in the dissemination of ICT in perinatal care. Moreover, disseminating campaigns should be supported by public and private health services, promoting routine assessments of emotional well-being during perinatal period. We tried to minimize this risk by offering both groups a reward for participating (i.e., feedback about their well-being), but maybe the effect of the institution was still larger. Another possible explanation for these findings is anonymity. The stigma of mental illness is a frequent issue during the perinatal period [70] and some perinatal women report confidentiality or privacy concerns regarding online programs for well-being [71]. In the HM-Web, women did not need to download any application that would be visible in the phone. In the HM-Web, women simply needed to access the website (which can be done from any device) and complete the evaluations. While this remains speculative at this stage, it is possible that this procedure was perceived as more anonymous than downloading and installing an app that would be visible in the phone, thus leading to an increased number of responses in the HM-Web.

While acknowledging the previous findings in favor of the HM-Web, it is interesting that the proportion of women who completed all five assessments was higher in the HM-App. This indicates, in line with our hypothesis, a higher fidelity to the app platform. Again, while the following conclusions are merely speculative, it is possible that the easier accessibility and widespread use of smartphones apps make these platforms more attractive for some people when it comes to repeated measurement. Indeed, there is previous literature to suggest that some women are interested in having web-based interventions adapted to smartphone apps [3], so this platform appears to be an attractive option for a number of users and should be considered when repeated measurement is planned. It is important to note, however, that retention rates were low both in the HM-Web and the HM-App (4.5% and 9.1%, respectively), which confirms that longitudinal studies result in high dropout rates [28], especially when a large number of questionnaires is administered like in the present study [29]. The results suggest that long assessments with a wide number of measures might be counterproductive, so strategies like questionnaire reduction or even single-item use for the measurement of constructs should be considered [8]. This could be combined with the inclusion of motivating practices, such as gamification or benefits for participating (i.e., access to an online chat with a mental health professional).

Regarding women's satisfaction with HM, we anticipated that the satisfaction with the HM-App would be higher when compared to the HM-Web. Our results do not support this hypothesis and indicated a good satisfaction for both HM versions. Previous research [3, 18, 72] has also showed that online platforms have high acceptability by perinatal women. HM was not an exception and both devices were perceived as easy to use and very well accepted, including no technical difficulties, straightforward questions, adequate response time, minimal impact on the individual's routine, and trust in the feedback received about emotional well-being. The only difference in HM satisfaction refers to the utility of reminders. Specifically, women who used the web were more grateful that e-mails were sent to them reminding them to respond to the evaluations. What these results suggest is that reminders are less necessary for the app version of the program, arguably because of the less extended assessment protocol and the frequent use of smartphones in our daily living.

Despite the general satisfaction with HM, its perceived impact in the mental well-being of participants and the future intention to use the platform and to recommend it to others was modest. As suggested by previous studies, screening programs are not sufficient for perinatal depression treatment and prevention [73, 74], so it is not surprising that a quarter of women in our sample did not perceive any improvement in their emotional well-being after using HM, which might explain their low interest in using the platform in the future and recommending it to others. Future screening programs should not only provide feedback about emotional status, but also offer other resources valued for perinatal women such as information, tips or the possibility of an online treatment via ICT if necessary. While these findings are important and suggest a need to improve screening programs for perinatal women using technology, it should be noted that all women in our sample considered the study of perinatal well-being a fundamental goal. Considering that women have considered HM and other online platforms for perinatal care to be easy and acceptable tools for the assessment of their well-being, future health campaigns should focus on implementing ICT protocols to perinatal mental health assessment and treatment in routine care.

Our study certainly has some limitations. Participant recruitment was different in the HM-Web and the HM-App, so that only the web was recommended by health care professionals. As discussed above, this could affect the final sample obtained in the web and the app (both numbers and their motivation to participate). Additionally, because of HM characteristics, only women who were able to understand and answer questions in Spanish were able to participate in the study, thus limiting the generalization of results to all perinatal women. Related to this, the majority of women were from Spain, so nationality comparison was not possible. It is possible that feasibility and satisfaction results of ICTs programs for perinatal mental health are higher in countries were the use of eHealth is more frequent (i.e., United States of America or United Kingdom). It is also important to note that our satisfaction results are based on the opinion of women who completed all evaluations, as women who did not respond to the last biopsychosocial assessment could not complete the satisfaction survey. In future research, we should include and better comprehend the opinions of participant who left the study, but this was not possible in the present investigation because of the characteristics of the study (i.e., the phone number or email address of women using the app were not collected to increase the sense of anonymity). Finally, there were some differences in the assessment protocol in the web and in the app, so differences in dropout rates should be considered with caution.

To sum up, our results show that online platforms (web-based and app-based) can be reliable and acceptable methods to deliver mental health assessment during the perinatal period. User's satisfaction was good for both devices, especially regarding ease of use, time devoted to the platform, and interference with daily life. The HM-Web obtained overall better results in terms of feasibility (i.e., number of registrations and percentage of women who completed each assessment), which suggests that perinatal mental health evaluations can be carried out successfully via web-pages. While the following is merely speculative, our results might also suggest that response rates will be higher if health care professionals are involved in dissemination. Interestingly, though, retention rates were in favor of the HM-App, so mobile applications might be suitable tools for longitudinal assessment. While acknowledging the previous feasibility findings, it is important to note that response rates were generally low, so strategies when performing repeated assessment using technology (i.e., gamification and benefits of participation) should be implemented in future research using technology for perinatal care.

References

1. International Telecommunication Union: ICT Facts and Figures (2017). https://www.itu.int/en/ITU-D/Statistics/Pages/facts/default.aspx
2. Barrera, A.Z., Kelman, A.R., Muñoz, R.F.: Keywords to recruit Spanish- and English-speaking participants: evidence from an online postpartum depression randomized controlled trial. J. Med. Internet Res. **16**, e6 (2014)
3. Haga, S.M., Drozd, F., Brendryen, H., Slinning, K.: Mamma mia: a feasibility study of a web-based intervention to reduce the risk of postpartum depression and enhance subjective well-being. JMIR Res. Protoc. **2**, e29 (2013)
4. Kim, H., Bracha, Y., Tipnis, A.: Automated depression screening in disadvantaged pregnant women in an urban obstetric clinic. Arch. Womens Ment. Health **10**, 163–169 (2007)
5. Donker, T., Cuijpers, P., Stanley, D., Danaher, B.: The future of perinatal depression identification can information and communication technology optimize effectiveness? (2015)
6. Eurostat: Internet use. Individuals using the Internet for seeking health-related information. http://ec.europa.eu/eurostat/tgm/table.do?tab=table&plugin=1&language=en&pcode=tin00101
7. Osma, J., Barrera, A.Z., Ramphos, E.: Are pregnant and postpartum women interested in health-related apps? Implications for the prevention of perinatal depression. Cyberpsychol. Behav. Soc. Netw. **19**, 412–415 (2016)
8. Suso-Ribera, C., Castilla, D., Zaragozá, I., Ribera-Canudas, M.V., Botella, C., García-Palacios, A.: Validity, reliability, feasibility, and usefulness of pain monitor, a multidimensional smartphone app for daily monitoring of adults with heterogeneous chronic pain. Clin. J. Pain **34**, 900–908 (2018)
9. Ashford, M.T., Olander, E.K., Ayers, S.: Computer- or web-based interventions for perinatal mental health: a systematic review. J. Affect. Disord. **197**, 134–146 (2016)
10. Bakker, D., Kazantzis, N., Rickwood, D., Rickard, N.: Mental health smartphone apps: review and evidence-based recommendations for future developments. JMIR Ment. Health **3**, 67 (2016)
11. Capon, H., Hall, W., Fry, C., Carter, A.: Realising the technological promise of smartphones in addiction research and treatment: an ethical review. Int. J. Drug Policy **36**, 47–57 (2016)
12. Martínez-Borba, V., Suso-ribera, C., Osma, J.: The use of information and communication technologies in perinatal depression screening. Cyberpsychol. Behav. Soc. Netw. **21**, 741–752 (2018)
13. Pospos, S., et al.: Web-based tools and mobile applications to mitigate burnout, depression, and suicidality among healthcare students and professionals: a systematic review. Acad. Psychiatry **42**, 109–120 (2017)
14. Rathbone, A., Clarry, L., Prescott, J.: Assessing the efficacy of mobile health apps using the basic principles of cognitive behavioral therapy: systematic review. J. Med. Internet Res. **19**, e399 (2017)
15. Richards, D., Richardson, T.: Computer-based psychological treatments for depression: a systematic review and meta-analysis. Clin. Psychol. Rev. **32**, 329–342 (2012)
16. Hamel, C., et al.: Screening for depression in women during pregnancy or the first year postpartum and in the general adult population: a protocol for two systematic reviews to update a guideline of the Canadian Task Force on Preventive Health Care. Syst. Rev. **8**, 1–13 (2019)
17. Barrera, A.Z., Wickham, R.E., Muñoz, R.F.: Online prevention of postpartum depression for Spanish- and English-speaking pregnant women: a pilot randomized controlled trial. Internet Interv. **2**, 257–265 (2015)

18. Danaher, B.G., et al.: MomMoodBooster web-based intervention for postpartum depression: feasibility trial results. J. Med. Internet Res. **15**, e242 (2013)
19. Jones, B.A., Griffiths, K.M., Christensen, H., Ellwood, D., Bennett, K., Bennett, A.: Online cognitive behaviour training for the prevention of postnatal depression in at-risk mothers: a randomised controlled trial protocol. BMC Psychiatry **13**, 265 (2013)
20. Le, H.-N., Perry, D.F., Sheng, X.: Using the internet to screen for postpartum depression. Matern. Child Health J. **13**, 213–221 (2009)
21. O'Mahen, H.A., et al.: Internet-based behavioral activation–treatment for postnatal depression (Netmums): a randomized controlled trial. J. Affect. Disord. **150**, 814–822 (2013)
22. Faherty, L.J., Hantsoo, L., Appleby, D., Sammel, M.D., Bennett, I.M., Wiebe, D.J.: Movement patterns in women at risk for perinatal depression: use of a mood-monitoring mobile application in pregnancy. J. Am. Med. Inform. Assoc. **24**, 746–753 (2017)
23. Jimenez-Serrano, S., Tortajada, S., Miguel Garcia-Gomez, J., Jiménez-Serrano, S., Tortajada, S., García-Gómez, J.M.: A mobile health application to predict postpartum depression based on machine learning. Telemed. E-Health **21**, 567–574 (2015)
24. Belisario, J.S.M., et al.: A bespoke mobile application for the longitudinal assessment of depression and mood during pregnancy: protocol of a feasibility study. BMJ Open **7**, e014469 (2017)
25. Tsai, A.C., et al.: Antenatal depression case finding by community health workers in South Africa: feasibility of a mobile phone application. Arch. Womens Ment. Health. **17**, 423–431 (2014)
26. Demirci, J., Bogen, D.: Feasibility and acceptability of a mobile app in an ecological momentary assessment of early breastfeeding. Matern. Child Nutr. **13**, 1–18 (2017)
27. Timmer, B.H.B., Hickson, L., Launer, S.: Ecological momentary assessment: Feasibility, construct validity, and future applications. Am. J. Audiol. **26**, 436–442 (2017)
28. Young, A.F., Powers, J.R., Bell, S.L.: Attrition in longitudinal studies: who do you lose? Aust. N. Z. J. Public Health **30**, 353–361 (2006)
29. Karyotaki, E., et al.: Predictors of treatment dropout in self-guided web-based interventions for depression: an 'individual patient data' meta-analysis. Psychol. Medici. **45**, 2717–2726 (2015)
30. Christensen, H., Griffiths, K.M., Farrer, L.: Adherence in internet interventions for anxiety and depression. J. Med. Internet Res. **11**, e13 (2009)
31. Becker, S., Miron-Shatz, T., Schumacher, N., Krocza, J., Diamantidis, C., Albrecht, U.-V.: mHealth 2.0: experiences, possibilities, and perspectives. JMIR mHealth uHealth **2**, e24 (2014)
32. Feather, J.S., Howson, M., Ritchie, L., Carter, P.D., Parry, D.T., Koziol-McLain, J.: Evaluation methods for assessing users' psychological experiences of web-based psychosocial interventions: a systematic review. J. Med. Internet Res. **18**, e181 (2016)
33. Beck, A., Steer, R., Brown, G.: Manual for the Beck Depression Inventory-II. Psychological Corporation, San Antonio (1996)
34. Sanz, J., Perdigón, A., Vázquez, C.: Adaptación española del Inventario para la Depresión de Beck-II (BDI-II): 2. Propiedades psicométricas en población general. Clin. Salud. **14**, 249–280 (2003)
35. Cox, J.L., Holden, J.M., Sagovsky, R.: Detection of postnatal depression: development of the 10-item edinburgh postnatal depression scale. Br. J. Psychiatry **150**, 782–786 (1987)
36. Garcia-Esteve, L., Ascaso, C., Ojuel, J., Navarro, P.: validation of the Edinburgh Postnatal Depression Scale (EPDS) in Spanish mothers. J. Affect. Disord. **75**, 71–76 (2003)
37. First, M., Spitzer, R., Gibbon, M., Williams, J.: Entrevista Clínica estructurada para los trastornos del Eje II del DSM-IV, Versión Clínica. MASSON, Barcelona (1999)

38. Eysenck, S.B.G., Eysenck, H.J., Barrett, P.: A revised version of the psychoticism scale. Pers. Individ. Diff. **6**, 21–29 (1985)

39. Ortet, G., Ibáñez, M., Moro, M., Silva, F.: Cuestionario revisado de Personalidad de Eysenck: versiones completa (EPQ-R) y abreviada (EPQ-RS), Madrid (2001)

40. Brown, T.A., White, K.S., Forsyth, J.P., Barlow, D.H.: The structure of perceived emotional control: psychometric properties of a revised anxiety control questionnaire. Behav. Ther. **35**, 75–99 (2004)

41. Osma, J., Barrada, J.R., Garciá-Palacios, A., Navarro-Haro, M., Aguilar, A.: Internal structure and clinical utility of the Anxiety Control Questionnaire-Revised (ACQ-R) Spanish version. Span. J. Psychol. **19**, E63 (2016)

42. Sandín, B., Chorot, P., Lostao, L., Joiner, T.E., Santed, M.A., Valiente, R.M.: Escalas PANAS de afecto positivo y negativo: validacion factorial y convergencia transcultural. Psicothema **11**, 37–51 (1999)

43. Watson, D., Clark, L.A., Tellegen, A.: Development and validation of brief measures of positive and negative affect: the PANAS scales. J. Pers. Soc. Psychol. **54**, 1063 (1988)

44. Morejón, A.J.V., García-Bóveda, R.J., Jiménez, R.V.-M.: Escala de autoestima de Rosenberg: fiabilidad y validez en población clínica española. Apunt. Psicol. **22**, 247–255 (2004)

45. Rosenberg, M.: Society and the Adolescent Self-image. Princeton University Press, Princeton (1965)

46. Spielberger, C., Cubero, N., Gorsuch, R., Lushene, R.: Cuestionario de ansiedad estado-rasgo: manual, Madrid (1982)

47. Spielberger, C.D., Gorsuch, R.L., Lushene, R.E.: The State-Trait Anxiety Inventory. Consulting Psychologists Press Inc., Palo Alto (1970)

48. Echeburúa, E., de Corral, P., Fernandez-Montalvo, J.: Escala de inadaptación (EI): propiedades psicométricas en contextos clínicos. Anál. Modif. Conduct. **26**, 325–340 (2000)

49. Rodríguez-Carvajal, R., Moreno-Jiménez, B., Garrosa, E.: Cuestionario de regulación emocional. Versión española. Autorizado por los autores de la versión original en inglés (Gross y John, 2003) (2006)

50. Gross, J., John, O.: Individual differences in two emotion regulation processes: implications for affect, relationships, and well-being. J. Pers. Soc. Psychol. **85**, 348–362 (2003)

51. Sandín, B., Chorot, P.: Cuestionario de Afrontamiento del Estrés (CAE): Desarrollo y validación preliminar. Rev. Psicopatol. Psicol. Clín. **8**, 39–53 (2003)

52. Mezzich, J., Ruipérez, M., Pérez, C., Yoon, G., Liu, J., Mahmud, S.: The Spanish version of the quality of life index: presentation and validation. J. Nerv. Ment. Dis. **188**, 301–305 (2000)

53. Beck, A., Steer, R.: Manual for the Beck Anxiety Inventory. The Psychological Corporation, San Antonio (1993)

54. Beck, A., Steer, R.: Manual. BAI. Inventario de Ansiedad de Beck (Adaptación española de Sanz, J.). Pearson Educación, Madrid (2011)

55. Diener, E., Emmons, R., Larsen, R., Grifin, S.: The satisfaction with life scale. J. Pers. Assess. **49**, 71–75 (1985)

56. Atienza, F.: Escala de Satisfacción con la vida. Psicothema **12**, 314–319 (2000)

57. González de Rivera, J., Morera, A.: La valoración de sucesos vitales: adaptación española de la escala de Holmes y Rahe. Psiquis (Mexico) **4**, 7–11 (1983)

58. Holmes, T.H., Rahe, R.H.: The social readjustment rating scale. J. Psychosom. Res. **11**, 213–218 (1967)

59. Landeta, O., Calvete, E.: Adaptación y validación de la escala multidimensional de apoyo social percibido. Ansiedad Estrés **8**, 173–182 (2002)

60. Zimet, G.D., Dahlem, N.W., Zimet, S.G., Farley, G.K.: The multidimensional scale of perceived social support. J. Pers. Assess. **52**, 30–41 (1988)
61. Carrobles, J.: Adaptación en población española de la Escala de Ajuste Marital de Locke-Wallace. In: Cáceres Carrasco, J. (ed.) Manual de Terapia de Pareja en Intervención en familias, pp. 105–106 (1989)
62. Locke, H.J., Wallace, K.M.: Short marital-adjustment and prediction tests: their reliability and validity. Marriage Fam. Living **21**, 251–255 (1959)
63. Rodríguez-Muñoz, M.F., Vallejo Slocker, L., Olivares Crespo, M.E., Izquierdo Méndez, N., Soto, C., Le, H.-N.: Propiedades psicométricas del Postpartum Depression Predictors Iinventory-revised-versión prenatal en una muestra española de mujeres embarazadas. TT - [Psychometric properties of postpartum depression predictors inventory-revised- prenatal version in a sample of Spanish pregnant women]. Rev. Esp. Salud. Publica **91**, e1–e8 (2017)
64. Beck, C., Records, K., Rice, M.: Further development of the postpartum depression predictors inventory-revised. J. Obstet. Gynecol. Neonatal Nurs. **35**, 735–745 (2006)
65. Villarreal, R., Blozis, S.A., Widaman, K.F.: Factorial invariance of a pan-hispanic familism scale. Hisp. J. Behav. Sci. **27**, 409–425 (2005)
66. Lane, T.S., Armin, J., Gordon, J.S.: Online recruitment methods for web-based and mobile health studies: a review of the literature. J. Med. Internet Res. **17**, e183 (2015)
67. Logsdon, M.C., Foltz, M.P., Stein, B., Usui, W., Josephson, A.: Adapting and testing telephone-based depression care management intervention for adolescent mothers. Arch. Womens Ment. Health **13**, 307–317 (2010)
68. Baker-Ericzén, M.J., Connelly, C.D., Hazen, A.L., Dueñas, C., Landsverk, J.A., Horwitz, S. M.: A collaborative care telemedicine intervention to overcome treatment barriers for Latina women with depression during the perinatal period. Fam. Syst. Health **30**, 224–240 (2012)
69. Fernández, M.: Herramienta metodológica para la evaluación de contenidos digitales para las gestantes. Interv. Eval. Matronas Hoy **3**, 14–25 (2015)
70. Maloni, J.A., Przeworski, A., Damato, E.G.: Web recruitment and internet use and preferences reported by women with postpartum depression after pregnancy complications. Arch. Psychiatr. Nurs. **27**, 90–95 (2013)
71. Hantsoo, L., Podcasy, J., Sammel, M., Epperson, C.N., Kim, D.R.: Pregnancy and the acceptability of computer-based versus traditional mental health treatments. J. Womens Health (Larchmt) **26**, 1106–1113 (2017)
72. Kim, H.G., Geppert, J., Quan, T., Bracha, Y., Lupo, V., Cutts, D.B.: Screening for postpartum depression among low-income mothers using an interactive voice response system. Matern. Child Health J. **16**, 921–928 (2012)
73. Miller, L., Shade, M., Vasireddy, V.: Beyond screening: assessment of perinatal depression in a perinatal care setting. Arch. Womens Ment. Health **12**, 329–334 (2009)
74. Kingston, D., et al.: Study protocol for a randomized, controlled, superiority trial comparing the clinical and cost-effectiveness of integrated online mental health assessment-referral-care in pregnancy to usual prenatal care on prenatal and postnatal mental health and infant. Trials **15** (2014)

Feasibility and Utility of Pain Monitor: A Smartphone Application for Daily Monitoring Chronic Pain

Irene Jaén[1]([⊠]), Carlos Suso-Ribera[1], Diana Castilla[2,3], Irene Zaragoza[3], and Azucena García-Palacios[1,3]

[1] Jaume I University, 12007 Castelló, Spain
{ijaen,susor,azucena}@uji.es
[2] University of Zaragoza, 44003 Teruel, Spain
castilla@uji.es
[3] CIBER of Physiopathology of Obesity and Nutrition CIBERobn,
CB06/03 Instituto de Salud Carlos III (Spain), Madrid, Spain
irenezaragoza@gmail.com

Abstract. The way monitoring is performed in health settings in general and chronic pain in particular is mostly based on traditional, episodic, onsite evaluation. This assessment method has important limitations and might be negatively impacting the effectiveness of treatments by providing non-ecological, delayed, and retrospective information about the patients' course over treatment. This pilot study explores the feasibility and discusses the utility of using technology (i.e., a smartphone app) for daily ecological momentary assessment of chronic pain patients. Twelve individuals attending a specialized pain clinic used the app twice daily for a month. Alarms were sent to the physicians in the presence of unwanted events (i.e., side effects). Feasibility was evidenced by excellent response rates in the patients (>80%) and the physicians (>93% of alarms were responded to). Utility of daily monitoring was evidenced when graphically representing patients' responses, in which the fluctuation of pain within and across days evidences the need for daily assessment. The utility of alarms will also be discussed, considering the number of alarms received (i.e., 96), which would have remained undetected or belatedly detected with traditional assessment. The study evidences the utility and feasibility of EMA using apps both from the patients' and the physicians' perspective. We believe these findings are not only important for pain settings, but also relevant for other health conditions.

Keywords: Ecological momentary assessment · Smartphone app · Feasibility · Utility

1 Introduction

Chronic pain is defined as pain that persists over a normal healing period, in contrast with acute pain. Specifically, pain was considered chronic when it persists more than 3–6 months [1]. Chronic pain affects approximately 20 to 30% of the population

© ICST Institute for Computer Sciences, Social Informatics and Telecommunications Engineering 2019
Published by Springer Nature Switzerland AG 2019. All Rights Reserved
P. Cipresso et al. (Eds.): MindCare 2019, LNICST 288, pp. 190–198, 2019.
https://doi.org/10.1007/978-3-030-25872-6_15

worldwide, so this disease has become a matter of social concern globally [2]. There is a wide range of interventions addressed to treat chronic pain, with medical treatments being the mainstream and psychological and physical therapy increasingly being used in multicomponent interventions [3, 4]. Despite the advances made in the treatment of this disease, many reviews have evidenced an only modest effectiveness of current interventions for patients with chronic pain [4, 5].

Some authors have suggested that the limited effectiveness showed in research could be partly explained by deficits in the assessment of pain [5]. For instance, the evaluation of treatment effectiveness is frequently made on a discrete basis, with a reduced number of measurement points frequently during onsite consultations only. This is problematic as pain intensity can vary naturally between and within days even when no treatment is proposed. Additionally, the assessment of pain course is usually performed retrospectively (i.e., "How intense was your pain during the past week"), which has been shown to be an unreliable measure of average daily pain because of recall bias [6, 7].

Ecological Momentary Assessment (EMA) is an excellent alternative to traditional, episodic evaluation due to several factors. First, with EMA pain can be measured in the moment it occurs, which attenuates the memory effects derived from recalled past pain experiences. Second, EMA allows assessing pain in a natural environment (i.e., not only during onsite consultations). Third, obtaining a measure of pain in a real time allows giving feedback to the patient (i.e., suggest to call the pain clinic if pain is not being reduced), which might, in turn, be used to improve the treatment. Last but not least, momentary data collection allows capturing the real course of pain trajectories, so that the conclusions about the effectiveness of treatments become a result of several measurement points and, thus, they become more reliable [8–10].

To date, EMA has been rare due to the use of ineffective or unreliable data collection methods, including paper diaries or telephone calls [11]. In the last years, however, the use of smartphone apps for research has increased drastically, which has renewed the interest in EMA. This is also the case of chronic pain, a field in which the use of smartphones for EMA is attracting the interest of researchers and clinicians [11–13]. Hundreds of pain apps currently exist. However, to date very few studies have reported the feasibility and utility of such devices for EMA in chronic pain.

Our team recently developed and tested the validity, reliability, and feasibility of Pain Monitor, a smartphone app used for EMA of pain severity and pain-related biopsychosocial factors [14]. The results obtained are very promising and suggest that the content assessed in traditional paper and pencil methods can be reliably measured with an app. However, the incorporation of smartphones to pain research is still on an early stage and there is a need to further investigate the applicability of this new monitoring procedure in health settings to be able to generalize the existent findings and to integrate their use in daily routine practice. Additionally, feasibility was only calculated from the patients' perspective, but not from the physicians' point of view (i.e., number of alarms sent by the app to the physicians in the presence of unwanted clinical events and number of alarms attended by the physicians). With the aforementioned purpose in mind, the aim of this study was to evaluate the utility and feasibility of the Pain Monitor app in a different setting (i.e., different hospital, patients, and region) and including the physicians' perspective.

App feasibility from the patients' perspective was calculated by dividing the number of completed measurements by the number of possible assessment points (i.e., sixty, twice a day for thirty days). Completion rates were also calculated separately for morning and evening assessments to explore whether time of day was an important variable explaining feasibility. App feasibility from the physicians' perspective will be computed by calculating the number of alarms responded by the number of alarms sent. Utility was explored by observing pain trajectories graphically and discussing how EMA could affect the conclusions regarding pain course and treatment effectiveness. Additionally, the utility of daily monitoring will be discussed when considering the alarms received in the presence of unwanted events. We expect to obtain good feasibility results, that is, with similar completion rates compared with the previous study with the same app (70–80%), as well as to observe graphical representations of pain trajectories that justify the utility of EMA in chronic pain [14].

2 Method

2.1 Pain Monitor App

Pain Monitor was originally developed and tested by a multidisciplinary team of psychologists, physicians, and nurses from the Vall d'Hebron Hospital and the Labpsitec group at the Jaume I University [14]. There are four groups of items in the app. The first one is administered the first day of use and includes sociodmographic and patient health and pain status information. Next, on a daily basis, patients are asked to respond to two different sets of questions: one in the morning and another in the evening. Both assessment points have some items in common (i.e., pain severity and mood), while other variables are assessed in the morning (i.e., interference of pain on sleep) or in the evening (i.e., interference of pain on daily activities). Specifically, daily assessment was predefined at 10:00 a.m. and 7:00 p.m. with a two-hour range in which patients can respond to each measurement. At the end of the study (after 30 days of daily evaluation), an end-of-study measurement is made with additional items (i.e., perceived change after treatment).

App content includes pain-related variables selected by experts following IMMPACT and recent review's recommendations on outcome and app assessment in chronic pain settings [15, 16], which has been adapted from traditional, well-established paper-and-pencil measures for their use in an app context. These include sociodemographic information, pain intensity (Brief Pain Inventory) [17], fatigue and mood (Profile Mood States) [18], anxiety and depression (Hospital Anxiety and Depression scale) [19], perceived heath status (Short Form-12) [20], catastrophizing (Pain Catastrophizing Scale) [21], acceptance (Chronic Pain Acceptance Questionnaire) [22], fear/avoidance of pain (Fear-Avoidance Beliefs Questionnaire) [23], activity level (Roland Morris Disability Questionnaire) [24], and coping strategies (Chronic Pain Coping Inventory-42 and Coping Strategies Questionnaire for coping) [25, 26].

The app has an alarm system which sends the participating physicians an e-mail in the presence of a predetermined undesired event (i.e., pain intensity is above 7 for more than 5 consecutive days, the patient is reporting nausea for more than 2 consecutive days, or the patient has stopped taking the medication for more than 2 consecutive days, to name some examples). The response to these alarms (i.e., call the patient and make a change in treatment or not taking any action) is determined by the participating physicians. The alarms are only notified to the physicians, but not the patients to reduce the risk of response expectation. However, all patients are informed at the beginning of the study that their responses might generate alarms and that physicians might call them.

The app is available for Android System (version 2.3 or higher) and can be downloaded for free at Play store (https://play.google.com/store/apps/details?id=painmonitor.srccode).

2.2   Sample and Procedure

This study was conducted with 12 participants with musculoskeletal pain who were being treated at the pain unit of *Hospital General Universitari de Castello* for the first time. Patients were over 18 years of age (mean= 49.83, $SD = 8.47$) with a mobile phone with Android operating system. Physical and psychological limitations or language problems which could prevent the use of the application were checked and resulted in study exclusion ($n = 3$). All participants had a chronic pain diagnosis (i.e., mostly back and neck pain over 3 months of duration) and began a medical treatment after this first consultation (see the results section for a more detailed description of clinical characteristics of the sample).

With respect to sociodemographic characteristics, the 25% of the sample was temporary on time off work, the 16.66% were active workers, the 16.66% were unemployed, the 16.66% had the incapacity to work, 16.66% were homemakers, and 16.66% were retired. Regarding the educational profile, 41.7% had primary studies, 23% had secondary studies, and 33% had coursed technical studies. Additionally, 66% of participants were married, 8.3% had a relationship, 8.3% were single, and 16.7% were widowed people.

All participants were identified by means of an alphanumeric code automatically generated by the app to ensure anonymity and confidentiality of data. This code was associated to the medical registry number so that the physicians could identify the patient. This file and the app data were saved following the Spanish law and data protection rules ("Ley Orgánica 15/1999, de 13 de diciembre, de Protección de Datos de carácter personal", "RD 1720/2007, de 21 de diciembre, por el que se aprueba el reglamento de desarrollo de LOPD (RLOPD)", and "Ley 34/2002, de 11 de Julio de Servicios de la Sociedad de la Información y de comercio electrónico"). In addition, all patients signing the informed consent were indicated that their participation was voluntary and would not affect the prospective treatment at the pain clinic.

2.3   Data Analysis

To evaluate the usability of Pain Monitor, the overall response rate will be calculated by dividing the number of completed assessments (both morning and evening responses) by the number of possible assessments (i.e., sixty). Additionally, morning and evening responses rates will be computed separately. A similar procedure was used for the physicians' responses to the alarms (i.e., alarms responded divided by alarms sent). Finally, pain intensity responses of a number of patients will be graphically displayed to observe different pain trajectories and to discuss the utility of EMA as opposed to episodic assessment.

3 Results

3.1 Clinical Characteristics of the Sample

Patients had a mean pain intensity of 7.67 ($SD = 1.72$; possible range = 0 to 10). The majority of patients had been experiencing pain for more than 5 years ($n = 9$). Only one patient had experienced pain for less than one year. Pain diagnoses, including comorbidities, were low back pain ($n = 11$), neck pain ($n = 6$), fibromyalgia ($n = 3$), and migraine ($n = 3$). None of the patients had pain due to arthritis or cancer.

3.2 Feasibility

Patient perspective. The results showed an overall response rate of 82% after 30 days of daily use of Pain monitor twice a day. In addition to this, results showed that morning assessment was answered 80% of times, while evening evaluations were completed 84% of times.

Physician perspective. In total, 96 alarms were sent. Of these, the physicians responded to 90 alarms, so 93.9% of them were responded to.

3.3 Utility

A graphical representation of the pain course over the study period is shown for three patients to discuss the utility of EMA using a smartphone. As seen in Fig. 1, morning-to-evening pain reports for this patient differed notably, so that pain levels were repeatedly higher in the evening. Additionally, as reported in Fig. 2, a patient reported unstable pain reports with some days experiencing very severe pain (i.e., on day 3) and weaker pain levels on the other days. Finally, in Fig. 3, a trend recovery trajectory is observed, with a decrease in pain reports starting with pain treatment onset, especially for evening pain intensity.

Regarding the utility of daily telemonitornig and alarms, the majority of the alarms (i.e., 75) included taking action (i.e., calling the patient) and only in 15 alarms that were responded to no further action was considered (i.e., recurrent symptom already known and treated for or symptom presumably not related to the pain treatment).

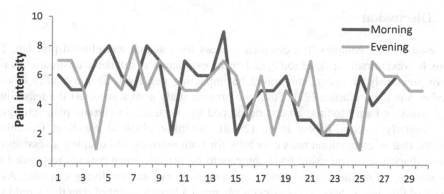

Fig. 1. Pain intensity responses of Patient A twice a day during 30 days of Pain Monitor app use.

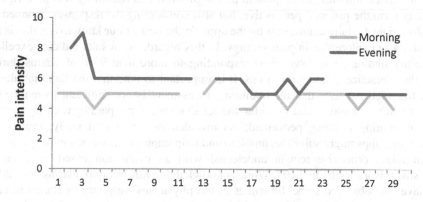

Fig. 2. Pain intensity responses of Patient B twice a day during 30 days of Pain Monitor app use.

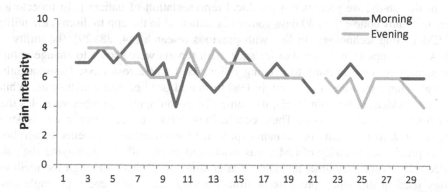

Fig. 3. Pain intensity responses of Patient C twice a day during 30 days of Pain Monitor app use.

4 Discussion

Assessment is a complex, but essential process for research and clinical practice. To date, however, traditional, episodic, and onsite evaluation is still the mainstream. As we have previously discussed, this might be impacting negatively in the quality of our studies and daily practice [27]. Thus, the present study goal was to test the feasibility and utility of Pain Monitor, an app developed by our team, in chronic pain settings.

Similarly to Suso-Ribera et al. (2018), we have obtained excellent feasibility results, that is, competition rates over 80% for both morning and evening assessments. Thus, diary assessment using EMA appears to be feasible since patients responded to the majority of the daily assessments (on average, 48 evaluations during a month). As a result of this, researchers and physicians obtained a large amount of data that would be very costly (or impossible) to collect by any traditional onsite assessments or other forms of EMA (i.e., paper diaries or phone calls).

An important finding in the present investigation is that feasibility was investigated not only form the patients' perspective, but also considering the responses obtained by the physicians to daily alarms sent by the app. To the best of our knowledge, this is the first study to explore this in pain settings. In this regard, our results indicate excellent feasibility findings, with physicians responding to more than 93% of alarms during their daily practice. Adding up to this, it is important to note that the fact that alarms were triggered suggests that the traditional assessment is not sufficient to reduce the patient symptomatology and provides further evidence for a paradigm change in the way monitoring is being performed. As revealed in the present study, the use of smartphone apps might solve this problem and help improve the detection of symptoms which might otherwise remain undetected with an evaluation based on a single assessment in a specific moment. While acknowledging this utility of alarms and EMA, we have also observed some difficulties in the physicians' response to alarms in days were there was a high workload, which suggests that there is a need to allocate a specific time during daily practice (i.e., 15 min daily outside the consultation hours as formally indicated by the physicians) to respond to the alarms.

In this study, we presented a graphical representation of patient pain trajectories over the study course (i.e., 30 days course) as indicated in the app to discuss the utility of EMA using technology. In line with previous research [14, 28, 29], the utility of EMA using apps seems clear. For instance, pain reports were shown to change within the same day (i.e., morning to evening differences) and across days. Consequently, taking a single measure of pain might lead to biased or imprecise conclusions. While this was evidenced for pain levels, the same discussion applies to other variables that can fluctuate, such as mood. Thus, conclusions extracted via episodic assessments might not show the reality of the pain experience for a number of patients. In addition to the previous, the utility of EMA was evidenced graphically by displaying the pain trajectories easily over time, including a large amount of data. Although the methodology used in this study prevents us from drawing causal inferences (a single case experimental design would be needed), the graphical representations presented in the study suggest that a more reliable conclusion about treatment effectiveness could be reached with EMA using technology.

The present study has certainly limitations. Because this is a pilot study to explore the feasibility and utility of using the app in clinical settings, before a larger implementation study is performed, the sample size is rather small. However, we consider the size to be sufficient to reach preliminary conclusions about feasibility and utility of the Pain Monitor app. It is also important to note that this is not a single case experimental study, so no conclusions about treatment effectiveness should be made. This was not a study goal at this stage and the step taken in the present investigation (i.e., ensuring that the use of the app for EMA is feasible and useful) was believed to be a necessary first step before the implementation of an experimental study.

The use of EMA with the support of smartphone apps in the health care system seems to be necessary to assess pain symptomatology. We believe, however, that this applies to other symptoms (i.e., mood) and a wide range of patients other than chronic pain individuals. The Pain Monitor app has demonstrated to be a useful and feasible tool to this purpose. In addition, Pain Monitor has not only demonstrated to be a feasible measure to assess pain from a patients' perspective, in the form of excellent completion rates, but also it demonstrated to be feasible when considering their daily use by physicians, as revealed by over 93% response rates to alarms. We believe that future research and health policies have to be directed towards the implementation of EMA using technology in routine medical practice.

References

1. Merskey, H., Bogduk, N.: Classification of chronic pain, 2nd edn. IASP Press, Seattle (1994)
2. Breivik, H., Collett, B., Ventafridda, V., Cohen, R., Gallacher, D.: Survey of chronic pain in Europe: prevalence, impact on daily life, and treatment. Eur. J. Pain 10(4), 287–333 (2006)
3. Gatchel, R.J., Peng, Y.B., Peters, M.L., Fuchs, P.N., Turk, D.C.: The biopsychosocial approach to chronic pain: scientific advances and future directions. Psychol. Bull. 133(4), 581 (2007)
4. Turk, D.C.: Clinical effectiveness and cost-effectiveness of treatments for patients with chronic pain. Clin. J. Pain 18(6), 355–365 (2002)
5. Dansie, E.J., Turk, D.C.: Assessment of patients with chronic pain. Br. J. Anaesth. 111(1), 19–25 (2013)
6. Gorin, A.A., Stone, A.A.: Recall biases and cognitive errors in retrospective self-reports: a call for momentary assessments. Handbook Health Psychol. 23, 405–413 (2001)
7. Schwarz, N.: Retrospective and concurrent self-reports: the rationale for real-time data capture. The science of real-time data capture: Self-reports in health research. In: Stone, A., Shiffman, S.S., Atienza, A., Nebeling, L. (eds.). Oxford University Press, New York (2007)
8. Shiffman, S., Stone, A.A., Hufford, M.R.: Ecological momentary assessment. Annu. Rev. Clin. Psychol. 4, 1–32 (2008)
9. Smyth, J.M., Stone, A.A.: Ecological momentary assessment research in behavioral medicine. J. Happiness Stud. 4(1), 35–52 (2003)
10. Stone, A.A., et al.: A comparison of coping assessed by ecological momentary assessment and retrospective recall. J. Pers. Soc. Psychol. 74(6), 1670 (1998)
11. May, M., Junghaenel, D.U., Ono, M., Stone, A.A., Schneider, S.: Ecological momentary assessment methodology in chronic pain research: a systematic review. J. Pain 19(7), 699–716 (2018)

12. Reynoldson, C., et al.: Assessing the quality and usability of smartphone apps for pain self-management. Pain Med. **15**(6), 898–909 (2014)
13. Rosser, B.A., Eccleston, C.: Smartphone applications for pain management. J. Telemedicine Telecare **17**(6), 308–312 (2011)
14. Suso-Ribera, C., Castilla, D., Zaragozá, I., Ribera-Canudas, M.V., Botella, C., García-Palacios, A.: Validity, reliability, feasibility, and usefulness of pain monitor. Clin. J. Pain **34** (10), 900–908 (2018)
15. Dworkin, R.H., et al.: Core outcome measures for chronic pain clinical trials: IMMPACT recommendations. Pain **113**, 9–19 (2005)
16. Alexander, J., Joshi, G.: Smartphone applications for chronic pain management: a critical appraisal. J. Pain Res. **9**, 731–734 (2016)
17. Cleeland, C.S., Ryan, K.M.: Pain assessment: global use of the Brief Pain Inventory. Ann. Acad. Med. Singapore **23**, 129–138 (1994)
18. McNair, D., Lorr, M., Droppleman, L.: Profile of Mood States. Educational and Industrial Testing Service, San Diego (1971)
19. Zigmond, A.S., Snaith, R.P.: The hospital anxiety and depression scale. Acta Psychiatr. Scand. **67**, 361–370 (1983)
20. Ware, J., Kosinski, M., Keller, S.D.: A 12-Item Short-Form Health Survey: construction of scales and preliminary tests of reliability and validity. Med. Care **34**, 220–233 (1996)
21. Sullivan, M.J.L., Bishop, S., Pivik, J.: The pain catastrophizing scale: development and validation. Psychol. Assess. **7**, 524–532 (1995)
22. Mccracken, L.M., Vowles, K.E., Eccleston, C.: Acceptance of chronic pain: component analysis and a revised assessment method. Pain **107**, 159–166 (2004)
23. Waddell, G., Newton, M., Henderson, I., Somerville, D., Main, C.J.: Fear-Avoidance Beliefs Questionnaire (FABQ) and the role of fear-avoidance beliefs in chronic low back pain and disability. Pain **52**, 157–168 (1993)
24. Roland, M., Morris, R.: A study of the natural history of back pain. Part I: development of a reliable and sensitive measure of disability in low-back pain. Spine **8**, 141–144 (1983)
25. Romano, J.M., Jensen, M.P., Turner, J.A.: The Chronic Pain Coping Inventory-42: reliability and validity. Pain **104**, 65–73 (2003)
26. Rosenstiel, A.K., Keefe, F.J.: The use of coping strategies in chronic low back pain patients: Relationship to patient characteristics and current adjustment. Pain **17**, 33–44 (1983)
27. Stone, A.A., Broderick, J.E., Kaell, A.T.: Single momentary assessments are not reliable outcomes for clinical trials. Contemp. Clin. Trials **31**(5), 466–472 (2010)
28. Garcia-Palacios, A., et al.: Ecological momentary assessment for chronic pain in fibromyalgia using a smartphone: a randomized crossover study. Eur. J. Pain **18**(6), 862–872 (2014)
29. Kratz, A.L., Murphy, S.L., Braley, T.J.: Ecological momentary assessment of pain, fatigue, depressive, and cognitive symptoms reveals significant daily variability in multiple sclerosis. Arch. Phys. Med. Rehabil. **98**(11), 2142–2150 (2017)

Discrimination of Bipolar Disorders Using Voice

Masakazu Higuchi[1]([✉]), Mitsuteru Nakamura[1], Shuji Shinohara[2],
Yasuhiro Omiya[3], Takeshi Takano[3], Hiroyuki Toda[4], Taku Saito[4],
Aihide Yoshino[4], Shunji Mitsuyoshi[2], and Shinichi Tokuno[1]

[1] Graduate School of Medicine, The University of Tokyo, Tokyo, Japan
{higuchi,m-nakamura,tokuno}@m.u-tokyo.ac.jp
[2] Graduate School of Engineering, The University of Tokyo, Tokyo, Japan
{shinohara,mitsuyoshi}@bioeng.t.u-tokyo.ac.jp
[3] PST Inc., Yokohama, Japan
{omiya,takano}@medical-pst.com
[4] Department of Psychiatry, National Defense Medical College, Tokorozawa, Japan
{toda1973,tsaito,aihide}@ndmc.ac.jp

Abstract. Several methods have been developed for screening mentally impaired patients using biomarkers, but these methods are invasive and costly. Self-administered tests are also used as screening methods. They are non-invasive and relatively simple, but they cannot eliminate the influence of reporting bias. On the other hand, the authors have conducted studies on technologies for inferring the mental state of persons from their voices. Analysis using voice has the advantage of being non-invasive and easy to perform. This study proposes a vocal index that will distinguish between a healthy person and a bipolar I or II patient using a polytomous logistic regression analysis with patients with bipolar disorder as subjects. When the subjects were classified using the prediction model obtained from the analysis, the subjects were categorized into three groups with an accuracy of approximately 67%. This result suggested that the vocal index could be a new evaluation index for discriminating between subjects with and those without bipolar disorder.

Keywords: Voice · Bipolar disorders ·
Polytomous logistic regression analysis

1 Introduction

In terms of the screening of patients with mental illness, methods have been developed that use biomarkers [1–3] such as saliva, blood, and heart rate; however, they are invasive and costly. Noninvasive methods include self-administered psychological tests [4–6] such as the General Health Questionnaire (GHQ), Beck Depression Inventory (BDI), and Young Mania Rating Scale (YMRS), which are used commonly. Although self-administered tests are relatively easy, they cannot completely eliminate reporting bias. Reporting bias occurs when certain

© ICST Institute for Computer Sciences, Social Informatics and Telecommunications Engineering 2019
Published by Springer Nature Switzerland AG 2019. All Rights Reserved
P. Cipresso et al. (Eds.): MindCare 2019, LNICST 288, pp. 199–207, 2019.
https://doi.org/10.1007/978-3-030-25872-6_16

pieces of information are selectively under or over-evaluated, either consciously or subconsciously, by the respondents [7].

On the other hand, a change in mood is empirically known to be manifested in the voice, with research studies having been conducted to infer depressive or stressed states of subjects using voices [8–11]. Assessment using the voice has a number of advantages. It is noninvasive, allows for easy and remote analysis, and does not require special, specific devices. Furthermore, it also has the potential to resolve several issues with detecting psychiatric disorders, including the reporting bias in self-administered psychological testing.

Bipolar disorder is a psychiatric disorder in which the patient goes through a cycle of manic and depressive episodes, with type I involving stronger manic states and type II involving milder ones [12]. Diagnosing bipolar disorder is often difficult, even for experts. In particular, it is difficult to distinguish depression caused by bipolar disorder from unipolar depression. The earlier the age of onset, the higher the likelihood of the first few episodes to be depressive [13]. Since the diagnosis of bipolar disorder requires a manic or hypomanic episode, many patients are initially misdiagnosed as having major depression [14]. Therefore, newer technology that can distinguish between major depression and bipolar disorder at an early stage is required. We have been conducting research on a voice index that can detect bipolar and major depressive disorders in patients [15,16]. In a study with only bipolar patients, Faurholt-Jepsen et al. presented that the manic state measured using the YMRS can be discriminated with high accuracy from vocal features [17]. Maxhuni et al. reported that it is possible to classify with high confidence the course of mood episodes or relapse in bipolar patients, using motor activity information including audio, accelerometer and self-assessment data [18]. However, neither study has conducted an analysis by separating type I and II bipolar disorders.

Therefore, this study only examined patients with bipolar disorder to propose a vocal evaluation index that will differentiate between type I and II bipolar disorders using healthy subjects as a control.

2   Methods

2.1   Subjects

The voices of patients who visited the National Defense Medical College Hospital for the treatment of bipolar disorder were studied, as well as those of healthy subjects, who lived their everyday lives without mental health issues. Of the patients, 25 had type I bipolar disorder (BPI) and 39 had type II bipolar disorder (BPII). The patients were diagnosed using the Mini-International Neuropsychiatric Interview (MINI) [19]. Moreover, the patients were interviewed by a doctor using Hamilton Depression Rating Scale (HAM-D) [20], and a self-administered psychological test, YMRS, was conducted. Fourteen healthy subjects (HE) were included.

2.2   Acquisition of Voices

Vocal data were acquired by recording the voices of the subjects, reading out a fixed sentence comprised of 17 Japanese phrases, after obtaining their consent. This reading aloud was conducted twice. The vocal recordings were conducted in the hospital consultation room for both the healthy subjects, and the patients. The voice was recorded using the pin microphone ME52W (Olympus, Tokyo, Japan) attached at the breast, approximately 10 cm away from the subject's mouth. The recording device used was the Portable Recorder R-26 (Roland, Shizuoka, Japan), with the recording format being 96 kHz and 24-bit linear PCM.

2.3   Analysis of Voice Data

Selection of Features. The vocal features extracted from voices of subjects. The feature extraction was conducted using the freeware openSMILE version 2.3 [21]. The openSMILE freeware comes with scripts that automatically extract vocals from various feature sets. In this study, the feature set used in emotion recognition (the large openSMILE emotion feature set) was extracted from each voice. From a single vocal data, 6, 552 vocal features were extracted. From these features, those that fit the model were selected. The procedure used was as follows:

1. Of the data, 75% were extracted from the HE, BPI, and BPII groups, respectively, using feature data of all subject's vocal data, with each used as a data set for training. The remaining 25% of the data were used as the data set for testing the model. The details for each data set are presented in Tables 1 and 2.
2. For feature f, the training data were divided into the HE_f, BPI_f, and $BPII_f$ groups, with the combination of each pair of groups being HE_f versus BPI_f, HE_f versus $BPII_f$, and BPI_f versus $BPII_f$. The classification performance of the two groups were calculated for all combinations using the area under the curve (AUC) of the receiver-operating characteristic (ROC). In this study, a feature in which the AUC was >0.9 for combinations HE_f versus BPI_f or HE_f versus $BPII_f$ was selected, or a feature of an AUC of >0.7 for the combination BPI_f versus $BPII_f$ was selected.
3. A correlation analysis was conducted for the features of the training data selected in step 2. With a feature pair in which the Pearson product-moment correlation coefficient exceeded 0.8, one of the features was eliminated.

Multivariate Analysis. By using the features of the selected training data as the explanatory variable and category information as objective variables, a regularized polytomous logistic regression analysis was conducted [22]. The polytomous logistic regression analysis is a multivariate analysis method that categorizes data into three groups or more, and is an extended version of the regular logistic regression analysis that categorizes data into two groups. From the model formula obtained from the analysis, the probability of each piece of data belonging to each group is estimated, with the data categorized into the group with the highest probability. The probability P_g in which the data x comprising of F pieces of features belonging to group $g \in \{HE, BPI, BPII\}$ is calculated using the following equation:

$$P_g = \frac{\exp\left(\alpha_g + \sum_{i=1}^{F} \beta_{ig} x_i\right)}{\sum_{j \in \{HE, BPI, BPII\}} \exp\left(\alpha_j + \sum_{i=1}^{F} \beta_{ij} x_i\right)}, \tag{1}$$

where the $\alpha_g, \beta_{1g}, \ldots, \beta_{Fg}$ are the model coefficient in the model formula for group g. For statistical processing, the statistical analysis freeware R version 3.4.2 [23] was used.

Evaluation. The model performance was evaluated by calculating the precision (the percentage of correctly predicted subjects among the subjects predicted as a group), recall (the percentage of correctly predicted subjects among the subjects in a group), and accuracy (the percentage of correctly predicted subjects among the total subjects) from the confusion matrix for both training and test data.

Table 1. Subjects' information of the training data set.

Category		Number of subjects	Age	HAM-D score	YMRS score
HE	Male	7	42.0 ± 4.6 (n/a 2)	-	-
	Female	4	28 (n/a 3)	-	-
BPI	Male	10	56.3 ± 11.1	5.4 ± 5.8	0.6 ± 1.3
	Female	9	57.9 ± 15.0	5.9 ± 7.3	0.8 ± 1.7
BPII	Male	12	52.0 ± 14.4	6.2 ± 6.0	1.6 ± 3.3
	Female	18	51.1 ± 12.4	7.2 ± 7.4	2.1 ± 2.8

"n/a" signifies the missing value of the sample.

Table 2. Subjects' information of the test data set.

Category		Number of subjects	Age	HAM-D score	YMRS score
HE	Male	3	47.0 ± 11.3 (n/a 1)	-	-
	Female	0	-	-	-
BPI	Male	3	45.3 ± 13.3	3.3 ± 3.5	1.3 ± 2.3
	Female	3	56.0 ± 14.9	1.0 ± 1.0	2.3 ± 4.0
BPII	Male	2	36.5 ± 9.2	8.0 ± 4.2	2.5 ± 0.7
	Female	7	55.3 ± 11.0	5.0 ± 4.2	2.7 ± 4.3

"n/a" signifies the missing value of the sample.

3   Results

3.1   Features of the Model

As a result of step 2 of feature selection, 402 pieces of data were collected from 6, 552 features. As a result of step 3 of the feature selection, 55 pieces of data were collected from 402 feature volumes. As a result of polytomous logistic regression analysis, a prediction model comprised of 28 features in total was obtained. For the individual model formulas, they were probability prediction formulas comprised of 6 features for the HE group, 13 features for the BPI group, and 11 features for the BPII group. Moreover, the model included features related to low to middle frequencies, Mel-frequency, signal power, zero crossing rate of time domain, and voiced sound.

3.2   Performance of the Model

Performance for Training Data. The confusion matrix in Table 3 was obtained as a result of conducting predictions on the training data using the prediction model. Over 90% recall was found in all the groups, with >90% precision found in all prediction groups, resulting in >95% accuracy found for the overall data.

Table 3. The confusion matrix of the training data according to prediction model.

		Prediction				
		HE	BPI	BPII	Recall	
	HE	10	0	1	90.9%	
Actual	BPI	0	18	1	94.7%	
	BPII	0	0	30	100%	
	Precision	100%	100%	93.8%	Accuracy	96.7%

The distribution of group discrimination probability of the subjects who belonging to each group is presented in Fig. 1. In all groups, the probability that the subjects were classified into the same group as the one they originally belonged tended to be higher than the probability that the data were classified into other groups.

Performance for Test Data. As a result of the prediction of test data using the prediction model, the confusion matrix of Table 4 was obtained. Over 50% recall was found in all the groups, with over 50% precision found in all prediction groups, resulting in >65% accuracy for the overall data.

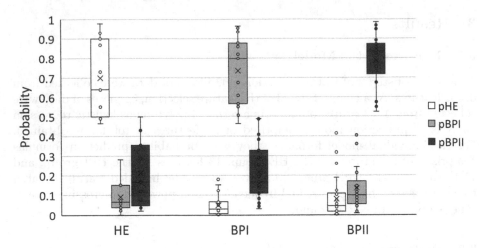

Fig. 1. The distribution of the group discrimination probability of the subjects used for training belonging to each group.

The distribution of the group discrimination probability of the subjects belonging to each group is presented in Fig. 2. In the HE group, the probability of the subjects being classified into the same group as the one they originally belonged to tended to be higher than the probability of the subjects being classified into other groups. Concerning the BPI and BPII groups, an overlap in distribution was observed between the probabilities of being classified into the BPI and BPII groups.

Table 4. The confusion matrix of test data using the prediction model.

		Prediction				
		HE	BPI	BPII	Recall	
	HE	3	0	0	100%	
Actual	BPI	1	3	2	50.0%	
	BPII	0	3	6	66.7%	
	Precision	75.0%	50.0%	75.0%	Accuracy	66.7%

4 Discussion

Concerning the prediction model performance, the overall accuracy was generally favorable for the training data. The accuracy for the test data was lower than that of the training data. Therefore, the prediction model was determined to be

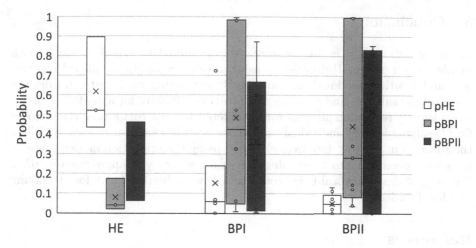

Fig. 2. The distribution of the group discrimination probability for testing subjects belonging in each group.

over-fitting, that is, a model optimized exclusively for learning data, and to be a model with inferior universality, that is, a model with low accuracy for data excluding the training data. Although the prediction model was over-fitting, it classified the training data, divided into three groups, with high accuracy, suggesting that the vocal features discriminate bipolar disorder. Moreover, if the BPI and BPII groups were merged, the prediction model may classify the healthy subjects and the patients with high accuracy.

Concerning the confusion matrix of the test data, the low recall in the BPI and BPII groups may be due to the similarities among the voices in the BPI and BPII patients. Even at the feature selection stage, the BPI and BPII groups could not be discriminated with an AUC of >0.8 for a single feature. Furthermore, this may indicate that the voices belonging to the two groups were similar; however, there were few subjects occasionally presenting equal probability of being classified into either of the BP groups. As shown in Tables 1 and 2, there was a difference in the numbers of males and females, age, HAM-D and YMRS score between the training and the test data. This can be attributed to the small sample size; moreover, it was impossible to match the training data and the test data sufficiently and may have affected the results.

In this study, audio data were collected in one setting. As such, the possibility of the data being impacted by the environment cannot be eradicated. In the future, it is necessary to collect audio data in other locations as well and to improve the prediction accuracy of the model.

In this study, analysis does not mention the details on the vocal features used in the model. Verifying which characteristics in the patient's voice were captured in the selected feature is another task for the future.

5   Conclusion

In this study, a vocal evaluation index was proposed to classify patients with bipolar type I or type II disorder by using patients with bipolar disorder as targets and healthy individuals as controls. By extracting vocal features from the voices of the subjects and selecting vocal features effective for a model, a polytomous logistic regression analysis was conducted to construct a prediction model for classifying healthy individuals and those with bipolar I or bipolar II. When the subjects in the test data were classified using the prediction model, the subjects were classified into three categories at an accuracy of approximately 67%. We suggest that the vocal index could be a new evaluation index for classifying bipolar disorders.

References

1. Izawa, S., et al.: Salivary dehydroepiandrosterone secretion in response to acute psychosocial stress and its correlations with biological and psychological changes. Biol. Psychol. **79**(3), 294–298 (2008)
2. Suzuki, G., et al.: Decreased plasma brain-derived neurotrophic factor and vascular endothelial growth factor concentrations during military training. PloS One **9**(2), e89455 (2014)
3. Garcia, R.G., Valenza, G., Tomaz, C.A., Barbieri, R.: Instantaneous bispectral analysis of heartbeat dynamics for the assessment of major depression. In: The Proceedings of Computing in Cardiology 2015, pp. 781–784. Nice (2015)
4. Goldberg, D.P.: Manual of the General Health Questionnaire. NFER Publishing, Windsor (1978)
5. Beck, A.T., Ward, C.H., Mendelson, M., Mock, J., Erbaugh, J.: An inventory for measureing depression. Arch. Gen. Psychiatry **4**(6), 561–571 (1961)
6. Young, R.C., Biggs, J.T., Ziegler, V.E., Meyer, D.A.: A rating scale for mania: reliability, validity and sensitivity. Br. J. Psychiatry **133**(5), 429–435 (1978)
7. Delgado-Rodriguez, M., Llorca, J.: Bias. J. Epidemiol. Community Health **58**(8), 635–641 (2004)
8. Cummins, N., Epps, J., Breakspear, M., Goecke, R.: An investigation of depressed speech detection: features and normalization. In: The Proceedings of the 12th Annual Conference of the International Speech Communication Association, Florence, pp. 2997–3000 (2011)
9. Mundt, J.C., Vogel, A.P., Feltner, D.E., Lenderking, W.R.: Vocal acoustic biomarkers of depression severity and treatment response. Biol. Psychiatry **72**(7), 580–587 (2012)
10. Tokuno, S., Mitsuyoshi, S., Suzuki, G., Tsumatori, G.: Stress evaluation by voice: a novel stress evaluation technology. In: The Proceedings of the 9th International Conference on Early Psychosis, Tokyo, pp. 17–19 (2014)
11. Jiang, H., et al.: Investigation of different speech types and emotions for detecting depression using different classifiers. Speech Commun. **90**, 39–46 (2017)
12. Diagnostic and statistical manual of mental disorders V. American Psychiatric Association (2013)
13. Bowden, C.L.: Strategies to reduce misdiagnosis of bipolar depression. Psychiatr. Serv. **52**(1), 51–55 (2001)

14. Muzina, D.J., Kemp, D.E., McIntyre, R.S.: Differentiating bipolar disorders from major depressive disorders: treatment implications. Ann. Clin. Psychiatry **19**(4), 305–312 (2007)
15. Nakamura, M., et al.: Feasibility study of classifying major depressive disorder and bipolar disorders using voice features. In: The Proceedings of WPA XVII World Congress of Psychiatry, Berlin (2017)
16. Higuchi, M., et al.: Classification of bipolar disorder, major depressive disorder, and healthy state using voice. Asian J. Pharm. Clin. Res. **11**(3), 89–93 (2018)
17. Faurholt-Jepsen, M., et al.: Voice analysis as an objective state marker in bipolar disorder. Transl. Psychiatry **6**, e856 (2016)
18. Maxhuni, A., Muñoz-Meléndez, A., Osmani, V., Perez, H., Mayora, O., Morales, E.F.: Classification of bipolar disorder episodes based on analysis of voice and motor activity of patients. Pervasive Mob. Comput. **31**, 50–66 (2016)
19. Sheehan, D.V., et al.: The mini-international neuropsychiatric interview (M.I.N.I.): the development and validation of a structured diagnostic psychiatric interview for DSM-IV and ICD-10. J. Clin. Psychiatry **59**(Suppl. 20), 22–33 (1998)
20. Hamilton, M.: A rating scale for depression. J. Neurol. Neurosurg. Psychiatry **23**, 56–62 (1960)
21. Eyben, F., Wöllmer, M., Schuller, B.: openSMILE - the Munich versatile and fast open-source audio feature extractor. In: The Proceedings of the 18th ACM International Conference on Multimedia, Firenze, pp. 1459–1462 (2010)
22. Friedman, J., Hastie, T., Tibshirani, R.: Regularization paths for generalized linear models via coordinate descent. J. Stat. Softw. **33**(1), 1–22 (2010)
23. R Core Team: R: A language and environment for statistical computing. R Foundation for Statistical Computing, Vienna. https://www.R-project.org/. Accessed 2 Dec 2018

Exploring Affect Recall Bias and the Impact of Mild Depressive Symptoms: An Ecological Momentary Study

Desirée Colombo[1(✉)], Carlos Suso-Ribera[1],
Javier Fernandez-Álvarez[2], Isabel Fernandez Felipe[1],
Pietro Cipresso[2,3], Azucena Garcia Palacios[1], Giuseppe Riva[2,3],
and Cristina Botella[1]

[1] Department of Basic Psychology, Clinic and Psychobiology,
Universitat Jaume I, 12071 Castellón, Spain
{dcolombo, susor, azucena, botella}@uji.es,
al260660@alumail.uji.es
[2] Department of Psychology, Università Cattolica del Sacro Cuore,
20100 Milan, Italy
{javier.fernandezkirszman, pietro.cipresso,
giuseppe.riva}@unicatt.it
[3] Applied Technology for Neuro-Psychology Lab,
IRCCS Istituto Auxologico Italiano, 20149 Milan, Italy
{p.cipresso, g.riva}@auxologico.it

Abstract. Traditional clinical and research assessments rely on retrospective questionnaires, that ask individuals to retrospectively summarize how they felt during the last period. Nevertheless, people are not accurate at recalling past experiences without altering the content, especially when they are required to report their affect. In this study, we adopted a smartphone-based ecological momentary assessment (EMA) to collect daily assessments of positive (PA) and negative (NA) affect throughout two weeks in a sample of healthy students (n = 47). Results showed that both PA and NA are subject to the recall bias; more specifically, people tended to overestimate both affects during the retrospective assessment. This bias was influenced by the presence of mild depressive symptoms as measured by the Beck Depression Inventory (BDI), which led participants to a greater overestimation of NA and higher underestimation of PA. While NA bias was more context-dependent, PA bias showed more stability across time.

Keywords: Ecological momentary assessment · Momentary affect · Recall bias

1 Introduction

Most of traditional assessment techniques both in research and clinical practice are retrospective, i.e. people are asked to summarize their affective experience or symptoms throughout the previous weeks [1]. However, people are not always able to recall past experiences without altering their content and, especially in depressed individuals,

© ICST Institute for Computer Sciences, Social Informatics and Telecommunications Engineering 2019
Published by Springer Nature Switzerland AG 2019. All Rights Reserved
P. Cipresso et al. (Eds.): MindCare 2019, LNICST 288, pp. 208–215, 2019.
https://doi.org/10.1007/978-3-030-25872-6_17

systematic biases can be observed, such as increased elaboration of negative information or greater recall of negative rather than positive stimuli [2]. This recall bias has been detected also in affect recall, pointing out a general tendency to retrospectively exaggerate both positive (PA) and negative (NA) affect [3–5]. Interestingly, clinically depressed individuals show greater inaccuracy for NA [6], which would be explained by different factors such as personal beliefs, memory salience, cognitive styles or past affective experiences [7, 8]. Nevertheless, no study has investigated the role of mild as opposed to moderate/severe depressive symptoms on affect recall bias, so the symptom severity level at which recall bias emerges is unclear.

Ecological momentary assessment (EMA) is an alternative approach to laboratory experiments to collect repeated daily self-reports [9] and/or objective data [10–13] by means of paper-and-pencil diaries or mobile devices, which can be performed in naturalistic settings and close-in-time to the real experience [14, 15]. Not surprisingly, an increasing number of researchers are adopting this approach to explore affect dynamics in daily life [16, 17]. Instead of using retrospective questionnaires, indeed, EMA allows to capture affect fluctuations with higher precision and accuracy and thus to delete the aforementioned recall bias of traditional retrospective assessments.

Here, we explored affect recall bias in a healthy population by comparing two-week EMA ratings of PA and NA collected with a mobile smartphone against affect retrospectively recalled using a paper-and-pencil approach. The aims of the study were to (1) investigate affect recall bias in healthy individuals, (2) explore the direction of such bias (i.e. retrospective affect overestimation and/or underestimation), and (3) deepen into the role that depressive symptoms may play in this phenomenon.

2   Methods

2.1   Participants

Participants were 48 students whose age ranged from 18 to 36 years ($M = 22.26$; $SD = 4.12$). The sample was mostly composed of women (71%). Recruitment was conducted via online advertisements at the Jaume I University (Castellon, Spain).

Participants were first contacted by telephone by one of the researchers and were provided with a web link to fulfil the baseline questionnaires. Subsequently, a face-to-face laboratory meeting was scheduled. Data from one of the participants was excluded because responses markedly deviated from other observations in the sample and within-individual inconsistencies were observed, which made us think of careless or random response style. Therefore, the final sample was composed of 47 participants.

2.2   Measures

At the beginning and at the end of the study, participants completed the Patient Health Questionnaire – 9 (PHQ-9) [18]. The PHQ-9 is a self-report tool for the assessment of depressive symptoms, based on DSM-IV depression diagnostic criteria. This questionnaire is composed of 9 items which refer to symptoms experienced during the past two weeks. At the end of the study, participants were also asked to fulfil the Positive and Negative Affect Schedule (PANAS) [19], a self-report measure of positive (10 items) and negative (10 items) affect. Specifically, participants were asked to rate PA and NA experienced during the past two weeks (i.e., to retrospectively report their affect throughout the duration of the study). The descriptive statistics of all these questionnaires are reported in Table 1.

Table 1. Questionnaires descriptive statistics.

Measure	Min-Max	Mean	St. Dev.
PHQ-9 (pre)	0–18	4.49	4.49
PHQ-9 (post)	0–18	3.53	3.53
PANAS-PA	16–44	29.87	6.72
PANAS-NA	0–41	18.64	6.88

2.3   Procedure

After the completion of baseline questionnaires, participants were invited to attend the laboratory in order to sign the informed consent. Participants were provided with an identification number to download and access "EMA Móvil", an Android mobile application created by our team to administer ecological assessments. This application can be easily monitored and programmed from a web platform, where items, type of answer, number of prompts and sampling method can be chosen. No programming skills are therefore required.

Over the following 14 days, the application prompted three daily assessments at random times within three-time intervals (9:30–14:00; 14:00–18:30; and 18:30–23:00). During each evaluation, participants were asked to complete single-items of momentary affect (PA: *"To what extent are you experiencing positive emotions in this moment?"*; NA: *"To what extent are you experiencing negative emotions in this moment?"*). Participants were just asked to enter the notification and to complete the questionnaire. To prevent backfilling, participants were given one hour to answer the current assessment. If they did not respond in time, the evaluation was marked as missing. At the end of the study, participants were asked to return to the laboratory to complete post-assessment questionnaires and receive a monetary compensation of 10 euros.

2.4   Data Analysis

EMA affect values were obtained by calculating the mean of PA and NA item scores across the study (42 possible assessments for each participant), while PANAS affect values were calculated by dividing the total PANAS score (positive and negative separately) administered at the end of the study by the total number of positive/negative affect items in the PANAS. The range scores for both forms of assessment (two weeks of daily, single-item assessments with an app and a single retrospective evaluation using the full-length scale at the end of the study) were the same (1 = lowes affect to 5 = highest affect).

To test the construct validity of the EMA affect items, we carried out a correlation between PA scores (Pearson correlation) and NA scores (Spearman correlation) obtained via EMA and the PANAS. We subsequently compared daily and retrospective PA means (paired-samples T-test) and NA means (Wilcoxon Signed Ranks Test) to test participants' ability to estimate PA and NA retrospectively.

To explore affect recall bias and distinguish between retrospective overestimation and underestimation of affect, we calculated delta scores between PA and NA measured via the PANAS and EMA. Positive delta scores would reflect affect overestimation during the retrospective assessment, while negative values would reveal retrospective underestimation of affect. We compared PA and NA delta scores (Wilcoxon Signed Ranks Test) and conducted four correlations to investigate the association between PA (Pearson correlation) and NA delta scores (Spearman correlation) and depressive symptoms measured by means of the PHQ-9 at the beginning and at the end of the study (i.e., to explore whether depressive symptoms were associated with the ability to estimate affect).

In the analyses, non-parametric tests were used when the assumptions for the use of parametric tests (i.e., normality of scores) were not met. Parametric tests were used elsewhere.

3   Results

Results showed a significant correlation between daily and retrospective PA measures and daily and retrospective NA measures, as showed in Table 2.

Table 2. Correlations between NA and PA measured via EMA or PANAS. Bivariate associations with NA (PANAS) were calculated with Spearman correlations. The remaining are calculated using Pearson correlations. $*p < .05$, $**p < .01$, $***p < .001$.

	Mean (SD)	Bivariate associations		
		NA (EMA)	PA (PANAS)	NA (PANAS)
PA (EMA)	2.75 (0.64)	.08	.36*	.043
NA (EMA)	1.47 (0.33)		−.32*	.48***
PA (PANAS)	2.99 (0.71)			−.22
NA (PANAS)	1.89 (0.74)			

The comparison of PA measured via EMA and with the PANAS evidenced significant mean difference in scores ($t = -2.25$, $p = .03$, 95% IC = -0.453, 0.025). Furthermore, the comparison of NA between assessment methods also resulted in statistically significant differences in rank scores ($Z = -4.11$, $p < .001$). Specifically, both PA and NA indicated higher scores when recalled retrospectively with the PANAS.

To further explore the observed recall bias and distinguish between retrospective affect overestimation or underestimation, we calculated delta scores between PA and NA measured by means of the PANAS and EMA. As shown in Fig. 1, a higher variability in the distribution of deltas was observed for PA. However, the analysis of differences in PA and NA delta scores did not result in a statistically significant difference in rank scores ($Z = -.810$, $p < .418$).

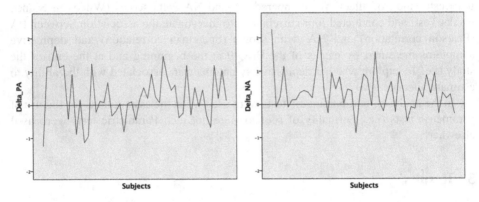

Fig. 1. Distribution of NA and PA delta scores across participants.

We finally investigated the role of depressive symptoms in affect recall bias. PA delta values negatively correlated with PHQ-9 scores measured both at baseline and the end of the study. NA delta scores positively correlated with PHQ-9 measured at the end of the study (Table 3 and Fig. 2).

Table 3. Correlations between delta scores and pre and post-PHQ-9. Bivariate associations with Delta NA are calculated using Spearman correlations. The remaining are Pearson correlations. *$p < .05$, **$p < .01$, ***$p < .001$.

	Mean (SD)	PHQ-9 (pre)	PHQ-9 (post)
Delta PA	2.75 (0.64)	−.530***	−.653***
Delta NA	1.47 (0.33)	.077	.300*

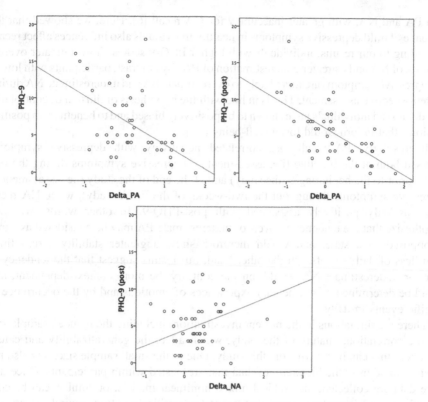

Fig. 2. Correlation between delta scores and pre/post PHQ-9.

4   Discussion

The aim of this study was to investigate affect recall bias in a healthy population by comparing two-week EMA affect assessments against the PANAS administrated via paper-and-pencil at the end of the study. To the best of our knowledge, this is the first investigation exploring the role of mild depressive symptomatology on affect recall bias in a healthy population.

Daily EMA measures and retrospective PANAS scores showed a significant correlation, suggesting the construct validity of our single items to assess daily PA and NA. Importantly, one of the main challenges when designing EMA protocols is adherence [20], that is, the percentage of completed assessments obtained from each participant. Our results suggest that the use of single items to assess PA and NA as opposed to long questionnaires is feasible and conceptually valid, which makes it an adequate solution to be adopted in EMA protocols.

According to previous literature [3–5], people tend to retrospectively exaggerate both PA and NA. Here, we replicated this result, as participants showed a general retrospective overestimation of both affects. We were also interested in exploring mild depressive symptomatology as a potential variable affecting affect recall. In their study, Ben-Zeev and colleagues found that clinical depression leads to the retrospective intensifications of both PA and NA, with greater inaccuracy for NA recall [6]. Here, we showed that the presence of mild depressive symptoms in healthy individuals also influences affect recall. According to our results, individuals with higher PHQ-9 scores show a greater overestimation of NA and a greater underestimation of PA. By contrast, participants with low or no depressive symptoms are more likely to overestimate PA and underestimate NA during the retrospective assessment. This is in line with the hypothesis of illusion of control that non-depressed individuals have shown to be positively biased and to benefit from positive illusions, that in turn would foster well-being [21].

Interestingly, PA recall bias correlated negatively with depressive symptoms assessed both at the baseline (i.e. assessment of depressive symptoms during the two weeks prior to the beginning of the study) and at the end of the study (i.e. assessment of depressive symptoms throughout the two-weeks of the EMA study), while NA recall bias was only positively associated with post-PHQ-9. In other words, we may hypothesize that the tendency to over- or underestimate PA may be considered as a trait as opposed to a state, and would therefore show a greater stability across time, regardless of daily events. On the other hand, our results suggest that the tendency to over- or underestimate NA would, on the contrary, be more context-dependent, and would be determined by momentary experiences of emotions and by the occurrence of specific events in daily life.

There are limitations in the present investigation, including the reduced sample size and the correlational nature of the study, which affect the generalizability and causal inferences that can be drawn from this study. Due to the small sample size, it is also not possible to address the hierarchy of data that are nested within participants. Once that more data are collected, hierarchical mixed nonlinear models, or similar, can be considered. A final important aspect that needs to consider revolves around the content validity. While it may be true that in our preliminary examination a proper correlation of PANAS and the single item exists, it is necessary to contrast this finding in larger populations in order to guarantee content validity. It may be the case that such a complex construct like affect may not be accurately grasped by means of a single item. Beyond these issues, future studies should also consider the impact that other variables have on affect recall, such as the presence of anxiety symptoms or high levels of stress, as well as focus on the development of standardized ad hoc items to be used in mobile devices for the daily assessment of affect.

Nevertheless, we believe that this study sheds new light into the importance and utility of EMA in the study of affect, as well as the need to study the influence of recall bias for a wider range of depressive severity scores, including milder cases as conducted in the present investigation. These findings are important for clinical purposes, as they indicate that recall bias can occur even when depressive symptoms are mild, especially for PA. Accordingly, the evaluation of affect should be preferably performed ecologically and repeatedly using EMA.

References

1. Shiffman, S., Stone, A.A., Hufford, M.R.: Ecological momentary assessment. Annu. Rev. Clin. Psychol. 4(1), 1–32 (2008)

2. Gotlib, I.H., Joormann, J.: Cognition and depression: current status and future directions. Annu. Rev. Clin. Psychol. **6**, 285–312 (2010)
3. Wirtz, D., Kruger, J., Scollon, C.N., Diener, E.: Psychol. Sci. **14**(5), 520–524 (2003)
4. Thomas, D.L., Diener, E.: Memory accuracy in the recall of emotions. J. Pers. Soc. Psychol. **59**(2), 291–297 (1990)
5. Kardum, I., Tićac Daskijević, K.: Absolute and relative accuracy in the retrospective estimate of positive and negative mood. Eur. J. Psychol. Assess. **17**(1), 69–77 (2001)
6. Ben-Zeev, D., Young, M.A., Madsen, J.W.: Retrospective recall of affect in clinically depressed individuals and controls. Cogn. Emot. **23**(5), 1021–1040 (2009)
7. Fredrickson, B.L.: Extracting meaning from past affective experiences: the importance of peaks, ends, and specific emotions. Cogn. Emot. **14**(4), 577–606 (2000)
8. Levine, L.J., Prohaska, V., Burgess, S.L., Rice, J.A., Laulhere, T.M.: Remembering past emotions: the role of current appraisals. Cogn. Emot. **15**(4), 393–417 (2001)
9. Suso-Ribera, C., Castilla, D., Zaragozá, I., Ribera-Canudas, M.V., Botella, C., García-Palacios, A.: Validity, reliability, feasibility, and usefulness of pain monitor, a multidimensional smartphone app for daily monitoring of adults with heterogeneous chronic pain. Clin. J. Pain **34**(10), 900–908 (2018)
10. Mohr, D.C., Zhang, M., Schueller, S.M.: Personal sensing: understanding mental health using ubiquitous sensors and machine learning. Annu. Rev. Clin. Psychol. **13**(1), 23–47 (2017)
11. Gaggioli, A., et al.: A mobile data collection platform for mental health research. Pers. Ubiquit. Comput. **17**(2), 241–251 (2013)
12. Gaggioli, A., et al.: Positive technology: a free mobile platform for the self-management of psychological stress. Annu. Rev. CyberTherapy Telemed. **199**, 25–29 (2014)
13. Cipresso, P., et al.: Is your phone so smart to affect your state? An exploratory study based on psychophysiological measures. Neurocomputing **84**, 23–30 (2012)
14. Stone, A.A., Shiffman, S., Atienza, A.A., Nebeling, A.: Historical roots and rationale of ecological momentary assessment (EMA). In: The Science of Real-Time Data Capture: Self-Reports in Health Research, pp. 3–10 (2007)
15. Csikszentmihalyi, M., Larson, R.: Validity and reliability of the experience-sampling method. J. Nerv. Ment. Dis. **175**(9), 526–536 (1987)
16. Ebner-Priemer, U.W., Trull, T.J.: Ecological momentary assessment of mood disorders and mood dysregulation. Psychol. Assess. **21**(4), 463–475 (2009)
17. Bylsma, L.M., Rottenberg, J.: Uncovering the dynamics of emotion regulation and dysfunction in daily life with ecological momentary assessment. In: Nyklíček, I., Vingerhoets, A., Zeelenberg, M. (eds.) Emotion Regulation and Well-Being. Springer, New York (2011). https://doi.org/10.1007/978-1-4419-6953-8_14
18. Kroenke, K., Spitzer, R.L., Williams, J.B.W.: The PHQ-9: validity of a brief depression severity measure. J. Gen. Intern. Med. **16**(9), 606–613 (2001)
19. Watson, D., Clark, L.A., Tellegen, A.: Development and validation of brief measures of positive and negative affect: the PANAS scales. J. Pers. Soc. Psychol. **54**(6), 1063–1070 (1988)
20. Colombo, D., Cipresso, P., Fernández Alvarez, J., Garcia Palacios, A., Riva, G., Botella, C.: An overview of factors associated with adherence and dropout to ecological momentary assessments in depression. Annu. Rev. CyberTherapy Telemed. (2018)
21. Taylor, S.E., Brown, J.D.: Positive illusions and well-being revisited: separating fact from fiction. Psychol. Bull. **116**(1), 21–27 (1994)

Full Body Immersive Virtual Reality System with Motion Recognition Camera Targeting the Treatment of Spider Phobia

Jacob Kritikos[1(✉)], Stavroula Poulopoulou[2], Chara Zoitaki[3],
Marilina Douloudi[4], and Dimitris Koutsouris[1]

[1] Biomedical Engineering Laboratory,
National Technical University of Athens, 15780 Athens, Greece
{jkritikos, dkoutsou}@biomed.ntua.gr
[2] Department of Digital Systems, University of Piraeus, 18534 Piraeus, Greece
stavroula.plplou2@gmail.com
[3] School of Electrical and Computer Engineering,
National Technical University of Athens, 15780 Athens, Greece
charazoitaki@gmail.com
[4] Department of Biology,
National Kapodistrian University of Athens, 15780 Athens, Greece
marilina.douloudi@gmail.com

Abstract. Exposure Therapy (ET) is one of the most widely-used methods for treating Specific Phobias, and, over the past few years, Virtual Reality (VR) has contributed significantly in this field, since the birth of what we call "Virtual Reality ET" (VRET). However, VR systems used in VRET so far do not fully integrate ET characteristics; the reason behind this is that they do not provide sufficient, or occasionally not any at all, interaction with the feared stimulus, which is a key factor for full ET implementation. Objective: The aim of our study is to propose a way to include natural interaction between the patient and the system during the treatment procedure. Method: We propose an addition to current session protocols for mental health professionals through which they can apply ET in full extent with the use of motion tracking sensors. Specifically, we added a Motion Recognition Camera, which tracks the patient's movements and places their physical body within the virtual environment, increasing their feeling of presence and making the system more immersive. Therefore, clinicians can assign interactive tasks for their patients to practice within a controlled virtual environment. Results: We present the feedback we received regarding the system's potential utility and efficiency by a group of psychiatry professionals who tried the system. Impact: With real-time interaction and VRET, patients stand a better chance to truly acquire the necessary skills to overcome their phobias.

Keywords: Virtual reality · Cognitive behavioral treatments ·
Exposure therapy · Anxiety disorders · Specific phobias ·
Motion tracking sensor · Motion recognition camera · Presence ·
Clinical treatment · Immersion

The original version of this chapter was revised: The missing reference has been added. The correction to this chapter is available at https://doi.org/10.1007/978-3-030-25872-6_23

P. Cipresso et al. (Eds.): MindCare 2019, LNICST 288, pp. 216–230, 2019.
https://doi.org/10.1007/978-3-030-25872-6_18

1 Introduction

Anxiety disorders share features of excessive worry and fear that cause behavioral disturbances to the suffering individuals. Approximately 1 in 5 adults will manifest some form of Anxiety Disorder at some point in their lives with rates being twice as high for minors [1–4]. Specific phobias are a type of anxiety disorder defined as the persistent fear of a stimulus, potentially an object or a situation, which renders the person unable to demonstrate self-control. Specific phobias along with agoraphobia and social phobia are one of the most common types of phobias, which in fact are considered as sub-types of a broader category, that of anxiety disorders, according to the Diagnostic and Statistical Manual of Mental Disorders, Fifth Edition (DSM-V). According to the American Psychiatric Association [1], the lifetime prevalence of specific phobias is approximately 7%–9% in the US and 6% in Europe, and can reach up to 12,5% [5]. Although a lot of research has been conducted in this field over the past few years, only a minority (8%) of people reported with specific phobias have received any treatment [6, 7].

The most well-known treatment of various cognitive and behavioral disorders is Cognitive Behavioral Therapy (CBT) [8, 9], since it appears as the preferred method by the majority of mental health professionals to treat phobias; this may be due to the fact that a number of scientists claim CBT has no possible side-effects, unlike medication [1, 10]. The basic principles of CBT focus on identifying, understanding and altering patients' thought and behavioral patterns. Patients are actively involved in their own recovery, which offers them a stronger sense of control; additionally, through therapy sessions, they obtain useful skills they ought to practice repeatedly in order to present the desirable progress [11].

The applications of CBT, along with its different forms, have been highly efficient so far; by evaluating previous studies, we can deduce that an average of 50% of patients managed to decrease their phobia-related anxiety [12–17]. Nonetheless, certain studies reviewing CBT results [18, 19] indicate that it is still unclear whether the phobia returns after a short period of time or not. For instance, a recent research [20] claims that the phobia does not return at least amid the first semester. Yet, some scientists disclose that CBT's benefits do not necessarily last long; specifically, another study [21] mentions that results lasted only for the first 20 days.

Exposure Therapy (ET) is a form of CBT treatment [22] developed to help people confront their fears in a safe environment. There are several variations of ETs, such as 'In VIVO ET', 'Virtual Reality ET' (VRET) [23], 'Imaginary ET' and 'Interoceptive ET' ([23, 24] but all of them follow the same basic procedure [25–27], which usually consists of the following steps:

Step 1: The cognitive sessions, where the patient is informed about their condition and their unreasonable thought patterns; next, the patient discusses any existent distressing thoughts and possible dreaded scenarios with the experts.
Step 2: The exposure sessions, where the patient is exposed to assorted phobic situations with graded difficulty through In VIVO ET or VRET. This step is repeated until the patient's anxiety levels decrease.
Step 3: The follow-up sessions appointed after a significant period of time in which clinicians evaluate the overall decrease in the patient's anxiety levels.

During In VIVO ET, patients are asked to confront the feared stimulus in real life. However, simulating every possible scenario in real life is expensive and time-consuming; for instance, in case a patient is suffering from aviophobia, they would have to buy an airplane ticket and go through the entire boarding process accompanied by their clinician, who usually charges by the hour [28, 29]. Also, in some cases, it could lead to undesired results since displeasing occurrences may further terrorize patients (e.g. turbulence during the flight in the early stages of ET [30]). In order to overcome such technical issues, VRET is starting to replace In VIVO ET.

In VRET, patients are exposed to virtual, life-like, anxiety-provoking environments instead of real stimuli [31–33]. Within them, they can practice tasks assigned by their clinician in a controllable, and therefore safe, virtual environment designed to appropriately stimulate their specific phobia, in the clinician's office. Due to that, patients feel more comfortable and confident; thus, they are more willing to confront situations that cause them discomfort and explore alternative ways of responding. Also, even though their actions occur in the virtual world, the knowledge acquired transfers to the real world [34]. Lastly, over the last few years, studies have found VRET to be as effective as In VIVO [31] in terms of triggering anxiety [46]. Therefore, treatment through VR systems could become a low-cost method of providing effective interventions at scale.

Overall, we can conclude that ET has two primary characteristics: [a] patients have to come in contact with the feared stimulus actively, and [b] patients have to master how to confront and respond to said stimuli without fear or anxiety. Current VRET applications provide contact with the feared stimulus, i.e. trigger fear through VR videos; however, they have not yet been able to allow patients to interact actively with the stimulus. At best, the only interaction that is currently available is via hand controllers through which complex tasks and exercises, such as touching and moving objects with the rest of their body (e.g. their feet) cannot be completed, due to the nature of hand controllers' design that only provides hand interaction. Therefore, certain scenarios cannot be simulated. Overall, VRET has managed to stimulate patients' anxiety through a virtual stimulus; yet, patients usually remain passive or interact poorly, which doesn't improve immersion, and consequently, the patient's feeling of presence in the virtual environment is decreased. Hence, in order for VRET to reach its full potential and implement ET as a whole, life-like interaction must be added to existing systems [31, 35, 36].

In this study, we present and propose a fully immersive VR System by adding a new tool, the Motion Recognition Camera (MRC), on top of the VR technology. The MRC tracks patients' movements, places their physical body within the virtual environment and gives them the impression that they are moving and interacting in full extent with that environment, as they would in the real world. This allows patients to practice tasks whilst in the virtual environment. By combining these technologies, we increase the user's immersion and presence. Additionally, we propose that Step 2 be separated into two different cycles regarding the exposure sessions: [a] Step 2-a in which VRET is applied as it currently is; patients come in contact with the phobic stimulus for the first time in a controlled environment and learn how to stay close to the stimulus without losing their composure, and [b] Step 2-b in which patients practice possible coping mechanisms, that differ from the ones originated from physical environment, like concepts of avoidance and fear anticipation [37] by directly interacting with the phobic stimulus, and by learning to control their reaction and regulate their anxiety response. In this study, we define Step 2-b as "Action Therapy", to emphasize the importance of confrontation, which needs to become a separate and independent part of the sessions.

So, our hypothesis is whether the proposed system can provide appropriate inter-action and confrontation with the phobic stimulus, which could improve current treatments in the future. We examined this hypothesis through a trial-run, with the medical staff of a psychiatric clinic as participants. After completing the study, the clinicians gave us their professional feedback on their experience with the proposed system as well as suggestions for its further improvement.

2   Materials

2.1   Hardware

The proposed system consists of the following equipment: [a] VR Goggles (VRG): "Gear VR" by Samsung; [b] a Mobile Phone: the "Galaxy S7" by Samsung; [c] a Motion Recognition Camera (MRC): the "Astra S" by ORBBEC; the specifications of the MRC are: Range: 0.6–8.0 m (Optimal 0.6–5.0 m), Depth Image Size: 640*480–30fps, RGB Image Size: 1280*960–30fps, Field of View: 60° horiz. x 49.5° vert. (73° diagonal). The MRC tracks the patient's movements, places their physical body in the virtual environment and gives them the impression that they are moving and interacting with their whole body in that environment in real time, as they would in the real world. This allows the patient to practice tasks assigned by their clinician in the virtual environment; [d] a Windows Desktop Computer.

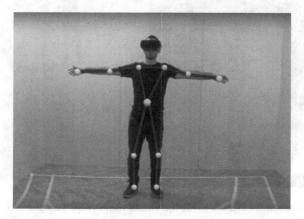

Fig. 1. The MRC is installed in front of the user to recognize the joints and place them inside the virtual environment.

2.2   Software

We created a C++ program and used the Orbbec Astra SDK, along with the Bluetooth Windows SDK, to assist us in body recognition and its dispatching from the Desktop Computer, which operates the MCR, to the Gear VR. Android Studio was used to create the Bluetooth receiver program; Unity 3D was used for creating the virtual environment depicted by the VRG; Blender 3D Computer Graphics was used for creating 3D objects, animated visual effects and materials, and Adobe Photoshop for designing images for the materials. Moreover, regarding the body tracking software, the Astra S MRC is designed for skeleton tracking (Fig. 1); consequently, it can recognize the entire body and movements of its limbs. The program we have written for the MRC tracks the joints (Fig. 2); then, the user's skeleton is represented in the virtual room as a set of spheres and lines (the spheres represent the joints and the lines represent the bones connecting joints).

2.3   System Setup

The outlined area is about 5 m^2 and will be referred to as the "Action Area". In the Action Area, the user wears the VRG and is able to observe the virtual environment. The user does not need to wear or hold any other equipment than the VRG, in order to move and interact with objects. The MRC is placed on a table at a 1 m distance from the Action Area, so as to record the user's movements and transfer them to the virtual environment.

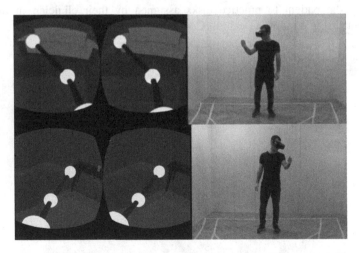

Fig. 2. Users can see their skeleton inside the virtual room. Top: The user's right arm. Bottom: The user's left arm.

3 Method

The proposed system was tested by twenty members of the Psychiatry Department of the Oncological Hospital of Kifisia staff (doctors, professors, nursing staff and the hospital's general manager), in Athens, Greece. All of the participants were familiar with the concept of using visual cues before (pictures, videos, standalone VR) as an effective way to stimulate fear emotions to phobic or non-phobic subjects. The aim of the session was for all participants to use the proposed system and answer a small questionnaire about their experience with it.

Q1: Do you believe that Exposure Therapy could benefit from the addition of interaction?

|_____|_____|_____|_____|_____|_____|
    NO   MAYBE-NO   MAYBE   MAYBE-YES   YES

Q2: Do you think that interaction with the Motion Recognition Camera in the Virtual Environment can give real life experience?

|_____|_____|_____|_____|_____|_____|
    NO   MAYBE-NO   MAYBE   MAYBE-YES   YES

Q3: Do you believe that coping mechanisms learnt in virtual situations and environments can be transferred to real-life situations?

|_____|_____|_____|_____|_____|_____|
    NO   MAYBE-NO   MAYBE   MAYBE-YES   YES

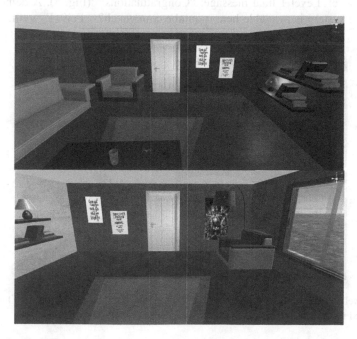

Fig. 3. Top: The virtual room of Level 1. Bottom: The virtual room of Level 2.

Furthermore, we present an implementation of Action Therapy. Spider phobia was used as a case study. The procedure consisted of one session with two levels of difficulty. During this session, two tasks were assigned to participants, aiming to help them in mastering new coping mechanisms, so as to confront their phobia, habituate with the phobic environment and eventually interact with the stimulus while remaining under control.

Level 1

Step 1: The user enters the Action Area, while the MRC is located at a 1 m distance. This is the area where the user can walk, move and react to the stimuli. *Step 2:* The user wears the VRG and enters the virtual environment (Fig. 3). *Step 3:* In the VR room, the user can observe their virtual arms, as well as walk and touch whatever objects are permitted. *Step 4:* The user reads the perspicuous instruction that appears at the top of the screen. This instruction describes the task the user is expected to fulfill in the level. Level 1 opening instruction: "Try to approach the spider" (Fig. 4). *Step 5:* The user performs the requested task. The aim of the first (easy) level is to allow users to observe the phobic object, to familiarize with it and thus exercise their response and composure when it appears in their personal space. In Level 1, the user must: [a] observe the virtual room: this helps users feel comfortable in the realm of the virtual environment, move more confidently in it and realize that their physical movements control their virtual ones in real time; [b] approach the spider in their own time whilst keeping their composure: the user can walk towards the table, where a white spider stands still; they can approach the spider whenever they feel ready and confident in themselves. The spider does not move at all, which gives users confidence and a strong sense of control. *Step 6:* The user reads the final instruction that appears at the top of the screen. This instruction congratulates them on successfully completing the task and marks the end of the first level. Level 1 final message: "Congratulations!" (Fig. 4). A demonstration video of the system is available here: youtube.com/watch?v=Fcj9uE_wv0I.

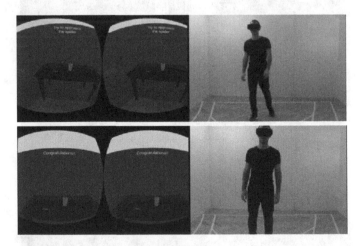

Fig. 4. Level 1: Top: The user's first goal is to try to approach the spider. Bottom: Once the user has managed to get close, the assignment is considered completed.

Level 2

Step 1: The user remains in the Action Area without taking the VRG off, since Level 2 starts automatically once Level 1 is completed. Step 2: The user enters a new virtual room. Step 3: The user reads the perspicuous instruction that appears at the top of the screen. This instruction describes the task the user is expected to complete during the level. Level 2 opening instruction: "Try hitting the spider 3 times". (Fig. 5) Step 4: The user performs the requested task. The aim of the second (hard) level is to allow users to touch the stimulus and learn how to remain calm, as well as confront the spider when it appears in their personal space. In Level 2 the user must: [a] approach the spider in their own time whilst keeping their composure: in this level, a black spider is hanging from the ceiling using its web, which gives it the ability to swing whenever the user hits it. The user can walk toward the spider when they feel ready and confident in themselves. The spider does not move unless the user hits it; this gives them time to relax and realize that the spider will not approach them unexpectedly; therefore, they have full control of the situation; [b] the user is requested to hit the spider three times and manage to stay close; the width of the spider's swing depends on the power of each hit, which increases the user's sense of control. They have to repeat the same action three times, so as to gradually realize that the spider cannot truly hurt them but instead, they can repel it if they want to; the user can even move a step back whenever the spider swings towards them; yet, it is crucial that they keep their composure and continue until they complete the task (Fig. 5). Step 5: After completing the task, the user reads the final instruction that appears at the top of the screen. This instruction congratulates them on successfully completing the task and marks the end of the second level: "Congratulations!". A demonstration video is available here: youtube.com/watch?v= qDBbSoOrUKY.

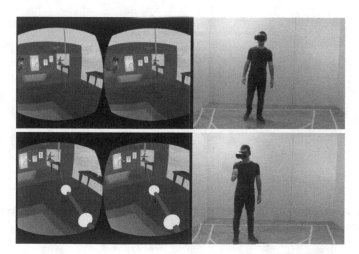

Fig. 5. Level 2: Top: The user sees a spider hanging from its web. Then, the instruction appears: "Try hitting the spider 3 times". Bottom: The user hits the spider.

4 Results

As we can see in Fig. 6, the clinicians reportedly mentioned that action is crucial for treating specific phobias, since 80% answered "MAYBE YES" or "YES". In Fig. 7, we can see that 80% of them answered "YES" or "MAYBE YES" to whether they think that the proposed system with MRC interaction can simulate real-life experiences. Last but not least, in Fig. 8, we can see a reduction of positive results, since 50% of the participating clinicians answered "MAYBE YES" or "YES" to whether coping mechanisms acquired in a virtual environment can be transferred to the real world. Only 2 out of 20 answered "YES".

Thereby, we conclude that not only is interaction necessary for the treatment process but also that the proposed system can simulate an appropriate interaction between the stimulus and the user through the VR simulation; however, according to the 20 clinicians, it is yet unclear whether virtual reality can actually assist patients in real life, despite the full body interaction.

Overall, the participants were initially thrilled with the opportunity to interact with the virtual environment. What was particularly interesting is that participants completed their task easily in the first level, where they were not asked to interact with the spider; nonetheless, during level 2, where participants were expected to interact with the stimulus, they were amazed by the possibility of interacting with the spider in such a straightforward way. Due to that, we can deduce that interaction with the feared object in the spectrum of a virtual environment could be far more efficient than the sole habituation of patients' anxiety through vivid virtual representations of the stimulus, i.e. images and videos. Also, even though participants were not familiar with the technology of the proposed system, no issues emerged during the simulations (Fig. 9).

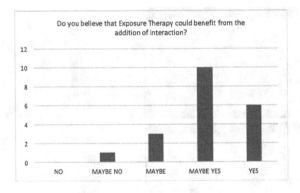

Fig. 6. The answers from the question Q1: "Do you believe that exposure therapy could benefit from the addition of interaction?".

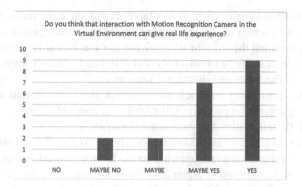

Fig. 7. The answers from the question Q2: "Do you think that interaction with the motion recognition camera in the virtual environment can give real life experience?".

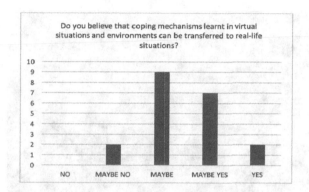

Fig. 8. The answers from the question Q3: "Do you believe that coping mechanisms learnt in virtual situations and environments can be transferred to real-life situations?".

5   Discussion

The present study investigated the possibility of expanding current ET treatments by adding another step, a new cycle of sessions in the procedure-, the one we refer to as "Action Therapy". The main intention of that step is to complement the visual stimuli already used in VRET by enhancing the confrontational capabilities of the patient towards their phobia during the treatment process. Our hypothesis is that the experience patients gain through the VR simulation could be more constructive and contribute significantly to their progress.

Thus, to determine whether the proposed Action Therapy could improve ET and be helpful to patients, we tested the proposed system on a group of 20 people consisting of professionals in the field of psychiatry. The aim of this trial was to introduce them to the system and, based on their experience, get their feedback on whether or not it could be beneficial for patients and add to their training.

Our hypothesis has been confirmed to a large extent since the majority of clinicians found the addition of action to the existing treatment procedure promising for patients. However, they presented their doubt whether coping mechanisms acquired during VR could be utilized in real-life; an indication that VR has to further improve to actually assist clinicians in the treatment of mental illnesses.

In spite of the promising feedback we received, there are limitations to take into consideration. Regarding the procedure, the trial was conducted on only a small group of 20 clinicians; therefore, the data was not extensive.

Another issue worthy of discussion is our choice to use the Motion Recognition Camera instead of other motion recognition tools, in order to add interaction to the VR system. Thanks to technological advances, there are various affordable commercial motion tracking devices available, from the motion recognition camera to wearable body tracking sensors, like gloves and suits with gyroscope trackers or accelerometer

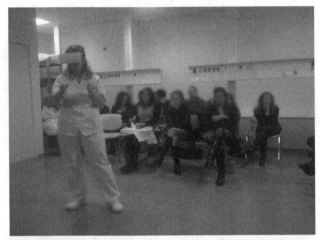

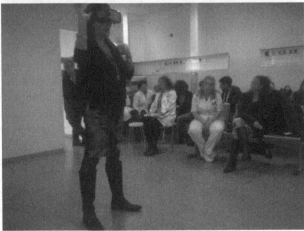

Fig. 9. Photos from the system trial-run at the Hospital: *(top)* The participant tries to hit the spider with her punches; *(bottom)* The participant observes her hands in the virtual room.

trackers, and hand controllers. The main reason we did not choose to use hand controllers is because they limit the interaction capability of the patient's body within the virtual environment, thus potentially rendering their movements unnatural, i.e. they have to press certain buttons instead of using their hands, so as to touch objects [38–40]. Regarding other wearable sensors, they would make the system's set up and operation more complicated, only to achieve the same result. Nevertheless, the MRC has some limitations as well, since it cannot track movements in all body parts (e.g. the fingers) due to its tracking range (0.6-8.0 m). However, the purpose of this study was not to extensively examine the differences between different types of motion tracking sensors, but to determine whether full-body interaction, in general, could benefit existing treatment protocols.

Finally, another interesting aspect of our study was that MRCs offer a remarkable feature: the tracking of the patient's physical movements is not only useful for placing their body in the virtual environment, but also for dispatching the information obtained by their movements in real time. Measurements of the patient's movements as they perform the assigned tasks can help draw further conclusions about the patient's performance, i.e. whether the patient completed the task effortlessly or not. This method could even help in the field of diagnostics, by comparing that data to those of healthy individuals.

6 Conclusion

Up to now, there has been no experimental indication stemming from clinical trial results that VRET is more effective than in VIVO ET. Nevertheless, previous studies have found them equally effective for patients. Considering the technical issues of In VIVO ET such as affordability, the time needed to implement it, as well as the fact that it is impossible for clinicians to acquire every phobic stimulus, VRET seems to be at least as helpful as In VIVO ET [41]. Acquisition costs of VR systems have dropped significantly, making it possible for VRET to be applied in a larger scale in clinicians' offices, either in private practice or clinics and hospitals.

Following, we propose that biomedical laboratories and tech-oriented research centers focus more on technologies that fit the needs of anxiety disorder field. Overall, VR applications related to anxiety disorders are still on an early stage of development, without any solid foundations built yet. Currently, this field seeks to adapt itself to the newly introduced technological tools [42–45]. At the same time, the technological tools themselves, also need to adapt to the respective safety regulations [30]. Our aim, through our research, focuses on encouraging the creation of systems precisely for the needs of this industry.

Finally, we suggest the proposed system could be an effective tool in other areas. By modifying the scenarios, it could be useful in the field of movement rehabilitation, for people with development disorders to control their movements and improve their social skills or in the area of forensic psychiatry, i.e. panic attacks, heart disease, epilepsy, or to people who take drugs with large psychological effects. The means of feedback currently in use are mainly subjective questionnaires. By adding cardiac rhythm, sweating and other sensors that track physiological changes to our system we can offer an objective evaluation based on the immediate bodily responses towards the stimuli without the interference of the possible manipulation of the questionnaires by the persons assessed.

Acknowledgements. We would like to thank the executive managers and members of the stuff of the General and Oncology Hospital of Kifissia for agreeing to provide the opportunity to present our work to them and receive their feedback.

At this point, we would like to discuss the expertise of the healthcare facility members we used as evaluators of our system a bit further. The medical staff of the facility we chose consists of experienced, well-trained, highly educated psychiatrists and healthcare attendants, who agreed to test our proposed system and provide their substantial feedback on its efficiency, as well as methods of enhancing it in the future. All of the members have graduated from reputable medical universities and have frequently assisted patients in treating their obsessive/irrational thought and behavioral patterns through exposure therapy sessions. Another important aspect of our preference in this particular psychiatric department is their constant quest for innovative diagnostic and therapeutic techniques. Our system and method are quite original; subsequently, they were highly interested in the new methods in which ET can be enhanced through VR technology. Taking the aforementioned facts into consideration, it is clear that our choice in this particular psychiatric department was everything but coincidental; we strongly believe that the clinic's specialists were the most fitting to evaluate the efficacy of our system in view of their experience and education.

References

1. American psychiatric association: diagnostic and statistical manual of mental disorders, 5th edn. (2013)
2. National Institute of Mental Health: Anxiety Disorder
3. National Institute of Mental Health: Mental Illness
4. Bandelow, B., Michaelis, S.: Epidemiology of anxiety disorders in the 21st century. Dialogues Clin. Neurosci. **17**(3), 327–335 (2015)
5. Kessler, R.C., Berglund, P., Demler, O., Jin, R., Merikangas, K.R., Walters, E.E.: Lifetime prevalence and age-of-onset distributions of DSM-IV disorders in the national comorbidity survey replication. Arch. Gen. Psychiatry **62**, 293–602 (2005)
6. Stinson, F.S.: The epidemiology of DSM-IV specific phobia in the USA: results from the national epidemiologic survey on alcohol and related conditions. Psychol. Med. **37**(March), 1047–1059 (2007)
7. Öst, L.G.: One-session treatment for specific phobias. Behav. Res. Ther. **27**, 1–7 (1989)
8. Scott, J., Beck, A.T.: Cognitive behavioural therapy. In: Essential Psychiatry, 4th edn. (2008)
9. Mayo-Wilson, E., Montgomery, P.: Media-delivered cognitive behavioural therapy and behavioural therapy (self-help) for anxiety disorders in adults. Cochrane Database Syst. Rev. (2013)
10. Treatment - (ADAA) Anxiety and Depression Association of America. https://www.adaa.org/finding-help/treatment
11. Otte, C.: Cognitive behavioral therapy in anxiety disorders: current state of the evidence. Dialogues Clin. Neurosci. **13**(4), 413–421 (2011)
12. Wittchen, H.-U., Mühlig, S., Beesdo, K.: Mental disorders in primary care. Dialogues Clin. Neurosci. **5**(2), 115–128 (2003)

13. Kerns, C.M., Read, K.L., Klugman, J., Kendall, P.C.: Cognitive behavioral therapy for youth with social anxiety: differential short and long-term treatment outcomes. J. Anxiety Disord. **27**(2), 210–215 (2013)
14. Riddle-Walker, L.: Cognitive behaviour therapy for specific phobia of vomiting (Emetophobia): a pilot randomized controlled trial. J. Anxiety Disord. **43**, 14–22 (2016)
15. Krebs, G.: Long-term outcomes of cognitive-behavioral therapy for adolescent body dysmorphic disorder. Behav. Ther. **48**(4), 462–473 (2017)
16. Rozental, A.: A randomized controlled trial of internet-based cognitive behavior therapy for perfectionism including an investigation of outcome predictors. Behav. Res. Ther. **95**, 79–86 (2017)
17. Warwick, H.: Complete recovery from anxiety disorders following cognitive behavior therapy in children and adolescents: a meta-analysis. Clin. Psychol. Rev. **52**, 77–91 (2017)
18. Peñate, W., Fumero, A., Viña, C., Herrero, M., Marrero, R.J., Rivero, F.: A meta-analytic review of neuroimaging studies of specific phobia to small animals. Eur. J. Psychiatry **31**, 1–44 (2017)
19. Twomey, C., O'Reilly, G., Meyer, B.: Effectiveness of an individually-tailored computerised CBT programme (Deprexis) for depression: a meta-analysis. Psychiatry Res. **256**, 371–377 (2017)
20. Ollendick, T.H., Öst, L.G., Ryan, S.M., Capriola, N.N., Reuterskiöld, L.: Harm beliefs and coping expectancies in youth with specific phobias. Behav. Res. Ther. **91**, 51–57 (2017)
21. Shiban, Y., Schelhorn, I., Pauli, P., Mühlberger, A.: Effect of combined multiple contexts and multiple stimuli exposure in spider phobia: a randomized clinical trial in virtual reality. Behav. Res. Ther. **71**, 45–53 (2015)
22. Treanor, M., Craske, M.G.: Exposure therapy. In: Encyclopedia of Mental Health, 2nd edn. (2015)
23. Rothbaum, B.O., Rizzo, A.S., McDaniel, D.D., Zanov, M.V.: Virtual reality exposure therapy. In: Encyclopedia of Mental Health, 2nd edn. (2015)
24. Society of Clinical Psychology: What is Exposure Therapy?. American Psychological Association: Division, vol. 12 (2013)
25. Waters, A.M.: Augmenting one-session treatment of children's specific phobias with attention training to positive stimuli. Behav. Res. Ther. **62**, 107–119 (2014)
26. Rizzo, A., Hartholt, A., Grimani, M., Leeds, A., Liewer, M.: Virtual reality exposure therapy for combat-related posttraumatic stress disorder. In: Computer, Long Beach California (2014)
27. Cardoş, R.A.I., David, O.A., David, D.O.: Virtual reality exposure therapy in flight anxiety: a quantitative meta-analysis. Comput. Hum. Behav. **72**, 371–380 (2017)
28. Bun, P., Gorski, F., Grajewski, D., Wichniarek, R., Zawadzki, P.: Low - cost devices used in virtual reality exposure therapy. Procedia Comput. Sci. **104**, 445–451 (2016)
29. Yiasemidou, M., Siqueira, J., Tomlinson, J., Glassman, D., Stock, S., Gough, M.: Take-home' box trainers are an effective alternative to virtual reality simulators. J. Surg. Res. **213**, 69–74 (2017)
30. Blakey, S.M., Abramowitz, J.S.: The effects of safety behaviors during exposure therapy for anxiety: critical analysis from an inhibitory learning perspective. Clin. Psychol. Rev. **49**, 1–15 (2016)
31. Krijn, M., Emmelkamp, P.M.G., Biemond, R., Schuemie, M.J., Van Der Mast, C.A.P.G.: Treatment of acrophobia in virtual reality: The role of immersion and presence. Behav. Res. Ther. **42**, 229–239 (2004)
32. Emmelkamp, P.M.G., Krijn, M., Hulsbosch, A.M., Vries, S., Schuemie, M.J.: Virtual reality treatment versus exposure in vivo: a comparative evaluation in acrophobia. Behav. Res. Ther. **40**, 509–516 (2002)

33. Carlin, A.S., Hoffman, H.G., Weghorst, S.: Virtual reality and tactile augmentation in the treatment of spider phobia: a case report. Behav. Res. Ther. **35**, 153–158 (1997)
34. Freeman, D.: Automated psychological therapy using immersive virtual reality for treatment of fear of heights: a single-blind, parallel-group, randomised controlled trial. Lancet Psychiatry **5**, 625–632 (2018)
35. Price, M., Anderson, P.: The role of presence in virtual reality exposure therapy. J. Anxiety Disord. **21**, 742–751 (2007)
36. Morina, N., Brinkman, W.-P., Hartanto, D., Emmelkamp, P.M.G.: Sense of presence and anxiety during virtual social interactions between a human and virtual humans. PeerJ **2**, e337 (2014)
37. Rudaz, M., Ledermann, T., Margraf, J., Becker, E.S., Craske, M.G.: The moderating role of avoidance behavior on anxiety over time: is there a difference between social anxiety disorder and specific phobia? PLoS ONE **12**, e0180298 (2017)
38. Da Gama, A.E.F., de Menezes Chaves, T., Fallavollita, P., Figueiredo, L.S., Teichrieb, V.: Rehabilitation motion recognition based on the international biomechanical standards. Expert Syst. Appl. **116**, 396–409 (2019)
39. Wang, X., Yan, K.: Immersive human-computer interactive virtual environment using large-scale display system. Future Gener. Comput. Syst. **96**, 649–659 (2017)
40. Chen, J., Qiu, J., Ahn, C.: Construction worker's awkward posture recognition through supervised motion tensor decomposition. Autom. Constr. **77**, 67–81 (2017)
41. Maples-Keller, J.L., Bunnell, B.E., Kim, S.J., Rothbaum, B.O.: The use of virtual reality technology in the treatment of anxiety and other psychiatric disorders. Harvard Rev. Psychiatry **25**, 103 (2017)
42. Morina, N., Ijntema, H., Meyerbröker, K., Emmelkamp, P.M.G.: Can virtual reality exposure therapy gains be generalized to real-life? A meta-analysis of studies applying behavioral assessments. Behav. Res. Ther. **74**, 18–24 (2015)
43. Turner, W.A., Casey, L.M.: Outcomes associated with virtual reality in psychological interventions: where are we now? Clin. Psychol. Rev. **34**, 634–644 (2014)
44. Suh, A., Prophet, J.: The state of immersive technology research: a literature analysis. Comput. Hum. Behav. **86**, 77–90 (2018)
45. Freeman, D.: Virtual reality in the assessment, understanding, and treatment of mental health disorders. Psychol. Med. **47**(14), 2393–2400 (2017)
46. Kritikos, J., Tzannetos, G., Zoitaki, C., Poulopoulou, S., Koutsouris, D.: Anxiety detection from Electrodermal Activity Sensor with movement & interaction during Virtual Reality Simulation. In: 9th International IEEE EMBS Conference on Neural Engineering, San Francisco, CA, USA, 20–23 March 2019, pp. 571–576 (2019). https://ieeexplore.ieee.org/document/8717170

Evaluation of a Self-report System for Assessing Mood Using Facial Expressions

Hristo Valev[1,2(✉)], Tim Leufkens[1,3], Corina Sas[2],
Joyce Westerink[1,3], and Ron Dotsch[1]

[1] Philips Research,
High Tech Campus 34, 5656 AE Eindhoven, The Netherlands
{hristo.valev,tim.leufkens,joyce.westerink,
ron.dotsch}@philips.com
[2] Lancaster University, Bailrigg, Lancaster LA1 4YW, UK
{hristo.valev,c.sas}@lancaster.ac.uk
[3] Eindhoven University of Technology Tu/e,
5600 MB Eindhoven, The Netherlands
{t.r.m.leufkens,j.h.d.m.westerink}@tue.nl

Abstract. Effective and frequent sampling of mood through self-reports could enable a better understanding of the interplay between mood and events influencing it. To accomplish this, we built a mobile application featuring a sadness-happiness visual analogue scale and a facial expression-based scale. The goal is to evaluate, whether a facial expression based scale could adequately capture mood. The method and mobile application were evaluated with 11 participants. They rated the mood of characters presented in a series of vignettes, using both scales. Participants also completed a user experience survey rating the two assessment methods and the mobile interface. Findings reveal a Pearson's correlation coefficient of 0.97 between the two assessment scales and a stronger preference for the face scale. We conclude with a discussion of the implications of our findings for mood self-assessment and an outline future research.

Keywords: Mood assessment · Self-report system · User interface

1 Introduction

Different approaches exist that can be used to measure mood, for example, using graphical discrete scales, such as Likert scale, continuous scales such as the visual analogue scale (VAS) or other abstract methods such as colors, pictures, etcetera.

Discrete scales such as the Likert scale [1] or a continuous scale such as the visual analogue scale (VAS) [2] are suitable for mood assessment as they are generally quite intuitive and have been widely used in practice. However, using such scales requires participants to transform the concept of mood onto a numerical or graphical scale. That may result in some information loss, which makes graphical scales less practical for mood assessment. Furthermore, graphical scales have no particular inherent inclination to represent mood [3].

Other approaches of measuring affect are through affective pictures [4–6], smileys [7, 8], colors [9, 10] or physiological data [11, 12]. Photographic Affect Meter (PAM),

P. Cipresso et al. (Eds.): MindCare 2019, LNICST 288, pp. 231–241, 2019.
https://doi.org/10.1007/978-3-030-25872-6_19

for example, is using affective pictures to measure affect. It consists of 16 images, spatially allocated in a two-dimensional space, according to their ratings valence and arousal. The authors in [7] use a discrete scale for valence and arousal represented through icons and sad/happy smileys, for the assessment of arousal and valence, respectively. [9] uses colors to span a two-dimensional emotion space. Different colors represent emotions while color shades represents the intensity of the emotions. All those approaches provide an easily accessible way of reporting mood, however, they are limited to the amount of emotional intensities they provide.

These abstract representations, while very expressive cannot translate well between people as they are highly subjective in nature. In order to have consistency in the measurements, we need a representation which is universally understood by different populations and provides enough variation to describe a broader space.

Facial expressions are inherently linked with emotions and are a visual tool for us to communicate our emotions to the surrounding world. They are embodied representations of our feelings and are as such intrinsically suitable for measuring mood. We are also well versed in using and recognizing facial expressions, which supports the universality of the representation. Research has identified distinct facial expressions, which are associated universally with a specific emotion [13, 14]. For those basic emotions there is a distinctly associated facial expression.

Lorish et al. introduced the concept of using a face scale to measure mood [3]. He argues that facial expressions are tuned to capture and represent mood, because facial feature variations are universal, valid indicators of mood [13, 14]. Kamashita et al. explored the reliability of such scales by comparing them to VAS [15]. The authors evaluated two facial expression-based scales with a VAS scale, which resulted in a 0.68–0.70 correlation between both assessments. Also, in a user experience questionnaire, participants preferred the face scales to VAS scales. This yields the insight, that there might be some interaction quality unique to such scales. Another study conducted by McKinley et al. explored the consistency of a facial expression-based scale [16]. Seven photographs of facial expressions with increasing intensities had to be positioned on a VAS scale. Six out of seven photograph placements were almost equidistant and fell within the expected intervals.

If we are to use and/or improve such a method, we need to make sure that it is reliable in the sense that assessing mood with facial expressions yield at least comparable results to established mood measurement methods and sensitive in the way that assessments provided with such a scale will effectively capture changes in the mood.

Increasing HCI research has focused on the impact of emotions and their awareness on emotional wellbeing and mental health [17]. Such a system would be particularly useful in the context of affective disorders, for example depression. Such conditions are characterized by disturbances in the mood as one of the main symptoms. Being able to frequently assess a person's mood could potentially provide us with a reasonable estimate of a person's state of well-being and enable, for example, the early detection of depressive episodes.

2   Method

We developed an android application, which features a bipolar sad-to-happy facial expression scale and a VAS scale. The facial expression scale is represented through an image of a face, which can be interacted with to display happier or sadder expressions by sliding your finger vertically along the display (see Fig. 1). The middle point of the scale is the neutral expression. Navigating upwards displays increasingly happier expressions, while downwards – sadder ones. The image space features 101 images, where 50 represent happiness, 50 – sadness and one – the neutral expression. The images were taken from the male facial expressions of sadness–happiness of the dynamic visual analogue mood scales (D-VAMS) project [18]. The scale is conceptualized as a brief, nonverbal mood assessment instrument to be used for self-reporting. A slider with 101 discrete points represents the VAS scale (see Fig. 2). Text anchored on both extremes denotes the respective emotions (i.e. sadness and happiness). Both scales aim to capture the valence of the provided assessment. When providing an assessment, both scales were initialized in the neutral position, i.e. the slider positioned in the middle and the face – to a neutral expression.

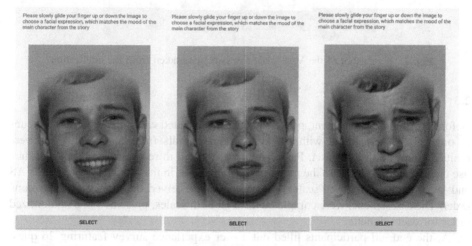

Fig. 1. Screenshots of the D-VAMS face scale assessment from the application.

2.1   Participants

We recruited 11 healthy participants via flyers. Eight women and three men took part in the study, with an average age of 29. The participants were recruited from a research environment. They have been handed and signed an informed consent form.

2.2 Assessment

The conducted experiment aimed to evaluate, whether a facial-expression based scale would yield a comparable performance to a VAS scale for mood assessment and whether the user experience between both scales would differ.

Participants were asked to read 30 vignettes and use a smartphone provided by the experimenter for the assessment. Half of the vignettes were taken from [19] and were labeled with a positive emotion. The negative vignettes were collected from various online blogs and forums. The vignettes were paraphrased to portray a story from third persons' perspective.

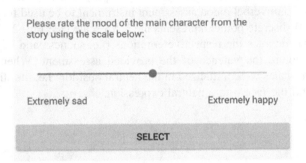

Fig. 2. Screenshot of the VAS scale assessment as taken from the application.

2.3 Procedure

Before starting the experiment, participants were presented with three training vignettes in order to be acquainted with the system. The results from the training set were omitted from the final dataset. Participants were asked to read each vignette and then use the application to assess the mood of the main actor in the vignette using both VAS and facial-expression based scales. All participants received the vignettes in the same order. The assessments were completed through both scales, presented in a randomized order for each vignette.

At the end, all participants filled out a user experience survey featuring 26 questions. The survey can be found in Appendix A. Eighteen questions evaluated the method and implementation. Those included the ease of use, suitability for mood-assessment, accuracy, satisfaction, user experience, responsiveness, intuitiveness and preference on unipolar Likert scales. Two questions evaluated the preference and speed of both implementations as bipolar Likert scales. Two yes/no questions prompted the participants if they would be able to use the interfaces without instructions. The survey also included four open-ended questions, which inquired about any potential difficulties participants might have had with the application or prompted them to share their insights as to how the assessment can be improved.

3 Results

The data was analyzed using python 3.6 with the numpy and pandas libraries. The plots were created using the seaborn library.

A Pearson's correlation coefficient was calculated between VAS and the facial expression scale assessments, which yielded a 0.97 correlation for all participants.

Figure 3 displays the results as a scatterplot, where the assessments obtained from the VAS and facial expression scale are plotted respectively on the Y- and X-axis. The lack of 'neutral' vignettes in the stimulus set explains the sparsity of assessments in the central region of the plot.

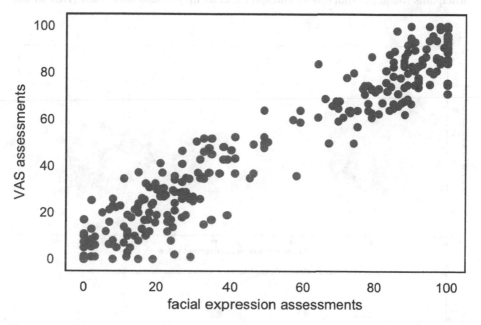

Fig. 3. Scatterplot of the assessments for each vignette and participant for the face scale and VAS.

The average time to complete an assessment with the VAS scale was 4.2 s, while using the face scale took 5.6 s. Figure 4 depicts the relationship between assessment values provided with each interface and the respective duration.

Table 1 features the part of results obtained from the user experience survey, which rated the method and implementation of each scale individually. The questions were represented through a five point Likert scale, where 1 was designated as a low/negative score and 5 – a high/positive one.

Albeit none of the results was statistically significant, due to the relatively low participant count, they still show consistent preference for the face scale on most aspects. Particularly interesting are the noticeable differences in the scores for satisfaction in the method section and user experience in the application section. On both accounts the face scale was preferred to VAS, with only two participants favoring the VAS on both accounts. Both participants also left the open-ended questions blank. Four participants found the slider more unresponsive, as they would have liked. This would

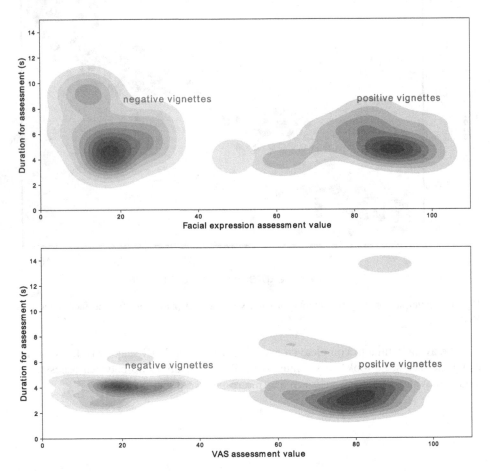

Fig. 4. KDEplot depicting the relationship between assessment values and duration with both interfaces. (The facial expressions values spread over the maximum value of 100, due to the gaussian kernel estimate used to model the data. The input is the assessment values and their respective durations. For the face scale assessments more often the maximum value was selected (see Fig. 1), which causes this effect.)

have partially influenced the user experience scores and the speed of assessment for the VAS scale. Only one participant pointed out, that they would need instructions before using the face scale.

Table 1. Features the part of results obtained from the user experience survey, which rated the method and implementation of each scale individually. The questions were represented through a five point Likert scale, where 1 was designated as a low/negative score and 5 – a high/positive one.

Method	Face (std)	VAS (std)	t-value (df = 10)	p-value
Ease of use	4.09 (1.0)	3.73 (0.96)	−0.83	0.42
Suitability for mood	3.73 (1.29)	3.64 (0.88)	−0.18	0.86
Accuracy	3.73 (0.96)	3.73 (0.62)	0	1
Satisfaction	4.0 (1.28)	3.18 (0.72)	−1.77	0.1
Application	Face (std)	VAS (std)	t-value (df = 10)	p-value
User experience	4.45 (0.89)	3.73 (1.19)	1.85	0.08
Ease of use	4.18 (1.19)	3.73 (0.75)	1.02	0.32
Responsiveness	4.36 (0.88)	3.6 (0.92)	1.84	0.08
Intuitiveness	4.0 (1.04)	4.09 (0.67)	−0.23	0.82
Assessment preference	3.91 (1.44)	3.73 (0.86)	0.34	0.73

The preferred method of assessment as well as which inter-face was considered faster for assessing were assessed on a bipolar Likert scale, where 1 favored the face scale and 5 – VAS. The results show that most participants found the VAS scale slightly faster than the face scale with a mean result of 2.9. This is also coherent with the results from Fig. 4, which established a 1.4 s difference on average for assessments between the VAS and the facial-expression scales.

However, most participants preferred the face scale for mood assessment with a mean score of 2. Two participants, which preferred the VAS scale in the previous section consistently, preferred the VAS scale here as well.

Several participants revealed in the open-ended questions section that a simple sadness-happiness scale is insufficient to capture mood for the presented vignettes.

One participant shared – *"I think there is more to the emotional spectrum than just happiness or sadness. Other emotions might be relevant to depression as well. Such as fear, disgust, anger, disappointment, frustration, satisfied, grateful, relaxed, nervous, challenged.*" Interestingly, one participant pointed out that they liked that the face scale featured a real face instead of a cartoon-like character – *"I like the use of a real person and not a cartoon or smiley-type of representation."*

4   Discussion

First, we would like to acknowledge that the study was conducted as a pilot and is aimed to give us some insight on the proposed assessment method. As several participants pointed out, such an approach featuring only sad and happy facial expressions are not sufficient for true mood assessment. The study was set up to assess only based on a sadness-happiness scale. An open question remains, how scales featuring multiple mood dimensions would perform. Future research will aim to assess interfaces featuring multiple facial expression and produce a more comprehensive tool for mood-assessment.

The high correlation obtained from both assessments points to a high consistency of results with an already established mood measurement method such as VAS. Surprisingly, this is despite the fact complex emotions, such as awe or compassion were present in the vignettes. We acknowledge that the vignettes were presented in the same order for all participants, which might have introduced a carry-over effect. This effect, however, would be consistently present in both assessments. The randomized order in which both scales were presented after each vignette ensured that participants would not be able to 'seek out' the corresponding value on the latter. Furthermore, the facial expression scale provided no numerical reference as to what value is currently selected. This made it more difficult to simply carry over values from one scale to another. The design, unfortunately, does not allow to establish whether either scale 'outperforms' the other. This is due to the mismatch of the emotions portrayed by the vignettes and the dimensions available on the scales. Furthermore, the negative vignettes have not been rated. It will be interesting, however, to evaluate a multidimensional facial-expression based scale with a validated set of stimuli. Such an approach could provide some insights as to how sensitive and accurate a facial expression-based scale is in capturing mood.

The slightly faster average time it took for each VAS assessment can be attributed to the scale space being completely visible. The participants could immediately select a value lying on the extremes, while the face scale needed to be 'browsed'. As the provided stimuli were emotionally charged, most of the assessments veered away from the neutral expression. Figure 4 visualizes the average time per vignette it took to complete an assessment with each scale with respect to the duration. Despite the fact that the facial expression scale had to be navigated, this didn't influence assessment time as there is no pronounced relationship, which links longer assessment times with assessments lying on the extremities of the scale. This means that the interface could be easily navigated, yielded negligible slowdown and hints that the scale can be used for frequent assessments. A potential application for this method would be as an ecological momentary assessment (EMA) tool [20]. A longitudinal approach employing such a scale might reveal if such a scale would be viable if it is to be used as frequently as multiple times per day.

Most participants preferred the face scale, despite the slightly longer time required to provide an assessment; however, some still found the VAS scale to be more adequate for mood-assessment. The face scale was preferred to VAS on most accounts. This could be due to the scale providing a better interaction experience or due to a 'novelty' factor. A real-world application would reveal if the preference for such a scale would remain if it is used daily.

It would also be interesting how such a scale would perform in a clinical population. It is known that clinical populations have an attentional bias towards sadder-looking faces and perceive more negative expression in ambiguous faces [21, 22].

The implications of such a use case could result in more frequent and reliable mood-tracking, which could open up opportunities for the design of intervention systems.

Such an approach could be further augmented by sensor data and enable a more comprehensive monitoring of patients.

5 Conclusion

This pilot study shows that assessing mood with a face scale provides similar results as assessing mood with a visual analogue scale. Additionally, most participants indicated to prefer a face scale to a visual analogue scale. The way the user interface was conceptualized resulted in slightly longer times required for assessment with a facial-expression based scale. However, most participants preferred such a scale in terms of ease of use, user experience and satisfaction.

Acknowledgment. This work has been supported by AffecTech: Personal Technologies for Affective Health, Innovative Training Network funded by the H2020 People Programme under Marie Skłodowska-Curie grant agreement No. 722022.

Appendix A

Participant information

What is your age? _____

What is your gender?   (M) □   □   (F)

Method-related questions

How would you rate the ease of use of the method working with the slider?	(difficult)	□ □ □ □ □	(easy)
How would you rate the ease of use of the method working with the image?	(difficult)	□ □ □ □ □	(easy)
How suitable was the slider for capturing mood?	(not suitable)	□ □ □ □ □	(suitable)
How suitable was the image for capturing mood?	(not suitable)	□ □ □ □ □	(suitable)
How accurate do you consider the slider is in capturing the mood?	(not accurate)	□ □ □ □ □	(accurate)
How accurate do you consider the image is in capturing the mood?	(not accurate)	□ □ □ □ □	(accurate)
How satisfying was the slider to work with?	(very dissatisfying)	□ □ □ □ □	(very satisfying)
How satisfying was the image to work with?	(very dissatisfying)	□ □ □ □ □	(very satisfying)
Which assessment method would you personally prefer?	(image)	□ □	(slider)
Which method, according to you, was faster to use for mood assessment?	(image)	□ □	(slider)

Do you have any comments regarding either of the mood capturing methods?

_____

Application-related questions

What was your experience using the image within the application?	(negative)	□ □ □ □ □	(positive)
What was your experience using the slider within the application?	(negative)	□ □ □ □ □	(positive)
How easy to use did you find working with the image within the application?	(difficult)	□ □ □ □ □	(easy)
How easy to use did you find working with the slider within the application?	(difficult)	□ □ □ □ □	(easy)
How responsive was the image assessment within the application?	(unresponsive)	□ □ □ □ □	(responsive)
How responsive was the slider assessment within the application?	(unresponsive)	□ □ □ □ □	(responsive)
How intuitive do you consider working with the image within the application is?	(not intuitive)	□ □ □ □ □	(very intuitive)
How intuitive do you consider working with the slider within the application is?	(not intuitive)	□ □ □ □ □	(very intuitive)
Do you think you would use the image for mood assessment?	(unlikely)	□ □ □ □ □	(likely)
Do you think you would use the slider for mood assessment?	(unlikely)	□ □ □ □ □	(likely)
Do you think you can use the image approach within the application for assessing mood without a clarification from a technical person?	(no)	□	(yes)
Do you think you can use the slider approach within the application for assessing mood without a clarification from a technical person?	(no)	□	(yes)

Is there some part of the functionality, which didn't work for you?

_____

Did you encounter any technical difficulties, while working with the application?

_____

Do you have any comments regarding the application?

References

1. Likert, R.: A technique for the measurement of attitudes. Arch. Psychol. **22**, 140 (1932)
2. Price, D.D., McGrath, P.A., Rafii, A., Buckingham, B.: The validation of visual analogue scales as ratio scale measures for chronic and experimental pain. Pain **17**(1), 45–56 (1983)
3. Lorish, C.D., Maisiak, R.: The face scale: a brief, nonverbal method for assessing patient mood. Arthritis Rheum. **29**(7), 906–909 (1986)
4. Pollak, J., Adams, P., Gay, G.: PAM: a photographic affect meter for frequent, in situ measurement of affect. In: Proceedings of the SIGCHI Conference on Human Factors in Computing Systems, pp. 725–734 (2011)
5. Watson, D., Clark, L.A.: PANAS-X Manual, pp. 1–27 (1999)
6. Watson, D., Clark, L.A.: JPSP Watson Clark Tellegen 1988, vol. 54, no. 6, pp. 1–8 (2004)
7. Broekens, J., Brinkman, W.P.: AffectButton: a method for reliable and valid affective self-report. Int. J. Hum. Comput. Stud. **71**(6), 641–667 (2013)
8. Rodriguez, I., Herskovic, V., Fuentes, C., Campos, M.: B-ePain: a wearable interface to self-report pain and emotions. In: UbiComp Adjunct, pp. 1120–1125 (2016)
9. Huang, S.T.-Y., Kwan, C.M.Y., Sano, A.: The moment: a mobile tool for people with depression or bipolar disorder. In: Proceedings of the 2014 ACM International Joint Conference on Pervasive Ubiquitous Computing: Adjunct Publication - UbiComp 2014, pp. 235–238 (2014)
10. Umair, M., Latif, M.H., Sas, C.: Dynamic displays at wrist for real time visualization of affective data, pp. 201–205 (2018)
11. Sas, C., Rees, M.: AffectCam : arousal – augmented SenseCam for richer recall of episodic memories. In: CHI 2013, pp. 1041–1046 (2013)
12. Sanches, P., Hook, K., Sas, C., Stahl, A.: Ambiguity as a resource to inform proto-practices: the case of skin conductance. TOCHI **26**(1) (2019). Eprints.Lancs.Ac.Uk
13. Ekman, P.: Universal-facial-expressions-of-emotion. Calif. Mental Health **8**(4), 151–158 (1970)
14. Ekman, P.: Facial expression and emotion. Am. Psychol. **48**(4), 384–392 (1993)
15. Kamashita, Y., Sonoda, T., Kamada, Y., Nishi, Y., Nagaoka, E.: Reliability, validity, and preference of an original faces scale for assessing the mood of patients with dentures. Prosthodont. Res. Pract. **6**, 93–98 (2007)
16. McKinley, S., Coote, K., Stein-Parbury, J.: Development and testing of a faces scale for the assessment of anxiety in critical ill patients. J. Adv. Nurs. **41**(1), 73–79 (2003)
17. Sanches, P., et al.: HCI and affective health taking stock of a decade of studies and charting future research directions, pp. 123–4567 (2019)
18. Barrows, P.D., Thomas, S.A.: Assessment of mood in aphasia following stroke: validation of the dynamic visual analogue mood scales (D-VAMS). Clin. Rehabil. **32**(1), 94–102 (2018)
19. Lagotte, A.: Eliciting discrete positive emotions with vignettes and films: a validation study (2014)
20. Stone, A.A., Shiffman, S.: Ecological momentary assessment (EMA) in behavioral medicine. Ann. Behav. Med. **16**(3), 199–202 (2018)
21. Joormann, J., Gotlib, I.H.: Is this happiness i see? Biases in the identification of emotional facial expressions in depression and social phobia. J. Abnorm. Psychol. **115**(4), 705–714 (2006)
22. Duque, A., Vázquez, C.: Mental health; researchers at Complutense University have reported new data on depression (Double attention bias for positive and negative emotional faces in clinical depression: evidence from an eye-tracking study). Ment. Heal. Wkly. Dig. **46**, 124 (2015)

Testing a Deactivated Virtual Environment in Pathological Gamblers' Anxiety

Michelle Semonella[1(✉)], Pietro Cipresso[1,2], Cosimo Tuena[1],
Alessandra Parisi[2], Michelle Toti[1], Aurora Elena Bobocea[3],
Pier Giovanni Mazzoli[3], and Giuseppe Riva[1,2]

[1] Applied Technology for Neuro-Psychology Lab,
Istituto Auxologico Italiano, Milan, Italy
semonellamichelle@gmail.com
[2] Department of Psychology, Catholic University, Milan, Italy
[3] U.O.S. Dipendenze Patologiche Fano DDP AV 1 - ASUR Marche, Fano, Italy

Abstract. In the last decades the use of Virtual Reality for exposure therapy has become a clinical standard and used in most disorders, including pathological gambling. Nonetheless, previous studies reported that exposure therapy might be not effective if the virtual environments present no interactions or break in presence, among other problems. We hypothesized that a virtual environment representing a gambling place but without lights and sounds or other stimuli promoting interactions, was not effective for gamblers. Thus we tested the anxiety level in a group of 20 pathological gamblers in this lights out virtual environment. Our results shown, by using Bayes Factor, that before and after an exposure to the lights out virtual gambling environments there was no difference in anxiety level. The study shed new light in designing and implementing virtual reality exposure therapy for future clinical applications.

Keywords: Gambling · Virtual reality · Anxiety · Exposure · Psychometrics · Gambling disorders · Addictions

1 Introduction

Pathological Gambling (PG) is a common psychiatric disorder that is associated with severe problem gambling. Who suffer of this has an urgent need to gamble interminably despite the numerous negative harmful consequences and desire to stop.

Another common feature shared by people who suffer from gambling addiction is impulsivity that can be defined as precipitately, non-inhibited, inappropriate, extremely risky behavior with potentially serious consequences (Durana et al. 1993).

Many evidences suggest that alterations in fronto-striatal circuits contribute to the tendency to behave impulsively (Fineberg et al. 2014).

Furthermore, is possible to distinguish two different components: the impulsive action and the impulsive choice (Evenden 1999).

The first can be defined as the diminished ability to inhibit motor responses, while the second one refers to tendency to selecting smaller immediate rewards instead of larger and long-term rewards.

© ICST Institute for Computer Sciences, Social Informatics and Telecommunications Engineering 2019
Published by Springer Nature Switzerland AG 2019. All Rights Reserved
P. Cipresso et al. (Eds.): MindCare 2019, LNICST 288, pp. 242–249, 2019.
https://doi.org/10.1007/978-3-030-25872-6_20

Indeed, the pathological player, as well as the patients who abuse substances, are characterized by dysfunctional behavior in decision-making processes and by the high dependence on reward that leads to the adoption of risky and loss strategies.

From recent studies has emerged an association between pathological gambling and deficits in frontal lobe function; in addition, the pathological gambler subjects show similar behavior to patients with bilateral VMPFC lesions (Bechara et al. 1994; Balodis et al. 2012) and SUD patients (Balconi et al. 2014).

Initially, Pathological Gambling was classified as "Impulse Control Disorder" (ICD), but in DSM-V was re-classified as an addictive disorder (DSM-V; American Psychiatric Association 2013).

Although there is still an open discussion about the classification of this disorder, some authors consider it more appropriate to think of pathological gambling as addiction (Fauth-Bühler et al. 2017). Many evidences seem to demonstrate as some core elements of addiction, such as tolerance and withdrawal, are relevant to PG and Drug dependence (DD).

At the neuronal level, Potenza et al. (2003) in their fMRI study, observed in pathological players compared to recreational ones, a change in the signal dependent on the level of oxygen in the blood (BOLD) in the frontal cortical regions, basal ganglion and the thalamic brain, only when people viewed gambling tapes and not during an happy or sad videotape.

Particularly, when were presented the most intense gambling stimuli, people who suffer from Pathological gambling compared who do not suffer it showed a relatively diminished of the BOLD signal in ventromedial prefrontal cortex (vmPFC). Furthermore, another fMRI study had demonstrated a less activation of vmPFC and in the ventral striatum during simulated gambling in individuals with PG as compared to those without (Reuter et al. 2005).

At the level of neurotransmitter systems, Roy et al. (1988) found higher levels of noradrenaline (particular relevant to aspects of arousal and excitement) in urine, blood or cerebrospinal fluid samples in the Pathological Gamblers as compared to those without PG; moreover studying serotonine, neurotransmitter particularly relevant to behavioral initiation and cessation and in mediating impulse control, Nordin and Eklundh (1999) observed in people with PG low levels of the serotonin metabolite 5-hydroxy indoleacetic acid.

During the last decades Virtual Reality became a new tool inside the field of therapy (Cipresso et al. 2018; Cipresso and Immekus 2017). There are several evidence, in research and clinical practice, that show how virtual reality can help, especially in exposure therapy (Repetto et al. 2013; Villani et al. 2012; Serino et al. 2014; Gaggioli et al. 2014; Cipresso et al. 2012, 2015, 2016, 2019). However, Pallavicini and Collegue hypothesized and verified that sometimes virtual reality is not always an effective stressor for exposure treatments (Pallavicini et al. 2013).

Due to this, it was hypothesized that a lights out virtual environment was not able to increase the level of anxiety in pathological gamblers, due to the missing interactions that represents the real activating elements to generate anxiety in these patients (Figs. 1 and 2).

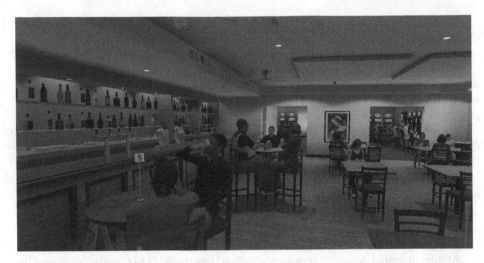

Fig. 1. Virtual environment representing a gambling place.

Fig. 2. Same virtual environment of Fig. 1, representing a gambling place, but without lights and sounds or other stimuli promoting interactions.

2 Procedure

Participants
The study will involve 20 adults without vestibular or balance disorders, and with a diagnosis of gambling disorder.

Procedure

Participants were patients recovered and patients who have been dismissed, both from Clinica Villa Silvia in Italy, with a diagnosis of Gambling. The psychiatrist of the Clinic invited them to take part of the study.

Patients were invited to Villa Silvia and they were kindly invited to take a seat, while explaining them what the study was about, showing them the tools of the study. In particular the participants were instructed in using the HTC VIVE virtual reality system and to navigate in a virtual environment. Also Near Infrared Spectroscopy (NIRS) was recorded, in order to detect frontal and pre-frontal activation during the virtual reality navigation.

After having explained them all the procedures, and having answered to all their doubts and questions, they were asked to sign the informed consent and to reply to the STAI-Y1 and STAI-Y2 questionnaires.

In the experiment, we first recorded the baseline having asked the participant to close his/her eyes and try to relax for 5 min. After the baseline, we put the HTC VIVE (with the NIRS on, there was no interferences using the helmet), and we asked the participant to navigate inside the environment without any specific task for 5 min.

Successively we asked to complete the last questionnaire STAI-Y2 in order to detect if the level of anxiety would have increased or not.

3   Data Analysis

In order to test our hypothesis, that the present virtual environment is not an activating environment and therefore would not elicit anxiety in former gamblers, we used Bayesian statistics provided by JASP Team: "JASP" (2018). In this sense, we used paired T-Test Bayes Factor (BF) to compare baseline state (Y1) STAI *vs.* post-exposure state STAI. R (Balodis ct al. 2012) and ggplot2 package (Bechara et al. 1994) were used for descriptive purposes of our sample (e.g. plots and descriptives). We excluded one participant, who did not accomplish the experimental session, whereas one participant did not filled out properly the state STAI after the exposure.

4   Results

Results are reported in relation to the hypothesis:

Null Hypothesis (H_0): there is no difference, in our sample, between the baseline and post-exposure of the STAI scores.
Alternative Hypothesis (H_1): baseline and post-exposure of the STAI scores are different in the sample.

First, we reported descriptive statistics (Table 1) of our sample.

Table 1. Descriptive statistics. Age, YoE (years of educations), STAI of state (Y1) for baseline and post-exposure and STAI of trait (Y2) are reported.

	N	Mean	SD	Median	Max	Min	Skewness	Kurtosis
Age	19	43.05	12.71	43	70	26	0.39	−1.01
YoE	4	13.25	4.11	13.5	18	8	−0.13	−1.89
Y2	19	49.16	9.66	52	65	29	−0.50	−0.81
Y1 baseline	19	35.95	11.67	32	61	20	0.55	−0.91
Y1 post	18	33.72	11.08	30	58	20	0.81	−0.62

The figure below (see Fig. 3) shows the scores of STAI in the clinical sample using boxplots.

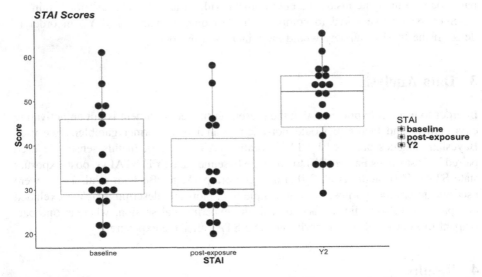

Fig. 3. Boxplots of Y1 baseline and Y1 post-exposure and Y2 are reported with each data point.

Results showed moderate evidence, as emerged from T-Test Bayes Factor, ($BF_{01} = 2.363$; err. = 0.005) that STAI scores are equal after the exposure to salient environment (see Figs. 4 and 5).

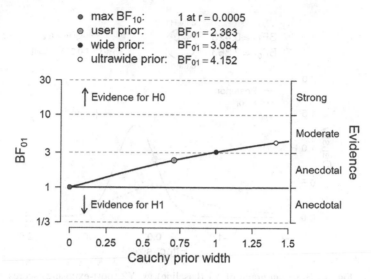

Fig. 4. The figure shows the robustness of the evidence for H_0.

Prior and posterior distributions are displayed in the Fig. 6. To summarize, Y1 (baseline) and Y2 (post-exposure) scores were statistically significantly similar before and after the immersion in the environment. Therefore, H0 was not rejected.

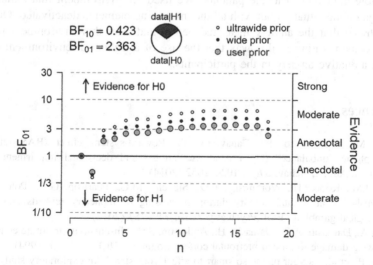

Fig. 5. Sequential analysis of each observation shows again a moderate evidence for H_0.

Prior and Posterior

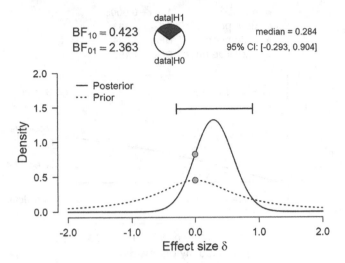

Fig. 6. Bayesian graph of Y1 (baseline) *vs.* Y2 (post-exposure) scores.

5 Conclusion

Anxiety generated by relevant scenes in virtual environment is considered a consolidated element in virtual reality exposure therapy. Nonetheless, the extend to which an environment can be really activating is less investigating.

In this study we wanted to demonstrate that to be activating an environment needed to be more than related to the patients. We used an environment that simulated the typical gambling situation but with all the interacting elements deactivated. Our results demonstrated that the anxiety measured before and after this environment was quite similar, demonstrating in this way that the use of a lights out environment does not produce a relative anxiety in the participants.

References

Balconi, M., Finocchiaro, R., Canavesio, Y.: Reward-system effect (BAS rating), left hemispheric "unbalance" (alpha band oscillations) and decisional impairments in drug addiction. Addict. Behav. **39**(6), 1026–1032 (2014)

Balodis, I.M., Kober, H., Worhunsky, P.D., Stevens, M.C., Pearlson, G.D., Potenza, M.N.: Diminished frontostriatal activity during processing of monetary rewards and losses in pathological gambling. Biol. Psychiatry **71**(8), 749–757 (2012)

Bechara, A., Damasio, A.R., Damasio, H., Anderson, S.W.: Insensitity to future consequences following damage to human prefrontal cortex. Cognition **50**(1–3), 7–15 (1994)

Cipresso, P., et al.: Is your phone so smart to affect your state? An exploratory study based on psychophysiological measures. Neurocomputing **84**, 23–30 (2012)

Cipresso, P.: Modeling behavior dynamics using computational psychometrics within virtual worlds. Front. Psychol. **6**, 1725 (2015)

Cipresso, P., Serino, S., Riva, G.: Psychometric assessment and behavioral experiments using a free virtual reality platform and computational science. BMC Med. Inform. Decis. Mak. **16** (1), 37 (2016)

Cipresso, P., Giglioli, I.A.C., Raya, M.A., Riva, G.: The past, present, and future of virtual and augmented reality research: a network and cluster analysis of the literature. Front. Psychol. **9**, 2086 (2018)

Cipresso, P., Immekus, J.C.: Back to the future of quantitative psychology and measurement: psychometrics in the twenty-first century. Front. Psychol. **8**, 2099 (2017)

Cipresso, P., Colombo, D., Riva, G.: Computational psychometrics using psychophysiological measures for the assessment of acute mental stress. Sensors **19**(4), 781 (2019)

Durana, J.H., Barnes, P.A., Johnson, J.L., Shure, M.B.: A neurodevelopmental view of impulsivity and its relationship to the superfactors of personality. In: The Impulsive Client, pp. 23–37 (1993)

Evenden, J.L.: Varieties of impulsivity. Psychopharmacology **146**(4), 348–361 (1999)

Fauth-Bühler, M., Mann, K., Potenza, M.N.: Pathological gambling: a review of the neurobiological evidence relevant for its classification as an addictive disorder. Addict. Biol. **22**(4), 885–897 (2017)

Fineberg, N.A., et al.: New developments in human neurocognition: clinical, genetic, and brain imaging correlates of impulsivity and compulsivity. CNS Spectr. **19**(1), 69–89 (2014)

Gaggioli, A., et al.: Experiential virtual scenarios with real-time monitoring (interreality) for the management of psychological stress: a block randomized controlled trial. J. Med. Internet Res. **16**(7), e167 (2014)

JASP Team: "JASP." (2018)

Nordin, C., Eklundh, T.: Altered CSF 5-HIAA disposition in pathologic male gamblers. CNS Spectr. **4**(12), 25–33 (1999)

Pallavicini, F., et al.: Is virtual reality always an effective stressors for exposure treatments? Some insights from a controlled trial. BMC Psychiatry **13**(1), 52 (2013)

Potenza, M.N., et al.: Gambling urges in pathological gambling: a functional magnetic resonance imaging study. Arch. Gen. Psychiatry **60**(8), 828–836 (2003)

R Core Team: R: A language and environment for statistical computing. R Foundation for Statistical Computing, Wien (2014)

Repetto, C., Gaggioli, A., Pallavicini, F., Cipresso, P., Raspelli, S., Riva, G.: Virtual reality and mobile phones in the treatment of generalized anxiety disorders: a phase-2 clinical trial. Pers. Ubiquitous Comput. **17**(2), 253–260 (2013)

Reuter, J., Raedler, T., Rose, M., Hand, I., Gläscher, J., Büchel, C.: Pathological gambling is linked to reduced activation of the mesolimbic reward system. Nat. Neurosci. **8**(2), 147 (2005)

Roy, A., Pickar, D., De Jong, J., Karoum, F., Linnoila, M.: Norepinephrine and its metabolites in cerebrospinal fluid, plasma, and urine: relationship to hypothalamic-pituitary-adrenal axis function in depression. Arch. Gen. Psychiatry **45**(9), 849–857 (1988)

Serino, S., Triberti, S., Villani, D., Cipresso, P., Gaggioli, A., Riva, G.: Toward a validation of cyber-interventions for stress disorders based on stress inoculation training: a systematic review. Virtual Real. **18**(1), 73–87 (2014)

Villani, D., Repetto, C., Cipresso, P., Riva, G.: May I experience more presence in doing the same thing in virtual reality than in reality? An answer from a simulated job interview. Interact. Comput. **24**(4), 265–272 (2012)

Wickham, H.: ggplot2: Elegant Graphics for Data Analysis. Springer, New York (2016). https://doi.org/10.1007/978-3-319-24277-4

Promoting Wellbeing in Pregnancy: A Multi-component Positive Psychology and Mindfulness-Based Mobile App

Claudia Carissoli[1], Giulia Corno[2,3], Stefano Montanelli[4],
and Daniela Villani[1(✉)]

[1] Department of Psychology, Università Cattolica del Sacro Cuore, Milan, Italy
{claudia.carissoli,daniela.villani}@unicatt.it
[2] LabPsiTec Universitat de Valencia, Valencia, Spain
giulia.me.corno@gmail.com
[3] I.R.C.C.S. Istituto Auxologico Italiano, Milan, Italy
[4] Department of Computer Science,
Università degli Studi di Milano, Milan, Italy
stefano.montanelli@unimi.it

Abstract. Pregnancy involves important changes for women of all ages: it is a time of physical and psychological change. Women may experience anxiety and negative emotions, which can negatively influence their wellbeing and make difficult their adaptation to the new role of mothers. Furthermore, poor mental well-being and difficulties in emotion regulation can negatively affect obstetric outcomes, development of the child and neonatal adaptation. The aim of this work is to present a new self-applied multi-component positive psychology- and mindfulness-based intervention (MPPMI) supported by a mobile App addressed to pregnant women. The core of this MPPMI is to combine traditional positive psychology activities with mindfulness-based exercises. The purpose of this MPPMI App (available in both Android and IOS versions) is to increase positive feelings, behaviors and cognitions and to learn strategies to better cope with anxiety to get adaptively and positively through pregnancy.

The intervention is composed by five modules, for a total length of five weeks, and each module includes three activities.

The future steps will be to carry out a pilot study to examine the program implementation and preliminary evaluate the effectiveness of the intervention on women's mental well-being, both at the end of the intervention and after childbirth.

Keywords: Pregnancy · Positive psychology · Multi-component intervention · Mindfulness · Mobile app · Wellbeing

1 Introduction

Pregnancy is a psychologically complex period in women's lives, and every pregnancy could be a phase of potential vulnerability. During pregnancy women change their status from daughter to mother in just a few months and this change requires a profound reconstruction of self [1]. In addition to biological changes, pregnancy leads to a

P. Cipresso et al. (Eds.): MindCare 2019, LNICST 288, pp. 250–262, 2019.
https://doi.org/10.1007/978-3-030-25872-6_21

search for a new identity at the individual, couple and social levels [2, 3]. All these changes can challenge women emotional adjustment and can lead to negative thoughts and emotions such as anxiety, stress and depression.

Women who present more difficulties in regulating their emotional states, lower self-compassion and who feel more isolated seem to be at higher-risk of developing post-partum depressive symptoms [4]. Furthermore, a wide consensus exists about the role of maternal emotional state in influencing the development of the child and the course of the pregnancy: negative emotions are often associated with various complications, such as preterm childbirth, low baby weight and difficulties in the fetal neurocognitive development and further poor emotional regulation abilities of the baby during infancy and childhood [5–12]. In contrast, positive affect has been associated with longer length of gestation, with reduced risks of delivering preterm [13] and of pregnancy-specific psychological stress [14] and with more self-reported social support [15].

As well-being of the mother is critical for optimal pregnancy outcomes, it is important to support and enhance mental well-being in pregnant women and provide women with coping strategies to increase their quality of life and to maximize infant health and development. Thus, the promotion of women's self-regulatory skills may help them to face the changes and challenges they are experiencing, allowing them to be aware of- and non-judgmentally accept their negative parenting-related emotions, to have a more compassionate attitude towards their experiences and difficulties, and to actively promote a positive mother-child relationship [4].

To reach these objectives a wide range of interventions have been tested (e.g., relaxation, mindfulness meditation, yoga therapy, breathing instructions, guided imagery, etc.), showing promising results [16–19]. Among these, on the one hand it is recognized the effectiveness of mindfulness-based interventions on women's prenatal well-being: a recent systematic review indicated potential benefits of mindfulness interventions on maternal prenatal well-being, especially in terms of decreased levels of negative affect, depression, and anxiety during pregnancy [20, 21] and increased self-acceptance. On the other hand, Positive Psychology Interventions (PPIs), defined as programs "aimed at increasing positive feelings, positive behaviors, or positive cognitions as opposed to ameliorating pathology or fixing negative thoughts of maladaptive behavior patterns" [22] have been confirmed as interventions leading to reliable and sustainable boosts in well-being [23–26]. Recently, PPIs have been implemented and experimentally demonstrated their effectiveness in reducing women's prenatal stress [14].

In order to target multiple domains of positive functioning, here we propose a multi-component positive psychology- and mindfulness-based intervention (MPPMI) [27], that is an intervention composed of a minimum of three positive psychology activities combined with mindfulness-based exercises, which to a large extent overlaps with principles of positive psychology [28].

Today, new technologies are becoming emergent tools to support these interventions. Thanks to their ubiquity, multimodality, interactivity and easiness of use, new technologies allow pregnant women to develop personal skills to manage their affective states and better deal with impending childbirth and motherhood [29, 30]. Specifically, both web-based and mobile app seem to be feasible options for supporting interventions aimed to promote well-being and prevent anxiety and post-partum depression, and there is preliminary evidence of their efficacy [31–36].

Starting from these premises, the App SerenaMente Mamma was developed: it is a mobile App containing a multi-component positive psychology- and mindfulness-based program addressed to promoting and enhancing women's prenatal mental well-being and preventing post-natal depression. The present contribution aims at describing the app contents and structure that will be tested through a pilot study.

2 The App SerenaMente Mamma

The app SerenaMente Mamma has been released for both Android and iOS plat-forms and it is conceived to work on mobile devices like smartphones and tablets. After the App installation, the final user, namely the pregnant woman, is initially expected to fulfill a baseline self-assessment before starting to browse contents. A post-assessment step is also expected at the end of the user experience, when the App contents have been completely exploited. The App is configured to communicate with a server-side software component released as a Java servlet service joint with a PostgreSQL database system where the assessment results are stored for subsequent analysis. It is important to note that data anonymity is enforced on the server-side component to ensure privacy preservation of the involved users/women.

The App contents are based on a brief self-help protocol characterized by five modules including fifteen exercises. Thus, the entire intervention lasts thirty-five days (five weeks), with three exercises/tasks to be completed every week (see Fig. 1).

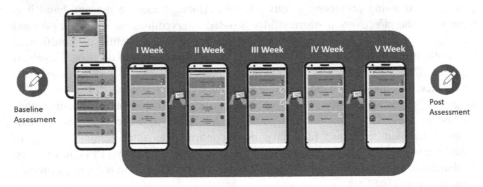

Fig. 1. Structure of *SerenaMente Mamma* App. After the baseline assessment, women can start the MPPMI: from the initial menu, they can have access to the first week module. At the end of each week, users are invited to rate the performed activities in order to unlock the contents of the following week. At the end of the intervention (after the fifth module) the final assessment is proposed. From that moment all contents are unlocked and freely re-usable.

Specifically, six of them are positive psychology-based exercises while the others are mindfulness-based guided meditation aimed to develop mindfulness abilities and self-awareness. It is also possible to replicate the exercises already completed following the five weeks, thus extending the duration of the intervention. Women can perform all the exercises on their own, wherever they want.

The App is available for Android and iOS devices. Users can install the app and use it after accepting the study conditions, presented after the first launch, and answering some questionnaires.

The modules are activated at a rate of one per week and after a week, the App automatically unlocks the next module, allowing users to complete the three weekly exercises proposed (see Fig. 2). To proceed to the next module, the app requests to rate user experience in terms of *perceived usefulness*, ("How much did you benefit from exercises practice?), *perceived ease of use* ("How difficult was the exercise?") and *pleasantness* ("How much did you like the exercise?") of the proposed activities.

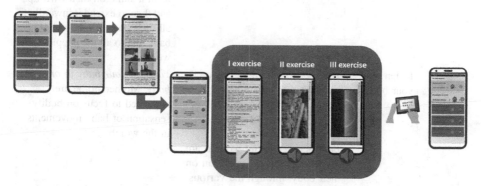

Fig. 2. First Week of SerenaMente Mamma App. After clicking on the first module, the App proposes a menu composed of four boxes. The first one contains some suggestions for a better practice. For example, the first module includes a description of the recommended positions of the body to favor meditation in pregnancy. Furthermore, the module proposes three exercises referred to mindfulness or positive psychology contents, which users have to rate to unlock and get access to the next module.

2.1   App Structure and Contents

Each module contains an introduction section ("Suggestions for practice" – "Consigli per la pratica") with text, images or audio which explains mindfulness or fundamental concept necessary for practice, with a simple language and images suitable for the specific users (see Table 1).

The first module is named **Savoring Life**: this module invites women to savor life, aiming to enhance and extend momentary pleasant experiences [37, 38]. This module aims to promote positive emotion and to decrease elements of negative affect [31], to enhance psychological wellbeing by engaging participants in three exercises: the "Three good things in life" [38], and "Inner connection" and "Inner meditation practice" [39].

The second module is named **Listen to your body**. This module provides a brief description of mindfulness and teaches participants to be connected to their body [40]. It proposes three exercises, to increased interoceptive awareness and acceptance [41] to better manage pain and discomfort. Three exercises are proposed: "Your body is changing", the "Body scan exercise" [40] and "You and your baby" in one body guided

Table 1. Modules structure and contents

Module	Name	Positive psychology-based exercises	Mindfulness-based exercises
1	Savouring life	*Three good things in life exercise*: participants identify three good things that went well each day and why	*Inner connection with you baby guided meditation*: mother to be are invited to think about their babies and to send loving thoughts to the unborn *Inner smile meditation*: mothers-to-be are requested form a smile on their own lips and then to extend it inwardly to all their body, to the unborn baby and to all the people in the world
2	Listen to your body	*Your body is changing*: women are invited to take a photo in front of a mirror every week or at the beginning of every month of pregnancy *Body scan exercise:* women are invited to focus the attention on their body, through the various regions of the body and to accept any discomfort or pain or any other bodily sensation. Body scan helps to understand the difference between thinking about a sensation and experiencing it [40]	*You and your baby in one body*. Mothers-to-be are requested to focus on bodily sensation of baby movements in the womb
3	People around you	*Connectedness exercise*: participants are asked to think about, identify and draw a graphic about their most important relationships and find an activity to do together *Gratitude exercise*: women are invited to write a letter or an email to a person they wanted to thank and to plan a visit to meet face to face this person	*Cuddling with my child in the womb and my partner*: women are invited to take a break of relaxing with their partner, to practice a guided meditation hugged
4	Optimism, a positive resource	*Best possible self-exercise*: participants visualize and write their ideal future life in as much detail as possible *Baby steps exercise*: participants write a list of goals and initial steps toward achieving their best possible self	*Inner smile*: see over

(*continued*)

Table 1. (*continued*)

Module	Name	Positive psychology-based exercises	Mindfulness-based exercises
5	Mind and body relax		*Breathing meditation* that invites to focus attention on breath and bodily movement (particularly of the chest and belly). When the mind wanders, the mother-to-be is invited to notice what distracted her and then return to observing her breathing. *Music relaxing exercise* *Rainbow guided imagery*: this exercise invites women to imagine herself in a quiet, peaceful and secure place to rest and to release anxieties, worries and thoughts, allowing her to come out of this imagery with a sense of comfort and refreshment; mothers-to-be are encouraged to imagine "a beautiful rainbow" and visualize the image's form, colour and flow, and to focus attention on how they are feeling. The voice guide suggested desired psychological states and emotions (e.g., "You feel calm, You feel relaxed, Your body is calm and relaxed, and also your baby is relaxed") to induce them

meditation. In particular, You and your baby in one body meditation is designed to create a state of direct connection with the baby to strengthen the relationship between mother and child in the womb, to prepare both for the childbirth [42].

Social support represents a protective factor against affective disorders during pregnancy [43]. Thus, the third module, **People around you**, encourages women to reflect on the relations with their loved ones and take steps to improve them. There are three simple exercises included: "Connectedness exercise", "Gratitude exercise" and "Cuddling with my child in the womb and my partner" [43].

The **Optimism** module is dedicated to developing and increasing a positive attitude toward the future. It includes "Best possible self-exercise" [44], "Inner smile meditation" and "Baby steps exercise" [44].

The fifth module, **Mind and Body Relax**, aims to teach relaxing and decentering technique to reduce reactivity and increase act with awareness [45]. Participants can learn how to manage their attention and to be more aware of the mind wandering; in terms of thought distancing, participants increase the ability to perceive thoughts as "events" in the minds, and simply observing the process of thought. Moreover, guided imagery is used to influence psychological and physiological states: the evoked images may mediate the communication between perception, emotion and physiological change and may induce a positive physiological process such as reducing the stress reaction and related stress symptoms (Schaub, 1995). This module proposes three practices: "Mindful breathing meditation" [42, 46], "Music relaxing exercise" [47, 48] and "Rainbow guided imagery" [49].

3   Method

3.1   Participants and Procedure

A pilot study will be performed to test the effectiveness of the SerenaMente Mamma app in promoting and enhancing women's prenatal well-being and preventing post-natal depression.

Women will be recruited from hospitals and perinatal services across Milan (Italy). Pregnant women up until gestational week 35, at least 18 years of age, able to read and write Italian, have access to the internet and have an electronic mailing account will be invited to participate to the study.

They can start the intervention from the second trimester of pregnancy. The reason for starting in the second trimester is that expectant mothers can be reached as early as possible, thus preventing prenatal depression and promoting a positive prenatal attachment to their baby [36].

3.2   Measures

In order to verify the effectiveness of the SerenaMente Mamma App in promoting and enhancing women's prenatal mental well-being and preventing post-natal depression, several questionnaires in App will be presented two times: (i) after acceptance of the study conditions (i.e., Baseline), (ii) at the end of the five-week intervention (i.e., Post Assessment). Finally, after the childbirth and within the first trimester of the child, the researchers will contact the new-mothers, that have voluntarily agreed to participate to the post-partum study, to propose to fill out a post-partum set of online questionnaires (i.e., Follow-up Assessment).

Firstly, a socio-demographic questionnaire aimed to assess women's age, nationality, marital status, education, current employment status and occupation, week of pregnancy and previous experience with relaxing or meditation techniques is proposed. Second, to investigate the MPPMI app effectiveness several validated self-report questionnaires (to be completed at Baseline, Post Assessment and Follow-up Assessment) are included.

The Flourishing Scale – FS [50, 51] consists in eight items on a 7-point Likert-type scale, which investigates the eudaimonic aspects of well-being (e.g., "I lead a purposeful and meaningful life," "My social relationships are supportive and reward-ing," "I am engaged and interested in my daily activities"). The total score is calculated by the sum of the item scores and can range from 8 to 56. Higher scores mean that the respondent rates herself as a very positive functioning individual.

Depression level is assessed using the Edinburgh Postnatal Depression Scale (EPDS) [52, 53], a widely used brief screening tool for depression. Participants are asked to think of their psychological conditions over the past seven days and to rate depressed mood, anhedonia, guilt, anxiety and suicidal ideation through 10 items on 4-point Likert scales (range 0–3). A sample item is 'I have blamed myself unnecessarily when things went wrong' with the following response format: 'yes, most of the time' (3), 'yes, some of the time' (2), 'not very often' (1), 'no, never' (0). The EPDS total score ranges from zero to 30, with higher values indicating more negative feelings.

Pregnancy-related anxiety (PRAS) [54] is a 10-item self-report scale that measures the frequency or extent to which pregnant women are worried or concerned about their health, their baby's health, labor and childbirth, and caring for a newborn. Responses are given on a four-point Likert scale ranging from 1 to 4, and the total scores range between 10 and 40.

The Maternity Social Support Scale (MSSS) [55] measures perceived social sup-port in pregnancy (family support, friendship network, help from spouse/partner, conflict with spouse/partner, feeling controlled by spouse/partner and feeling loved by spouse/partner). It is a six-item questionnaire, on a five-point Likert scale. The total possible score for the scale is 30, with higher scores indicating increased support. A cut-off score of 24 has been recommended (Webster et al., 2000a).

Emotional well-being is assessed through the WHO-5[1] [56], a short instrument consisting of five positively formulated items: 'I have felt cheerful and in good spirits', 'I have felt calm and relaxed', 'I have felt active and vigorous', 'I woke up feeling fresh and rested' and 'My daily life has been filled with things that interest me'. The degree to which these feelings were present in the last 2 weeks is scored on a 6-point Likert-type, from 0 (not present) to 5 (constantly present). Item scores are summated and transformed to a 0–100 scale, with lower scores indicating poorer well-being. Based on previous studies, a cut-off <50 is recommended as threshold for further testing for depression [57, 58], while one study found a WHO-5 index score <28 to provide the best screening performance in terms of sensitivity and specificity WHO [59].

In addition to these instruments, during the Post Assessment, women are asked to fill out a qualitative questionnaire about their user experience with the App. To rate the perceived app quality,, an adapted version of the MARS [60, 61] is used. The MARS adapted version contains 28 items in 3 sections: classification, app quality, and satis-faction. Each MARS item uses a 5-point scale (1-Inadequate, 2-Poor, 3-Acceptable, 4-Good, 5-Excellent). The 28-item app quality section rates apps on four subscales: engagement, functionality, aesthetics, and information quality. The subjective quality section contains 4 items evaluating the user's overall satisfaction. The MARS is scored by calculating the mean scores of the app quality subscales and the total mean score.

---

[1] Italian versions available here: https://www.psykiatri-regionh.dk/who-5/Documents/WHO5_Italian.pdf.

4 Discussion

Pregnancy is a challenging time that can impact women's and children's well-being and development [62]. Although psychological research on pregnancy has mainly focused on detecting and treating disorders related to the perinatal period, an increasing number of studies have investigated positive aspects and protective factors of well-being during the prenatal period [4, 14]. Their results show the relevance and beneficial effects of cultivating maternal prenatal positive affect, positive life events, optimism, social support, and mindfulness on women's and infants' well-being. Therefore, to develop programs that promote and enhance women's prenatal well-being is a priority.

This work describes a novel, multi-component positive psychology and mindfulness-based intervention (MPPMI) for pregnant women – "SerenaMente Mamma"-, which has been developed in a mobile App format. The App "SerenaMente Mamma" presents different strengths. First, the intervention contents have a solid theoretical base. PPIs and mindfulness-based interventions have shown to be effective in maximizing well-being in general populations and an increasing number of studies have shown that PPIs and mindfulness-based interventions are valid tools in supporting pregnant women mental well-being [14, 20, 31, 63]. Second, the mobile App format offers different important advantages, as it reaches many people in a cost-effective manner, offering anonymity and allowing women to access the contents at the most convenient time and place for them. Third, the self-paced nature of the intervention has the advantage of empowering women, increasing their perception of being responsible for their own mental well-being and the health of the baby.

5 Future Directions

The future steps are to examine program implementation, including number of pregnant women registered for the program, potential barriers and women's user experiences, and to preliminary assess the effectiveness of the proposed intervention in a pilot study with a follow-up assessment in order to investigate whether the effects of the intervention on women's mental well-being can be maintained over time. In order to carry out the proposed pilot study, the collaboration with hospitals and perinatal clinics will be necessary.

6 Conclusion

Recently research on antenatal care has expanded to a new positive perspective, which examines the potential benefits of positive and protective factors that can influence the course of pregnancy, women's perinatal well-being and childbirth. In the wake of this positive perspective of prenatal care, the proposed work aims to present a novel mobile App-based MPPMI addressed to support women's perinatal mental well-being. If shown to be effective, this App could be an affordable and valid tool to promote and improve well-being pregnant women, and it could be translated in other languages in order to improve its accessibility. Finally, we believe that the present work will contribute to bridging the research gap on promoting women's well-being during the prenatal period and provide a starting point for developing simple and cost-effective interventions for pregnant women around the world.

Acknowledgments. We want to thank to Manuel Tocchi and Giuseppe Doda for their support in developing the App.

References

1. Barclay, L., Everitt, L., Rogan, F., et al.: Becoming a mother-an analysis of women's experience of early motherhood. J. Adv. Nurs. **25**, 719–728 (1997). https://doi.org/10.1046/j.1365-2648.1997.t01-1-1997025719.x
2. Stern, D.N., Bruschweiler-Stern, N.: The Birth of a Mother: How the Motherhood Experience Changes you Forever. BasicBooks, New York (1998)
3. Bibring, G.L.: Some considerations of the psychological processes in pregnancy. Psychoanal. Study Child **14**, 113–121 (1959). https://doi.org/10.1080/00797308.1959.11822824
4. Haga, S.M., Ulleberg, P., Slinning, K., et al.: A longitudinal study of postpartum depressive symptoms: multilevel growth curve analyses of emotion regulation strategies, breastfeeding self-efficacy, and social support. Arch. Womens Ment. Health **15**, 175–184 (2012). https://doi.org/10.1007/s00737-012-0274-2
5. Drury, S.S., Scaramella, L., Zeanah, C.H.: The neurobiological impact of postpartum maternal depression. Child Adolesc. Psychiatr. Clin. N Am. **25**, 179–200 (2016). https://doi.org/10.1016/j.chc.2015.11.001
6. Edwards, E.S., Holzman, J.B., Burt, N.M., et al.: Maternal emotion regulation strategies, internalizing problems and infant negative affect. J. Appl. Dev. Psychol. **48**, 59–68 (2017). https://doi.org/10.1016/j.appdev.2016.12.001
7. Hoffman, S., Hatch, M.C.: Depressive symptomatology during pregnancy: evidence for an association with decreased fetal growth in pregnancies of lower social class women. Health Psychol. **19**, 535–543 (2000). https://doi.org/10.1037/0278-6133.19.6.535
8. Dunkel-Schetter, C.: Maternal stress and preterm delivery. Prenat. Neonatal Med. **3**, 39–42 (1998)
9. Dayan, J., Creveuil, C., Herlicoviez, M., et al.: Role of anxiety and depression in the onset of spontaneous preterm labor. Am. J. Epidemiol. **155**, 293–301 (2002)
10. Davis, E.P., Glynn, L.M., Schetter, C.D., et al.: Prenatal exposure to maternal depression and cortisol influences infant temperament. J. Am. Acad. Child Adolesc. Psychiatry **46**, 737–746 (2007). https://doi.org/10.1097/chi.0b013e318047b775
11. Buitelaar, J.K., Huizink, A.C., Mulder, E.J., et al.: Prenatal stress and cognitive development and temperament in infants. Neurobiol. Aging **24**, S53–S60 (2003)
12. O'Connor, T.G., Heron, J., Glover, V.: Antenatal anxiety predicts child behavioral/emotional problems independently of postnatal depression. J. Am. Acad. Child Adolesc. Psychiatry **41**, 1470–1477 (2002). https://doi.org/10.1097/00004583-200212000-00019
13. Voellmin, A., Entringer, S., Moog, N., et al.: Maternal positive affect over the course of pregnancy is associated with the length of gestation and reduced risk of preterm delivery. J. Psychosom. Res. **75**, 336–340 (2013). https://doi.org/10.1016/j.jpsychores.2013.06.031

14. Matvienko-Sikar, K., Dockray, S.: Effects of a novel positive psychological intervention on prenatal stress and well-being: a pilot randomised controlled trial. Women Birth **30**, e111–e118 (2017). https://doi.org/10.1016/j.wombi.2016.10.003

15. Bos, S.C., Macedo, A., Marques, M., et al.: Is positive affect in pregnancy protective of postpartum depression? Rev. Bras Psiquiatr. **35**, 5–12 (2013). https://doi.org/10.1016/j.rbp.2011.11.002

16. Sutter-Dallay, A.L., Giaconne-Marcesche, V., Glatigny-Dallay, E., Verdoux, H.: Women 1with anxiety disorders during pregnancy are at increased risk of intense postnatal depressive symptoms: a prospective survey of the MATQUID cohort. Eur. Psychiatry **19**, 459–463 (2004)

17. Adewuya, A.O., Ola, B.A., Aloba, O.O., Mapayi, B.M.: Anxiety disorders among Nigerian women in late pregnancy: a controlled study. Arch. Womens Ment. Health **9**, 325–328 (2006). https://doi.org/10.1007/s00737-006-0157-5

18. Andersson, L., Sundström-Poromaa, I., Wulff, M., et al.: Depression and anxiety during pregnancy and six months postpartum: a follow-up study. Acta Obstet. Gynecol. Scand. **85**, 937–944 (2006). https://doi.org/10.1080/00016340600697652

19. Heron, J., O'Connor, T.G., Evans, J., et al.: The course of anxiety and depression through pregnancy and the postpartum in a community sample. J. Affect Disord. (2004). https://doi.org/10.1016/j.jad.2003.08.004

20. Matvienko-Sikar, K., Lee, L., Murphy, G., Murphy, L.: The effects of mindfulness interventions on prenatal well-being: a systematic review. Psychol. Health **31**, 1415–1434 (2016). https://doi.org/10.1080/08870446.2016.1220557

21. Carissoli, C., Gasparri, D., Riva, G., Villani, D.: Promoting psychological well-being in pregnancy with a mobile app: a quasi experimental controlled study (Manuscript under review)

22. Lyubomirsky, S.: The How of Happiness: A Scientific Approach to Getting the Life You Want. The Penguin Press, New York (2008)

23. Bolier, L., Haverman, M., Westerhof, G.J., et al.: Positive psychology interventions: a meta-analysis of randomized controlled studies. BMC Public Health **13**, 119 (2013). https://doi.org/10.1186/1471-2458-13-119

24. Hone, L.C., Jarden, A., Schofield, G.M.: An evaluation of positive psychology intervention effectiveness trials using the re-aim framework: a practice-friendly review. J. Posit. Psychol. **10**, 303–322 (2015). https://doi.org/10.1080/17439760.2014.965267

25. Schueller, S.M.: Identifying and analyzing positive interventions: a meta-analysis. In: 5th Annual European Conference on Positive Psychology, Rijeka, Croatia, p. 296 (2008)

26. Sin, N.L., Lyubomirsky, S.: Enhancing well-being and alleviating depressive symptoms with positive psychology interventions: a practice-friendly meta-analysis. J. Clin. Psychol. **65**, 467–487 (2009). https://doi.org/10.1002/jclp.20593

27. Hendriks, T., Warren, M.A., Schotanus-Dijkstra, M., et al.: How WEIRD are positive psychology interventions? a bibliometric analysis of randomized controlled trials on the science of well-being. J. Posit. Psychol. 1–13 (2018). https://doi.org/10.1080/17439760.2018.1484941

28. Ivtzan, I., Young, T., Martman, J., et al.: Integrating mindfulness into positive psychology: a randomised controlled trial of an online positive mindfulness program. Mindfulness (N Y) **7**, 1396–1407 (2016). https://doi.org/10.1007/s12671-016-0581-1

29. Tripp, N., Hainey, K., Liu, A., et al.: An emerging model of maternity care: smartphone, midwife, doctor? Women Birth **27**, 64–67 (2014). https://doi.org/10.1016/j.wombi.2013.11.001

30. Carissoli, C., Villani, D., Riva, G.: An emerging model of pregnancy care: the introduction of new technologies in maternal wellbeing. In: Villani, V., Cipresso, P., Gaggioli, A., Riva, G. (eds.) Integrating Technology in Positive Psychology Practice, pp. 162–192. IGI Global, Hershey (2016)

31. Corno, G., Etchemendy, E., Espinoza, M., et al.: Effect of a web-based positive psychology intervention on prenatal well-being: a case series study. Women Birth **31**, e1–e8 (2018). https://doi.org/10.1016/J.WOMBI.2017.06.005

32. Daly, L.M., Horey, D., Middleton, P.F., et al.: The effect of mobile application interventions on influencing healthy maternal behaviour and improving perinatal health outcomes: a systematic review protocol. Syst. Rev. **6**, 26 (2017). https://doi.org/10.1186/s13643-017-0424-8

33. Fonseca, A., Alves, S., Monteiro, F., et al.: Be a mom, a web based intervention to prevent postpartum depression: results from a pilot randomized controlled trial. In: 48th Annual Congress of the European Association for Behavioral and Cognitive Therapies. Sofia, Bulgaria (2018)

34. Lee, E., Denison, F., Hor, K., Reynolds, R.: Web-based interventions for prevention and treatment of perinatal mood disorders: a systematic review. BMC Pregnancy Childbirth **16**, 38 (2016). https://doi.org/10.1186/s12884-016-0831-1

35. Drozd, F., Haga, S.M., Brendryen, H., Slinning, K.: An internet-based intervention (Mamma Mia) for postpartum depression: mapping the development from theory to practice. JMIR Res. Protoc. **4**, e120 (2015). https://doi.org/10.2196/resprot.4858

36. Haga, S.M., Drozd, F., Lisøy, C., et al.: Mamma Mia–a randomized controlled trial of an internet-based intervention for perinatal depression. Psychol. Med. 1–9 (2018). https://doi.org/10.1017/S0033291718002544

37. Peterson, C.: A Primer in Positive Psychology. Oxford University Press, New York (2006)

38. Schueller, S.M., Parks, A.C.: The science of self-help: translating positive psychology research into increased individual happiness. Eur. Psychol. (2014). https://doi.org/10.1027/1016-9040/a000181

39. Hofmann, S.G., Grossman, P., Hinton, D.E.: Loving-kindness and compassion meditation: potential for psychological interventions. Clin. Psychol. Rev. **31**, 1126–1132 (2011). https://doi.org/10.1016/j.cpr.2011.07.003

40. Williams, M., Penman, D.: Mindfulness: A Practical Guide to Finding Peace in a Frantic World. Hachette Digital, London (2011)

41. Dreeben, S.J., Mamberg, M.H., Salmon, P.: The MBSR body scan in clinical practice. Mindfulness (N Y) (2013). https://doi.org/10.1007/s12671-013-0212-z

42. Duncan, L.G., Bardacke, N.: Mindfulness-based childbirth and parenting education: promoting family mindfulness during the perinatal period. J. Child Fam. Stud. **19**, 190–202 (2010). https://doi.org/10.1007/s10826-009-9313-7

43. Dunkel Schetter, C.: Psychological science on pregnancy: stress processes, biopsychosocial models, and emerging research issues. Annu. Rev. Psychol. **62**, 531–558 (2011). https://doi.org/10.1146/annurev.psych.031809.130727

44. Layous, K., Katherine Nelson, S., Lyubomirsky, S.: What is the optimal way to deliver a positive activity intervention? the case of writing about one's best possible selves. J. Happiness Stud. **14**, 635–654 (2013). https://doi.org/10.1007/s10902-012-9346-2

45. Feldman, G., Greeson, J., Senville, J.: Differential effects of mindful breathing, progressive muscle relaxation, and loving-kindness meditation on decentering and negative reactions to repetitive thoughts. Behav. Res. Ther. (2010). https://doi.org/10.1016/j.brat.2010.06.006

46. Pan, W.-L., Gau, M.-L., Lee, T.-Y., et al.: Mindfulness-based programme on the psychological health of pregnant women. Women Birth (2018). https://doi.org/10.1016/J.WOMBI.2018.04.018

47. Daykin, N., Mansfield, L., Meads, C., et al.: What works for wellbeing? a systematic review of wellbeing outcomes for music and singing in adults. Perspect. Public Health **138**, 39–46 (2018). https://doi.org/10.1177/1757913917740391

48. Chang, S.-C., Chen, C.-H.: Effects of music therapy on women's physiologic measures, anxiety, and satisfaction during cesarean delivery. Res. Nurs. Health **28**, 453–461 (2005). https://doi.org/10.1002/nur.20102

49. Overholser, J.C.: The use of guided imagery in psychotherapy: modules for use with passive relaxation training. J. Contemp. Psychother. **21**, 159–172 (1991). https://doi.org/10.1007/BF00973115

50. Diener, E., Wirtz, D., Tov, W., et al.: New well-being measures: short scales to assess flourishing and positive and negative feelings. Soc. Indic. Res. **97**, 143–156 (2010). https://doi.org/10.1007/s11205-009-9493-y

51. Giuntoli, L., Ceccarini, F., Sica, C., Caudek, C.: Validation of the Italian versions of the flourishing scale and of the scale of positive and negative experience. SAGE Open **7**, 215824401668229 (2017). https://doi.org/10.1177/2158244016682293

52. Benvenuti, P., Ferrara, M., Niccolai, C., et al.: The Edinburgh postnatal depression scale: validation for an italian sample. J. Affect. Disord. **53**, 137–141 (1999). https://doi.org/10.1016/S0165-0327(98)00102-5

53. Cox, J.L., Holden, J.M., Sagovsky, R.: Detection of postnatal depression. Development of the 10-item Edinburgh postnatal depression scale. Br. J. Psychiatry **150**, 782–786 (1987). https://doi.org/10.1192/BJP.150.6.782

54. Rini, C.K., Dunkel-Schetter, C., Wadhwa, P.D., Sandman, C.A.: Psychological adaptation and birth outcomes: the role of personal resources, stress, and sociocultural context in pregnancy. Health Psychol. **18**, 333–345 (1999)

55. Webster, J., Linnane, J.W.J., Dibley, L.M., et al.: Measuring social support in pregnancy: can it be simple and meaningful? Birth **27**, 97–101 (2000). https://doi.org/10.1046/j.1523-536x.2000.00097.x

56. Bech, P.: Measuring the dimension of psychological general well-being by the WHO-5. Qual Life Newsl. **32**, 15–16 (2004)

57. Awata, S., Bech, P., Yoshida, S., et al.: Reliability and validity of the Japanese version of the World Health Organization-five well-being index in the context of detecting depression in diabetic patients. Psychiatry Clin. Neurosci. **61**, 112–119 (2007). https://doi.org/10.1111/j.1440-1819.2007.01619.x

58. de Wit, M., Pouwer, F., Gemke, R.J.B.J., et al.: Validation of the WHO-5 well-being index in adolescents with type 1 diabetes. Diabetes Care **30**, 2003–2006 (2007). https://doi.org/10.2337/dc07-0447

59. Löwe, B., Spitzer, R.L., Gräfe, K., et al.: Comparative validity of three screening questionnaires for DSM-IV depressive disorders and physicians' diagnoses. J. Affect. Disord. **78**, 131–140 (2004)

60. Domnich, A., Arata, L., Amicizia, D., et al.: Development and validation of the Italian version of the mobile application rating scale and its generalisability to apps targeting primary prevention. BMC Med. Inform. Decis. Mak. **16**, 83 (2016). https://doi.org/10.1186/s12911-016-0323-2

61. Stoyanov, S.R., Hides, L., Kavanagh, D.J., et al.: Mobile app rating scale: a new tool for assessing the quality of health mobile apps. JMIR mHealth uHealth **3**, e27 (2015). https://doi.org/10.2196/mhealth.3422

62. Smith, J.A.: Identity development during the transition to motherhood: an interpretative phenomenological analysis. J. Reprod. Infant Psychol. **17**, 281–299 (1999). https://doi.org/10.1080/02646839908404595

63. Carissoli, C., Villani, D., Triberti, S., Riva, G.: User experience of BenEssere Mamma, a pregnancy app for women wellbeing. Annu Rev. CyberTherapy Telemed. **14**, 195–198 (2016)

Beyond Cognitive Rehabilitation: Immersive but Noninvasive Treatment for Elderly

Elisa Pedroli[1(✉)], Pietro Cipresso[1,2], Silvia Serino[3], Michelle Toti[1],
Karine Goulen[4], Mauro Grigioni[5], Marco Stramba-Badiale[4],
Andrea Gaggioli[1,2], and Giuseppe Riva[1,2]

[1] Applied Technology for Neuro-Psychology Lab, IRCCS Istituto Auxologico
Italiano, Milan, Italy
{e.pedroli,p.cipresso}@auxologico.it,
michelletoti5@gmail.com
[2] Department of Psychology, Università Cattolica del Sacro Cuore, Milan, Italy
{andrea.gaggioli,giuseppe.riva}@unicatt.it
[3] MySpace Lab, Department of Clinical Neurosciences,
University Hospital Lausanne (CHUV), Lausanne, Switzerland
silvia.serino@gmail.com
[4] Department of Geriatrics and Cardiovascular Medicine,
IRCCS Istituto Auxologico Italiano, Milan, Italy
{goulene,stramba_badiale}@auxologico.it
[5] National Center of Innovative Technologies in Public Health,
Istituto Superiore di Sanità, Rome, Italy
mauro.grigioni@iss.it

Abstract. With the rapid increase of the aging population in Italy, the number
of subjects with cognitive deficits also increases. Two of the most damaged
cognitive domains since the first phase of decline are Executive Functions and
Spatial Memory. The general aim of this study is to evaluate the efficacy of a
novel VR-based mixed training protocol for improving executive functions and
spatial memory in patients with cognitive decline. To achieve this objective, the
neuropsychological performance of two groups of a subjects with cognitive
decline were compared before and at the end of the training period. One group
underwent a classic rehabilitation protocol, the other underwent the new VR-
based protocol. The results showed an improve in executive functioning in the
VR group after the training period.

Keywords: Cognitive decline · Rehabilitation · Virtual reality ·
CAVE · Executive functions · Spatial memory

1 Introduction

1.1 Cognitive Decline

Nowadays, about 19% of the European population are 65 or more years old and
probably will reach 150 million by 2080 [1]. With increasing age, health problems also
increase, including cognitive impairments [2, 3]. Before developing dementia, subjects

P. Cipresso et al. (Eds.): MindCare 2019, LNICST 288, pp. 263–273, 2019.
https://doi.org/10.1007/978-3-030-25872-6_22

can go through different stages of impairments. Different definitions have been given to these initial stages of cognitive impairment; i.e. Cognitive Frailty [4] or Mild Cognitive Impairment [2]. Regardless of the definition, these problems lead to a reduction in the autonomy of the subjects and their quality of life, impacting the ability to live safely and independently [5].

It is widely accepted the need to act promptly by targeting rehabilitation programs to prevent the negative consequences of decline. Accordingly, each rehabilitation programs should be implemented in pre-clinical or early stage of the cognitive impairment. Prompt interventions could improve the ability of the elderly individuals and preserve their autonomy, thus avoiding an early hospitalization [6].

Two of the most damaged cognitive domains since the first phase of decline are executive functions [7, 8] and spatial memory [9–11]. Both executive functions and spatial memory deficits are complex phenomena that the classical assessment and rehabilitation protocols are not able to detect and manage adequately [12]. A more ecological and customized procedure could help clinicians to improve the quality of the clinical care [12]. VR is an important technology for the improvement and amelioration of the classical paper &pencil protocols used both for assessment and rehabilitation sessions. VR can make more neuropsychological practice more engaging, generalizable, and ecological thanks to its ability to measure behavior in valid, safe, and controlled environments objectively and automatically; dynamic learning also may increase patients' engagement [13, 14]. In the last decade, VR-based protocols have been developed for many neurological diseases, for both motor [15, 16] and cognitive [17, 18] impairments.

In this regard, there is a growing urgency to identify the most effective strategies to prevent cognitive decline using all the tools available. The modern pharmacological treatments are not able to reduce symptoms or slow down the unavoidable progression of the cognitive impairment [19]. Therefore, there is increased interest for computerized or virtual reality-based cognitive rehabilitation programs that is assumed to improve, or at least stabilize, performance in a given cognitive domain (i.e. near transfer effect [20]). These kinds of protocols are based on the principles of neuronal plasticity and cognitive ability restoration, but also generalized effects beyond immediate training contexts are expected (i.e. far transfer effects) [21]. Here we present an innovative VR-based training for the rehabilitation of Executive Functions and Spatial Memory and some preliminary data from a larger trial that is still taking place.

2   Materials and Methods

2.1   Sample

In this preliminary phase of the trial we recruited 14 elderly subjects from the Department of Geriatrics and Cardiovascular Medicine of the IRCCS Istituto Auxologico Italiano located in Milan (Italy). The presence of cognitive decline was assessed by Mini-Mental State Examination (MMSE) [22] and only individuals who had a score between 23 and 26 were included in the study. Participants were randomly assigned to "VR training" ("VR Group"; n = 7) or "Control Group" ("NN-VR Group"; n = 7).

Exclusion criteria for the groups were: (1) presence of visual and balance deficits which may interfere with the use of VR technology; and (2) the additional presence of psychiatric disorders or other neurological conditions, such as traumatic brain injuries or strokes.

The VR Group included six men and one woman, while the NN-VR Group included four women and three men. The demographic information are show in the Table 1 There were no significant differences between two groups in terms of age [t(12) = 0.818; p = 0. 429] or education [t(12) = −0.899; p = 0.386].

Table 1. Demographic information.

	Age		YoE		MMSE	
	Mean	SD	Mean	SD	Mean	SD
VR group	78,86	4,22	13	4,08	25,99	2,10
NN-VR group	81,29	6,63	11	4,24	24,63	1,63

Note: YoE = Years of Educations, MMSE = Mini-Mental State Examination; SD = Standard Deviation.

All participants provided written informed consent, which was approved by the Ethical Committee of IRCCS Istituto Auxologico Italiano. The study was conducted in compliance with the Helsinki Declaration of 1975, as revised in 2008.

2.2 Rehabilitation Protocol

The protocol includes an assessment (T0), 5 weeks off, a second assessment (T1), 10 training sessions and one last evaluation (T2). During the assessment, a complete neuropsychological battery was performed. The cognitive rehabilitation sessions were held twice a week for at least 30 min each one, for five weeks. Accordingly to literature, we created two different highly-ecological virtual rehabilitation protocols for Executive Functions and Spatial Memory [23]. Both protocols could be implemented using low-end and high-end virtual reality systems [24]. NN-VR Group underwent a protocol for executive functions and spatial memory designed with traditional cognitive rehabilitative activities using paper & pencil materials.

Cognitive Assessment. A complete and extensive cognitive assessment was conducted to analyze a wide range of cognitive domains. All participants underwent a detailed neuropsychological assessment conducted by an experienced neuropsychologist three time. The neuropsychological assessments analyze several cognitive domains: executive functions, selective attention, short and long-term spatial and verbal memory, and visuo-spatial abilities. the neuropsychological battery was composed of: (a) phonemic verbal fluency and categorical verbal fluency test [25], (b) Frontal Assessment Battery (FAB) [26], (c) the Digit Span Test [27], (d) the Corsi Span Block Test [27], (e) Story recall [28], (f) Corsi Supra-span Block Test [28], and (g) Clock Drowing Test [29].

All scores obtained from the neuropsychological battery were corrected for age, education level and, when necessary, gender according to Italian normative data.

Executive Functions Training. The training environment is a virtual supermarket developed with Unity according to our needs (Fig. 1). The tasks were based on a VR-based assessment for the Executive Functions "Virtual Multiple Errands Test" (VMET), developed by Riva and colleagues [13, 30]. To move around and buy products in the shop patients could use a X-Box controller connected to the system. To complete the tasks the patients must buy several products on shelves following precise rules. First, the patient and the clinician analyze the task and the rules in order to understand and plan the different steps needed to solve the task. Then, patient start the shopping session in the virtual environment and the clinician helps patient only to avoid main errors and for technical support. At the end of the task a brief discussion about the outcome of the task is done. The software automatically records every object taken from the shelves and the path taken by the patient.

For the VR-based rehabilitation protocol, 10 different tasks with increasing difficulty are developed.

Spatial Memory Training. A virtual city (Fig. 1) was developed for the memory training. Patients can move around in the city using the X-Box controller connected to the system. The tasks are divided in encoding and retrieval phases. In the first phase patients start from the center of the city and have to explore the environment in order to find one, two or three objects located in different predefined place. In the retrieval phase, patients are asked to remember and reach the place where the objects were located before. Also, patient have to respect the order in which he found the objects in the previous phase. Here, the starting point is different for each session and is one of the target points where the patient does not return. In the first five tasks the clinician shows an allocentric map of the city and shows the patient the starting point of the retrieval phase in order to simplify the use of allocentric representation. If the patient gets lost during the task the software provides a cue, a green path that connects the present position of the subject to the forgotten point. Moreover, the system automatically records the path taken by the patient, when all target points have been achieved, and if the cue has been used. This task is developed to improve individuals' ability in storing, retrieving and synchronizing different spatial information, starting from results obtained from a previous trial with patients with dementia [31–33].

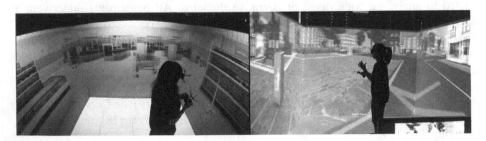

Fig. 1. The virtual environments: supermarket and city.

VR System. The virtual-based training took place inside a Cave Automatic Virtual Environment (CAVE) of Istituto Auxologico Italiano, CAVE is a room-sized cube with three walls and a floor. The 3D visualization occurs thanks to the combination of four stereoscopic projectors (Full HD 3D UXGA DLP), and the screens with a projectable area of 266 cm × 200 cm. A cluster system composed of two HPZ620 Graphics Workstations, mounting Nvidia Quadro K6000 GPU with dedicated Quadro Sync cards, is responsible for the rendering of the projection surfaces, user tracking and functional logic. Also, CAVE is equipped with a Vicon motion tracking system, with four infrared cameras, which allows the tracking of specific reflective markers positioned on target objects and a correct reading of the simulated spaces and distances with a 1:1 scale ratio, thus enhancing the feeling of being immersed in the virtual scene.

2.3 Statistical Analysis

Given the limited sample size a Wilcoxon test was done to compare the delta scores of the VR and NN-VR groups separately. The first delta scores (D1) were calculated by subtracting the results of the first evaluation to those of the second one. The second delta scores (D2) were calculated by subtracting the results of the second evaluation to those of the third one. Also, a comparison between D1 and D2 of each group was done with Mann-Whitney U test. This procedure was done for each of the analyzed outcome measures. Two separate hypotheses were done; in each group we hypnotize that D1 is less than D2. When the comparison was made between the groups, we expect that the values of D2 of the control group are less than the control group. All statistical analyses were performed using JASP for Windows, version 0.9.2. A $p < 0.05$ was considered statistically significant.

3 Results

3.1 Pre-post Comparison Within Groups

For each outcome measures the delta score were calculated. for the Frontal Assessment Battery, the score of each sub-test were analyzed separately, except for the "Prehension Behavior" in which all the patients obtained the maximum score. In the Table 2 the descriptive statistics were presented.

Accordingly to the results, a significant difference emerged for the Frontal Assessment Battery. This result indicates that there is an improvement aft virtual treatment there that is not found in the NN-VR group (Table 3). The graphical representation of these data are showed in the Figs. 2 and 3. Also for the Go-No-Go task it is possible to observe an improvement in scores for patients in VR-based group, although it was not statistically significant (Table 3).

Table 2. Descriptive analysis of Delta scores.

	D1				D2			
	NN-VR group		VR-group		NN-VR group		VR-group	
	Mean	SD	Mean	SD	Mean	SD	Mean	SD
CORSI_SUPRASPAN	1,12	5,54	0,49	6,9	1,3	3,61	3,41	7,9
FAB	0,86	2,8	−1,29	2,06	−0,04	1,98	2,47	2,17
PH_FLU	1	6,22	1,43	6,27	−0,14	6,15	1,71	3,68
CAT_FLU	1,57	8,22	2,14	3,13	1,14	10,98	0,71	6,08
DIGIT_SPAN	0,57	1,51	0,29	1,38	0,29	1,41	0	1,16
CORSI_SPAN	0,17	0,98	0,17	0,75	0,14	0,76	−0,14	0,38
FAB_SIM	0	1,16	0,14	1,07	0	1,16	0,57	0,79
FAB_PVF	−0,14	0,38	−0,14	0,69	0	0,58	0,14	0,38
FAB_MS	0,86	1,46	0,14	1,57	−0,14	0,69	0,43	1,13
FAB_CI	0,14	0,9	−0,71	1,25	0	0,58	0,71	1,6
FAB_GNG	0	0,58	−0,71	1,11	0,29	1,11	0,71	1,11
CLOCK	1	1,61	1,79	4,17	−0,29	1,58	−0,97	1,72
STORY	2,39	5,6	−1,61	6,9	2,22	5,36	1,54	5,3

FAB = Frontal Assessment Battery; PH_FLU = phonemic verbal fluency, CAT_FLU = categorical verbal fluency, SIM = Similarities, PVF = Phonological Verbal Fluency, MS = Motor Series, CI = Conflicting Instructions, GNG = Go-No Go Task.

Table 3. Results of Wilcoxon test.

D1 vs D2	NN-VR-group		VR-group	
	W	p	W	p
CORSI_SUPRA_SPAN	9,00	0,422	11,00	0,344
FAB	17,50	0,751	1,00	0,016*
PH_FLU	15,00	0,594	15,50	0,633
CAT_FLU	6,00	0,200	15,00	0,600
DIGIT_SPAN	16,00	0,664	16,00	0,667
CORSI_SPAN	5,00	0,572	7,50	0,885
FAB_SIM	6,00	0,710	2,00	0,172
FAB_PVF	2,00	0,386	1,50	0,293
FAB_MS	17,00	0,932	4,50	0,500
FAB_CI	2,00	0,814	1,00	0,211
FAB_GNG	6,00	0,392	3,00	0,069
CLOCK	17,00	0,929	16,50	0,915
STORY	14,00	0,534	10,00	0,500

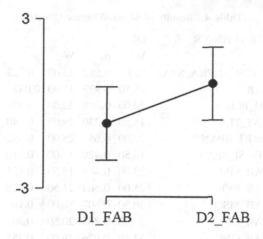

Fig. 2. Difference between D1 and D2 in the NN-VR Group.

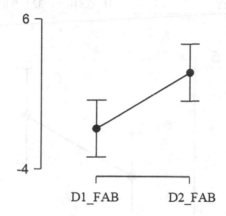

Fig. 3. Difference between D1 and D2 in the VR Group.

3.2   Between Groups Comparison

First, no significant results emerged from the analysis of D1 in the two groups for none of the outcome measures. As for the previous analysis, a significant difference emerged by analyzing FAB in D2. The results are highlighted in the Table 4 and in the Fig. 4.

Table 4. Results of Mann-Whitney U test.

VR vs NN-VR	D1		D2	
	W	p	W	p
CORSI_SUPRA_SPAN	22,00	0,582	15,00	0,223
FAB	35,50	0,933	11,00	0,047*
PH_FLU	22,00	0,398	22,00	0,398
CAT_FLU	18,50	0,239	29,00	0,740
DIGIT_SPAN	27,00	0,652	25,00	0,552
CORSI_SPAN	16,50	0,429	33,00	0,910
FAB_SIM	23,00	0,446	15,50	0,127
FAB_PVF	25,00	0,564	21,50	0,328
FAB_MS	30,50	0,807	18,00	0,196
FAB_CI	31,50	0,885	20,50	0,301
FAB_GNG	34,50	0,926	19,00	0,255
CLOCK	20,00	0,303	30,00	0,781
STORY	31	0,816	32	0,847

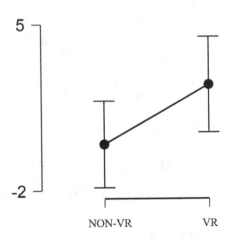

Fig. 4. Difference between NN-VR and VR in the FAB at D2.

4   Discussion

Here we presented the preliminary data of a larger project funded by the Italian government. The trial and patient's recruitment are still ongoing at the IRCCS Istituto Auxologico Italiano.

The aim of this study is to evaluate the efficacy of a novel VR-based mixed training protocol for both executive functions and spatial memory. The new training was compared with the classic rehabilitation tasks used for the stimulation of these cognitive domains. status of elderly individuals enrolled in the trails, especially as regards the targeted cognitive functions (i.e., executive functions and spatial memory).

The data are preliminary but encouraging. It was found an improvement in one of the two target cognitive domains: executive functions. The score of the Frontal Assessment Battery showed improvement in the VR group after the training period. This improvement is not highlighted in NN-VR group.

Also, the D2 scores are significantly different between the two groups. The FAB's score is higher in the experimental group after the treatment, thus indicating an improvement in the executive functions after our new VR training.

The greatest limitation that we can highlight in this work is the small sample size, and the representativity of the sample.

At the moment, we have only 14 subjects, but the number will be expanded in the coming months. The other limitation is related to the gender balance. In the VR group there is only one female subject. During the further recruitment this factor will be balanced.

At the same time, a motor rehabilitation program was developed. A stationary bike was integrated in the CAVE to promote the dual-task ability and another task to improve balance [34, 35].

Moreover, within the project a low-end device for a similar training is developing. The purpose of this new implementation is providing a program for home rehabilitation. The system will be designed to be used together by the patient and the caregiver at home without the therapist's support. Extending the training beyond the duration of the hospital journey could guarantee greater stability of improvements over time.

Acknowledgments. This work is supported by the Italian funded project "High-end and Low-End Virtual Reality Systems for the Rehabilitation of Frailty in the Elderly" (PE-2013-02355948).

References

1. Eurostat: Population structure and ageing—statistics explained (2018). http://ec.europa.eu/eurostat/statistics-explained/index.php/Population_structure_and_ageing. Accessed 29 Jan 2018
2. Petersen, R., et al.: Mild cognitive impairment: a concept in evolution. J. Intern. Med. **275**(3), 214–228 (2014)
3. Petersen, R.: Mild cognitive impairment as a diagnostic entity. J. Intern. Med. **256**(3), 183–194 (2004)
4. Kelaiditi, E., et al.: Cognitive frailty: rational and definition from an (IANA/IAGG) international consensus group. J. Nutr. Health Aging **17**(9), 726–734 (2013)
5. Maselli, M., et al.: Can physical and cognitive training based on episodic memory be combined in a new protocol for daily training? Aging Clin. Exp. Res., 1–9 (2018)
6. Forte, R., et al.: Enhancing cognitive functioning in the elderly: multicomponent vs resistance training. Clin. Interv. Aging **8**, 19 (2013)
7. Won, C.W., et al.: Modified criteria for diagnosing "cognitive frailty". Psychiatry Invest. **15**(9), 839 (2018)
8. Delrieu, J., et al.: Neuropsychological profile of "cognitive frailty" subjects in MAPT study. J. Prev. Alzheimer's Dis. **3**(3), 151 (2016)

9. Albert, M., et al.: The diagnosis of mild cognitive impairment due to Alzheimer's disease: recommendations from the National Institute on Aging-Alzheimer's Association workgroups on diagnostic guidelines for Alzheimer's disease. Alzheimer's Dementia **7**(3), 270–279 (2011)
10. Serino, S., et al.: Detecting early egocentric and allocentric impairments deficits in Alzheimer's disease: an experimental study with virtual reality. Front. Aging Neurosci. **7**(88), 1–10 (2015)
11. Lee, J.-Y., et al.: Spatial memory impairments in amnestic mild cognitive impairment in a virtual radial arm maze. Neuropsychiatric Dis. Treat. **10**, 653 (2014)
12. Pedroli, E., et al.: Exploring virtual reality for the assessment and rehabilitation of executive functions. Int. J. Virtual Augmented Reality (IJVAR) **2**(1), 32–47 (2018)
13. Serino, S., et al.: The role of virtual reality in neuropsychology: the virtual multiple errands test for the assessment of executive functions in Parkinson's disease. In: Ma, M., Jain, L.C., Anderson, P. (eds.) Virtual, Augmented Reality and Serious Games for Healthcare 1. ISRL, vol. 68, pp. 257–274. Springer, Heidelberg (2014). https://doi.org/10.1007/978-3-642-54816-1_14
14. Sugarman, H., et al.: Use of novel virtual reality system for the assessment and treatment of unilateral spatial neglect: a feasibility study. In: International Conference on Virtual Rehabilitation (ICVR). IEEE, Switzerland (2011)
15. Mirelman, A., et al.: V-TIME: a treadmill training program augmented by virtual reality to decrease fall risk in older adults: study design of a randomized controlled trial. BMC Neurol. **13**(1), 15 (2013)
16. Langhorne, P., Coupar, F., Pollock, A.: Motor recovery after stroke: a systematic review. Lancet Neurol. **8**(8), 741–754 (2009)
17. Pedroli, E., et al.: Assessment and rehabilitation of neglect using virtual reality: a systematic review. Front. Behav. Neurosci. **9**(226), 1–15 (2015)
18. Denmark, T., et al.: Using virtual reality to investigate multitasking ability in individuals with frontal lobe lesions. Neuropsychol. Rehabil. **29**, 1–22 (2017)
19. Zucchella, C., et al.: The multidisciplinary approach to Alzheimer's disease and dementia: a narrative review of non-pharmacological treatment. Front. Neurol. **9**(1058) (2018)
20. Lampit, A., Hallock, H., Valenzuela, M.: Computerized cognitive training in cognitively healthy older adults: a systematic review and meta-analysis of effect modifiers. PLoS Med. **11**(11), 1–18 (2014)
21. Vance, D.E., Crowe, M.: A proposed model of neuroplasticity and cognitive reserve in older adults. Activities Adapt. Aging **30**(3), 61–79 (2006)
22. Magni, E., et al.: Mini-mental state examination: a normative study in italian elderly population. Eur. J. Neurol. **3**(3), 198–202 (1996)
23. Pedroli, E., et al.: An immersive cognitive rehabilitation program: a case study. In: Masia, L., Micera, S., Akay, M., Pons, J. (eds.) Converging Clinical and Engineering Research on Neurorehabilitation III. ICNR 2018. Biosystems & Biorobotics, vol. 21, pp. 711–715. Springer, Cham (2019). https://doi.org/10.1007/978-3-030-01845-0_142
24. Pedroli, E., Serino, S., Stramba-Badiale, M., Riva, G.: An innovative virtual reality-based training program for the rehabilitation of cognitive frail patients. In: Oliver, N., Serino, S., Matic, A., Cipresso, P., Filipovic, N., Gavrilovska, L. (eds.) MindCare/FABULOUS/IIOT 2015-2016. LNICST, vol. 207, pp. 62–66. Springer, Cham (2018). https://doi.org/10.1007/978-3-319-74935-8_8
25. Novelli, G., et al.: Tre test clinici di ricerca e produzione lessicale. Taratura su soggetti normali. Archivio di psicologia neurologia e psichiatria **47**(4), 477–506 (1986)

26. Appollonio, I., et al.: The Frontal Assessment Battery (FAB): normative values in an Italian population sample. Neurol. Sci. **26**(2), 108–116 (2005)
27. Monaco, M., et al.: Forward and backward span for verbal and visuo-spatial data: standardization and normative data from an Italian adult population. Neurol. Sci. **34**(5), 749–754 (2012)
28. Spinnler, H., Tognoni, G.: Standardizzazione e taratura italiana di test neuropsicologici. Masson Italia Periodici, Milano (1987)
29. Mondini, S., et al.: Esame neuropsicologico breve. Raffaello Cortina Editore, Milano (2003)
30. Cipresso, P., et al.: Virtual multiple errands test (VMET): a virtual reality-based tool to detect early executive functions deficit in Parkinson's disease. Front. Behav. Neurosci. **8** (405), 1–11 (2014)
31. Serino, S., Riva, G.: How different spatial representations interact in virtual environments: the role of mental frame syncing. Cognit. Process. **16**(2), 191–201 (2015)
32. Serino, S., Riva, G.: What is the role of spatial processing in the decline of episodic memory in Alzheimer's disease? The "mental frame syncing" hypothesis. Front. Aging Neurosci. **6** (33), 1–7 (2014)
33. Serino, S., et al.: A novel virtual reality-based training protocol for the enhancement of the "mental frame syncing" in individuals with Alzheimer's disease: a development-of-concept trial. Front. Aging Neurosci. **9**(240), 1–12 (2017)
34. Pedroli, E., et al.: Characteristics, usability, and users experience of a system combining cognitive and physical therapy in a virtual environment: positive bike. Sensors **18**(7), 2343 (2018)
35. Gaggioli, A., et al.: "Positive Bike"-an immersive biking experience for combined physical and cognitive training of elderly patient. Ann. Rev. Cybertherapy Telemed. **15**, 196–199 (2017)

Correction to: Full Body Immersive Virtual Reality System with Motion Recognition Camera Targeting the Treatment of Spider Phobia

Jacob Kritikos, Stavroula Poulopoulou, Chara Zoitaki,
Marilina Douloudi, and Dimitris Koutsouris

Correction to:
Chapter "Full Body Immersive Virtual Reality System
with Motion Recognition Camera Targeting the Treatment
of Spider Phobia" in: P. Cipresso et al. (Eds.): *Pervasive*
Computing Paradigms for Mental Health, **LNICST 288,**
https://doi.org/10.1007/978-3-030-25872-6_18

The original version of this chapter was published without the reference "Anxiety detection from Electrodermal Activity Sensor with movement & interaction during Virtual Reality Simulation", https://ieeexplore.ieee.org/document/8717170, which has now been included.

The correction chapter has been updated with the changes.

The updated version of this chapter can be found at
https://doi.org/10.1007/978-3-030-25872-6_18

© ICST Institute for Computer Sciences, Social Informatics and Telecommunications Engineering 2019
Published by Springer Nature Switzerland AG 2019. All Rights Reserved
P. Cipresso et al. (Eds.): MindCare 2019, LNICST 288, p. C1, 2019.
https://doi.org/10.1007/978-3-030-25872-6_23

Author Index

Aguilar, Héctor   83
Altamirano, Luis   83

Bobocea, Aurora Elena   242
Botella, Cristina   43, 129, 147, 208
Bretón, Juana María   147
Bretón-Lopez, Juana   129

Carissoli, Claudia   250
Castelnuovo, Gianluca   29
Castilla, Diana   147, 190
Cattivelli, Roberto   29
Chirico, Alice   1
Chiu, Caleb   12
Cipresso, Pietro   102, 208, 242, 263
Colombo, Desirée   43, 208
Corno, Giulia   250

Di Lernia, Daniele   71
Díaz-García, Amanda   129, 147
Díaz-Sanahuja, Laura   129
Dotsch, Ron   231
Douloudi, Marilina   216

Felipe, Isabel Fernandez   208
Fernández-Álvarez, Javier   43, 147, 208

Gaggioli, Andrea   1, 263
García-Palacios, Azucena   43, 129, 147,
    157, 190
Ghiretti, Roberta   29
Giusti, Emanuele Maria   29
González-Robles, Alberto   147
Goulen, Karine   263
Grigioni, Mauro   263

Higuchi, Masakazu   168, 199

Iennaco, Daniela   117

Jaén, Irene   190
Jiménez, Liliana   83

Koutsouris, Dimitris   216
Kritikos, Jacob   216

Lam, Megan   12
Lee, Juwon   12
Leufkens, Tim   231
Longobardi, Teresa   117
López-Flores, Fernando   83

Maldonato, Mauro   117
Manzoni, Gian Mauro   29
Martínez, Ariadna   83
Martínez-Borba, Verónica   176
Martínez-Miranda, Juan   83
Mauri, Giancarlo   29
Mazzoli, Pier Giovanni   242
Mira, Adriana   129, 147
Mitsuyoshi, Shunji   168, 199
Molinari, Guadalupe   157
Montanelli, Stefano   250
Morganti, Francesca   55

Nakamura, Mitsuteru   168, 199

Omiya, Yasuhiro   168, 199
Osma, Jorge   176

Palacios, Azucena Garcia   208
Palacios-Isaac, Antonio   83
Parisi, Alessandra   242
Pedroli, Elisa   102, 263
Pietrabissa, Giada   29
Poulopoulou, Stavroula   216

Ramos, Roberto   83
Repetto, Claudia   117
Riva, Giuseppe   43, 71, 102, 117, 208, 242,
    263
Romero, Sonia   129
Rosales, Giovanni   83

Saito, Taku   199
Sas, Corina   231

Semonella, Michelle   102, 242
Serino, Silvia   71, 117, 263
Shinohara, Shuji   168, 199
So, Mirai   168
Spatola, Chiara   29
Sperandeo, Raffaele   117
Stramba-Badiale, Marco   263
Suso-Ribera, Carlos   157, 176, 190, 208

Takano, Takeshi   168, 199
Toda, Hiroyuki   199
Tokuno, Shinichi   168, 199
Toti, Michelle   102, 242, 263
Tuena, Cosimo   102, 242

Uraguchi, Tomotaka   168

Valev, Hristo   231
Villani, Daniela   250

Westerink, Joyce   231

Yoshino, Aihide   199

Zaragoza, Irene   190
Zoitaki, Chara   216
Zoppis, Italo   29

Printed in the United States
By Bookmasters